Diagnostic and Therapeutic Endoscopy

Diagnostic and Therapeutic Endoscopy

Editor: Christoph Fox

FOSTER
ACADEMICS
www.fosteracademics.com

www.fosteracademics.com

FOSTER
ACADEMICS

Cataloging-in-Publication Data

Diagnostic and therapeutic endoscopy / edited by Christoph Fox.
p. cm.
Includes bibliographical references and index.
ISBN 978-1-63242-626-0
1. Endoscopy. 2. Diagnosis. 3. Endoscopic surgery. I. Fox, Christoph.
RC78.7.E5 D53 2019
616.075 45--dc23

Foster Academics,
118-35 Queens Blvd., Suite 400,
Forest Hills, NY 11375, USA

ISBN 978-1-63242-626-0 (Hardback)

Printed and bound in China.

Contents

Preface IX

Chapter 1 **Efficacy of the Ovesco Clip for Closure of Endoscope Related Perforations** 1
Phonthep Angsuwatcharakon, Piyapan Prueksapanich, Pradermchai Kongkam, Thawee Rattanachu-ek, Jaksin Sottisuporn and Rungsun Rerknimitr

Chapter 2 **Effectiveness and Safety of Endoscopic Treatment of Benign Biliary Strictures Using a New Fully Covered Self Expandable Metal Stent** 7
Mihir S. Wagh, Disaya Chavalitdhamrong, Koorosh Moezardalan, Shailendra S. Chauhan, Anand R. Gupte, Michael J. Nosler, Chris E. Forsmark and Peter V. Draganov

Chapter 3 **Diagnostic Yield and Safety of Endoscopic Ultrasound Guided Fine Needle Aspiration of Central Mediastinal Lung Masses** 13
Enrique Vazquez-Sequeiros, Michael J. Levy, Manuel Van Domselaar, Fernando González-Panizo, Jose Ramon Foruny-Olcina, Daniel Boixeda-Miquel, Diego Juzgado-Lucas and Agustin Albillos

Chapter 4 **The Current State of Diagnosis and Treatment for Early Gastric Cancer** 19
Tomoyuki Yada, Chizu Yokoi and Naomi Uemura

Chapter 5 **Narrow Band Imaging with Magnification Can Pick up Esophageal Squamous Cell Carcinoma More Efficiently than Lugol Chromoendoscopy in Patients after Chemoradiotherapy** 28
Itsuko Asada-Hirayama, Shinya Kodashima, Mitsuhiro Fujishiro, Satoshi Ono, Keiko Niimi, Satoshi Mochizuki, Maki Konno-Shimizu, Rie Mikami-Matsuda, Chihiro Minatsuki, Chiemi Nakayama, Yu Takahashi, Nobutake Yamamichi and Kazuhiko Koike

Chapter 6 **Endoscopic Papillary Large Balloon Dilation Reduces the Need for Mechanical Lithotripsy in Patients with Large Bile Duct Stones** 34
Mohammad F. Madhoun, Sachin Wani, Sam Hong, William M. Tierney and John T. Maple

Chapter 7 **Endomicroscopy of the Pancreaticobiliary System** 42
Shajan Peter, Ji Young Bang, Klaus Mönkemuller, Shyam Varardarajulu and C. Mel Wilcox

Chapter 8 **Endoscopic Ultrasound-Guided Celiac Plexus Neurolysis in Pancreatic Cancer: A Prospective Pilot Study of Safety Using 10 mL versus 20 mL Alcohol** 48
Julia K. LeBlanc, Susan Rawl, Michelle Juan, Cynthia Johnson, Kurt Kroenke, Lee McHenry, Stuart Sherman, Kathy McGreevy, Mohammad Al-Haddad and John DeWitt

Chapter 9 **Peroral Endoscopic Myotomy for the Treatment of Achalasia** 54
Dennis Yang and Mihir S. Wagh

Chapter 10 **The use of Endobronchial Ultrasound in the Diagnosis of Subacute Pulmonary Histoplasmosis** 62
Katarine von Lang Egressy, Mohammed Mohammed and J. Scott Ferguson

Chapter 11 **Is It Possible to Predict the Presence of Intestinal Angioectasias?** 68
Tiago Cúrdia Gonçalves, Joana Magalhães, Pedro Boal Carvalho, Maria João Moreira, Bruno Rosa and José Cotter

Chapter 12 **Treatment of Internal Hemorrhoids by Endoscopic Sclerotherapy with Aluminum Potassium Sulfate and Tannic Acid** 74
Yuichi Tomiki, Seigo Ono, Jun Aoki, Rina Takahashi, Shun Ishiyama, Kiichi Sugimoto, Yukihiro Yaginuma, Yutaka Kojima, Michitoshi Goto, Atsushi Okuzawa and Kazuhiro Sakamoto

Chapter 13 **Capsule Endoscopy for Obscure Gastrointestinal Bleeding in Patients with Comorbid Rheumatic Diseases** 81
Neal Shahidi, George Ou, Jessica Tong, Ricky Kwok, Cherry Galorport, Joanna K. Law and Robert Enns

Chapter 14 **Narrow Band Imaging with Magnification Endoscopy for Celiac Disease: Results from a Prospective, Single-Center Study** 88
L. De Luca, L. Ricciardiello, M. B. L. Rocchi, M. T. Fabi, M. L. Bianchi, A. de Leone, S. Fiori and D. Baroncini

Chapter 15 **Increased Incidence of Benign Pancreatic Pathology following Pancreaticoduodenectomy for Presumed Malignancy over 10 Years despite Increased use of Endoscopic Ultrasound** 94
Shadi S. Yarandi, Thomas Runge, Lei Wang, Zhijian Liu, Yueping Jiang, Saurabh Chawla, Kevin E. Woods, Steven Keilin, Field F. Willingham, Hong Xu and Qiang Cai

Chapter 16 **Postcolonoscopy Followup Recommendations: Comparison with and without Use of Polyp Pathology** 100
Shiva K. Ratuapli, Suryakanth R. Gurudu, Mary A. Atia, Michael D. Crowell, Sarah B. Umar, M. Edwyn Harrison, Jonathan A. Leighton and Francisco C. Ramirez

Chapter 17 **Spiral Enteroscopy Utilizing Capsule Location Index for Achieving High Diagnostic and Therapeutic Yield** 107
Rohan Mandaliya, Jason Korenblit, Brendan O'Hare, Anastasia Shnitser, Ramalinga Kedika, Rebecca Matro, Dina Halegoua-De Marzio, Anthony Infantolino and Mitchell Conn

Chapter 18 **Colonoscopy Practice in Lagos, Nigeria: A Report of an Audit** 114
C. A. Onyekwere, J. N. Odiagah, O. O. Ogunleye, C. Chibututu and O. A. Lesi

Chapter 19 **Transpancreatic Precut Sphincterotomy for Biliary Access: The Relation of Sphincterotomy Size to Immediate Success Rate of Biliary Cannulation** 120
Lien-Fu Lin

Chapter 20 **Efficacy, Safety, and Long-Term Follow-Up Results of EUS-Guided Transmural Drainage for Pancreatic Pseudocyst** 127
Shin Kato, Akio Katanuma, Hiroyuki Maguchi, Kuniyuki Takahashi, Manabu Osanai, Kei Yane, Toshifumi Kim, Maki Kaneko, Ryo Takaki, Kazuyuki Matsumoto, Tomoaki Matsumori, Katsushige Gon and Akiko Tomonari

Chapter 21 **Multicenter Randomized Trial of 10-French versus 11.5-French Plastic Stents for Malignant Biliary Obstruction** 133
Mihir S. Wagh, Mario de Bellis, Evan L. Fogel, James T. Frakes, John F. Johanson, Tahir Qaseem, Douglas A. Howell, Glen A. Lehman and Stuart Sherman

Chapter 22 **Long-Term Endoscopic Follow-Up of Patients with Chronic Radiation Proctopathy after Brachytherapy for Prostate Cancer** 139
Masahiro Ohtani, Hiroyuki Suto, Takuto Nosaka, Yasushi Saito, Yoshihiko Ozaki, Ryoko Hayama, Tatsushi Naito, Kazuto Takahashi, Kazuya Ofuji, Hidetaka Matsuda, Katsushi Hiramatsu, Tomoyuki Nemoto, Hiroki Shioura, Hirohiko Kimura, Yoshitaka Aoki, Osamu Yokoyama and Yasunari Nakamoto

Chapter 23 **Improved Bowel Preparation with Multimedia Education in a Predominantly African-American Population** 146
Shashank Garg, Mohit Girotra, Lakshya Chandra, Vipin Verma, Sumanjit Kaur, Allawy Allawy, Alessandra Secco, Rohit Anand and Sudhir K. Dutta

Chapter 24 **Factors Significantly Contributing to a Failed Conventional Endoscopic Stone Clearance in Patients with "Difficult" Choledecholithiasis: A Single-Center Experience** 153
Emmanuel Christoforidis, Konstantinos Vasiliadis, Konstantinos Tsalis, Dimitrios Patridas, Konstantinos Blouhos, Manousos-Georgios Pramateftakis, Moysis Moysidis and Charalampos Lazaridis

Chapter 25 **Endoscopic Submucosal Dissection Outcomes for Gastroesophageal Tumors in Low Volume Units: A Multicenter Survey** 160
Ahmad Najib Azmi, Christopher J. L. Khor, Khek-Yu Ho, Rapat Pittayanon, Rungsun Rerknimitr, Thawee Ratanachu-ek, Doreen S. C. Koay, Jianyi Calvin Koh, Shiaw-Hooi Ho, Khean-Lee Goh and Sanjiv Mahadeva

Chapter 26 **Endoscopic Ultrasound Guided Rendezvous Drainage of Biliary Obstruction Using a New Flexible 19-Gauge Fine Needle Aspiration Needle** 167
Zhouwen Tang, Efehi Igbinomwanhia, Sherif Elhanafi and Mohamed O. Othman

Chapter 27 **The Role of EUS-BD in the Management of Malignant Biliary Obstruction: The Indonesian Perspective** 173
Dadang Makmun, Achmad Fauzi, Murdani Abdullah and Ari Fahrial Syam

Chapter 28 **Extended Cystogastrostomy with Hydrogen Peroxide Irrigation Facilitates Endoscopic Pancreatic Necrosectomy** 181
Mohamed O. Othman, Sherif Elhanafi, Mohammed Saadi, Christine Yu and Brian R. Davis

Chapter 29 **Use of 4-Fr versus 6-Fr Nasobiliary Catheter for Biliary Drainage: A Prospective, Multicenter, Randomized, Controlled Study** 186
Tomofumi Tsuboi, Masahiro Serikawa, Tamito Sasaki, Yasutaka Ishii, Yoshifumi Fujimoto, Atsushi Yamaguchi, Takashi Ishigaki, Akinori Shimizu, Keisuke Kurihara, Yumiko Tatsukawa, Eisuke Miyaki and Kazuaki Chayama

Chapter 30 **Therapeutic Endoscopy Can Be Performed Safely in an Ambulatory Surgical Center: A Multicenter, Prospective Study** 193
Shaffer R. S. Mok, Henry C. Ho, John P. Gaughan and Adam B. Elfant

Chapter 31 **Endoscopic Ultrasound Elastography for Evaluation of Lymph Nodes: A Single Center Experience** 203
Ahmed Youssef Altonbary , Hazem Hakim and Ahmed Mohamed El-Shamy

Chapter 32 **Unsuspected Small-Bowel Crohn's Disease in Elderly Patients Diagnosed by Video Capsule Endoscopy** 208
Che-Yung Chao, Carl Frederic Duchatellier and Ernest G. Seidman

Chapter 33 **Outcomes of the use of Fully Covered Esophageal Self-Expandable Stent in the Management of Colorectal Anastomotic Strictures and Leaks** 215
Chad J. Cooper, Angel Morales and Mohamed O. Othman

Permissions

List of Contributors

Index

Preface

Over the recent decade, advancements and applications have progressed exponentially. This has led to the increased interest in this field and projects are being conducted to enhance knowledge. The main objective of this book is to present some of the critical challenges and provide insights into possible solutions. This book will answer the varied questions that arise in the field and also provide an increased scope for furthering studies.

Therapeutic endoscopy is an endoscopic procedure during which a treatment is carried out using an endoscope. Diagnostic endoscopy can become therapeutic in case of upper gastrointestinal bleeding or for finding polyps during colonoscopy. Disorders such as strictures, bleeding and polyps are some of the disorders treated endoscopically. Some of the different types of endoscopic therapy include injection sclerotherapy, endoscopic haemostasis, dilatation, stenting, argon plasma coagulation, polypectomy, percutaneous endoscopic gastrostomy, etc. Significant research and development is being undertaken in clinical and therapeutic endoscopy for the treatment of Barrett's oesophagus, gastro-oesophageal reflux disease and gastric stapling. This book brings forth some of the most innovative concepts and elucidates the unexplored aspects of clinical and therapeutic endoscopy. The ever-growing need of advanced technology for the diagnosis and treatment of medical conditions is the reason that has fueled research in this field in recent times. Students, researchers, experts and all associated with this field will benefit alike from this book.

I hope that this book, with its visionary approach, will be a valuable addition and will promote interest among readers. Each of the authors has provided their extraordinary competence in their specific fields by providing different perspectives as they come from diverse nations and regions. I thank them for their contributions.

Editor

Efficacy of the Ovesco Clip for Closure of Endoscope Related Perforations

Phonthep Angsuwatcharakon,[1,2] Piyapan Prueksapanich,[1] Pradermchai Kongkam,[1] Thawee Rattanachu-ek,[3] Jaksin Sottisuporn,[4] and Rungsun Rerknimitr[1]

[1]*Department of Medicine, Faculty of Medicine, King Chulalongkorn Memorial Hospital, Chulalongkorn University, Bangkok 10330, Thailand*
[2]*Department of Anatomy, Faculty of Medicine, King Chulalongkorn Memorial Hospital, Chulalongkorn University, Bangkok 10330, Thailand*
[3]*Center of Excellence, Laparoscopic Endoscopic Surgery, Department of Surgery, Rajavithi Hospital, Bangkok 10400, Thailand*
[4]*NKC Institute of Gastroenterology and Hepatology, Faculty of Medicine, Prince of Songkla University, Songkhla 90110, Thailand*

Correspondence should be addressed to Rungsun Rerknimitr; ercp@live.com

Academic Editor: Patrick J. O'Dwyer

Aim. To study the efficacy and other treatment outcomes of Ovesco clip closure of iatrogenic perforation. *Methods*. Retrospective study from 3 tertiary-care hospitals in Thailand. Patients with iatrogenic perforation who underwent immediate endoscopic closure by Ovesco clip were included. Patients' demographic data, perforation size, number of Ovesco clips used, fasting day, length of hospital stay, success rates, and complication rate were recorded. Technical success was defined as closure achievement during endoscopic procedure and clinical success was defined as the patient can be discharged without the need of additional surgical or radiological intervention. *Results*. There were 6 iatrogenic perforations in 2 male and 4 female patients. The median age was 59 years (range 39–78 years). The locations of perforation were 5 duodenal walls and 1 rectosigmoid junction. The median perforation size was 13 mm (range 10–40 mm). The technical success was 100% and the clinical success was 83.3%. The success rates per locations were 100% in colon and 80% in duodenum, respectively. The median fasting time was 5 days (range 1–10 days) and the median length of hospital stay was 10 days (range 2–22 days). There was no mortality in any. *Conclusion*. Ovesco clip seems to be an effective and safe tool for a closure of iatrogenic perforation.

1. Introduction

Iatrogenic perforation during gastrointestinal endoscopy is generally needed surgical management [1] because surgery provides a complete closure as well as an opportunity for a clearance of the spillage content. However, surgical interventions carry significant morbidity and mortality especially in patients with comorbid illness [2, 3]. Early detection and closure are the key factors for a favorable outcome [4, 5]. Immediate closure during endoscopy may reduce the risk of further spillage of gastrointestinal content [6, 7] and should be the optimal time-point to carry; however, the reliable device is needed for this purpose.

Ovesco clip (Tübingen, Germany), an over-the-scope clip (OTSC), is made from nitinol which is biocompatible and has self-memory shape. The clip is mounted on an applicator cap. When using, the cap will be affixed to the tip of the scope. There is a threat connecting between the clip and hand wheel. The manner of deployment is similar to variceal band ligation. Ovesco has been approved in Europe since 2009 and in the US since 2010 [8]. Ovesco provides the secure closure strength as tight as hand suture in ex vivo porcine model [9] because it can grasp all layers of visceral wall and this in turn leads to a full thickness healing [10]. Among leakage indications of Ovesco, acute perforation has the most success rate when compared with other postoperative leakages or

TABLE 1: Patients characteristics and treatment of perforation.

Age/gender	Diagnosis	Cause of perforation	Size (mm)	Location	Treatment	NPO/LOS (days)
78/F	Bowel habit change	Colonoscope	10	Rectosigmoid junction	1 OTSC	1/3
56/F	Distal cholangiocarcinoma failed biliary cannulation	Needle-knife dilation of choledochoduodenostomy	15	Medial duodenal wall	1 OTSC, PTBD	10/22
70/F	Choledocholithiasis	Duodenoscope	10	Lateral duodenal wall	1 OTSC, ERCP with stone removal	7/15
60/M	Choledocholithiasis	Duodenoscope	13	Lateral duodenal wall	1 OTSC	1/2
58/F	Choledocholithiasis	Duodenoscope	13	Lateral duodenal wall	1 OTSC	3/8
39/M	Chronic pancreatitis with pancreatic duct stone and stricture after pancreatic stenting	Duodenoscope	40	Lateral duodenal wall	2 OTSCs with 1 band ligation	8/12

NPO, nil per oral; LOS, length of stay; OTSC, over-the-scope clip.

fistulas because acute perforation contains fresh ulcer edge with less fibrosis [11, 12]. We aim to evaluate the performance of OTSC for perforation closure in the tertiary-care hospitals in Thailand.

2. Methods

Endoscopy database from 3 tertiary-care hospitals in Thailand including King Chulalongkorn Memorial Hospital, Rajavithi Hospital, and Songklanagarind Hospital were retrospectively reviewed. Patients with iatrogenic perforation who received endoscopic closure by Ovesco clip were included in this study.

The procedures of endoscopic perforation closure were as follows. Once perforation was detected during endoscopy procedure, the insufflation was switched from air to CO_2 where applicable, broad-spectrum antibiotic was administered intravenously, and the vital signs were closely monitored. The Ovesco clip cap was mounted at the tip of the end-viewing scope; the thread connected between the cap and control wheel was inserted through the accessory channel. The twin-grasper was used only when the perforation edges were apart. During closure, the perforation edge was suctioned into an applicator cap and then the clip was deployed. Enterogram using water soluble contrast media was performed to confirm the complete closure. After procedure, patients were admitted to the hospital and closely observed. Duration of fasting depended on endoscopists' discretion. Technical success is defined as successful closure of perforation confirmed by enterogram and clinical success is defined as the patient can be discharged without the need of surgical or radiological intervention.

3. Results

There were 6 iatrogenic perforations (Table 1) caused by colonoscope ($n = 1$), needle-knife creation of choledochoduodenostomy tract ($n = 1$), and duodenoscope ($n = 4$). Locations of perforation were rectosigmoid colon (1), medial duodenal wall (1), and lateral duodenal wall (4). There were 2 male and 4 female patients with median age of 59 years (range 39–78 years). The median size of perforation was 13 mm (range 10–40 mm). Five patients (83.3%) required 1 Ovesco clip (Figure 1) and one patient needed 2 Ovesco clips and 1 rubber band to achieve a complete closure. Technical success and clinical success rates of endoscopic closure were 100% and 83.3%, respectively. The median fasting time was 5 days (range 1–10 days) and the median length of stay was 10 days (range 2–22 days).

One patient was diagnosed with chronic pancreatitis with pancreatic duct obstruction from stone and stricture. He had been placed with a pancreatic stent for 3 months and was scheduled for ERCP and stent exchange. A 40 mm perforation was detected during duodenoscope insertion. After the application of two Ovesco clips with omental patch, the perforation could not be completely closed as confirmed by the presence of contrast leakage during enterogram (Figure 2). One rescue band was attempted and successfully closed the perforation (Figure 3). He had no fever or abdominal pain and could resume oral intake by day 8 after closure. The intraperitoneally misplaced Ovesco clips were incidentally found by computed tomography on day 9. After surgical consultation, the patient underwent laparoscopy on day 11 which found that 2 Ovesco clips were dislodged intraperitoneally and wrapped by the omentum; laparoscopic removal of 2 Ovesco clips without need of duodenal repair was done. He was discharged on day 12, the next day after laparoscopy. He underwent ERCP at another 3 months for pancreatic stent exchange without any complication. In another patient with rectosigmoid perforation, a repeated colonoscopy was successful within the next month after a successful endoscopic closure by an Ovesco clip. In a patient who underwent an EUS-guided choledochoduodenostomy for failed biliary cannulation, a percutaneous transhepatic biliary drainage was performed immediately after closure, and the second ERCP with internal stenting was performed one day later. In another 4 patients with lateral duodenal wall perforations, the perforation was detected right after finishing ERCP and no further intervention was needed after closure in one patient. Biliary cannulation, endoscopic sphincterotomy, and stone removal were continued immediately after closure

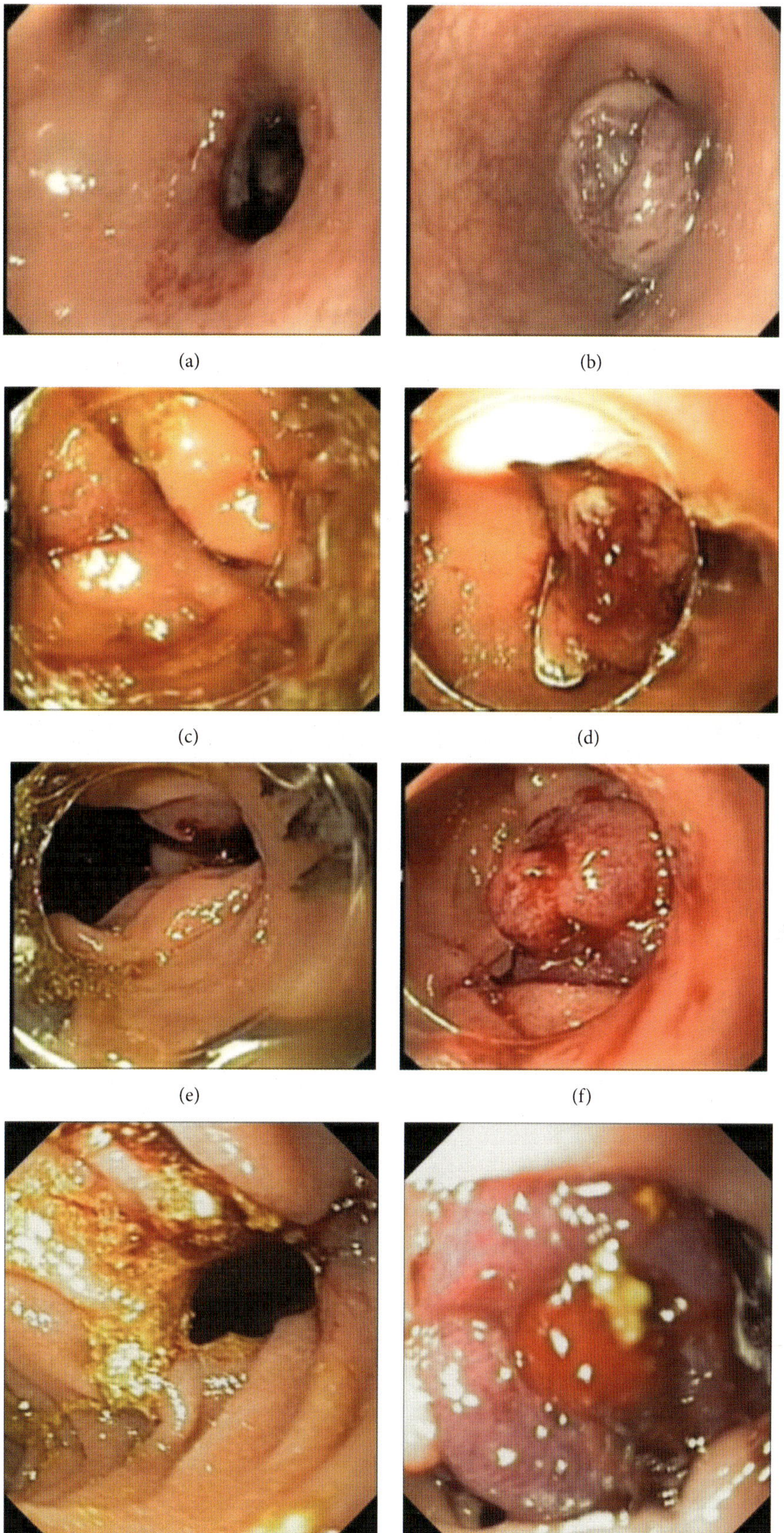

(a) (b) (c) (d) (e) (f) (g) (h)

FIGURE 1: Continued.

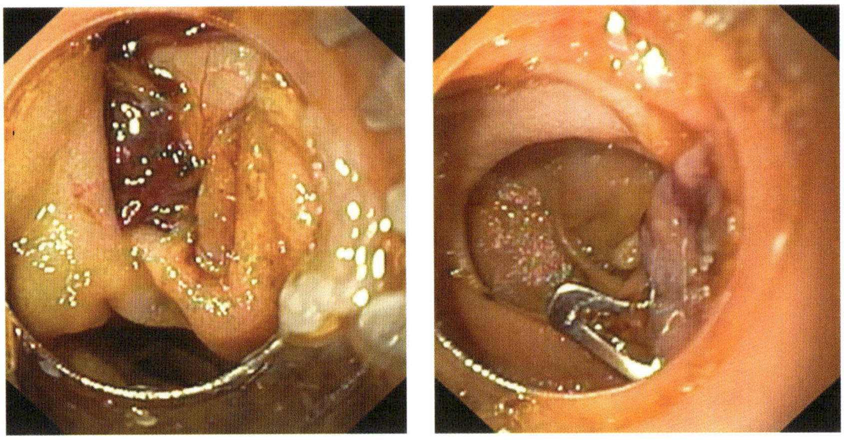

(i) (j)

Figure 1: Endoscopic pictures of patients with successful closure by one Ovesco clip. (a) Rectosigmoid perforation; (b) after Ovesco clip closure of rectosigmoid perforation; (c) medial duodenal wall perforation; (d) after Ovesco clip closure of medial duodenal wall perforation; (e, g, i) lateral duodenal wall perforations; (f, h, j) after Ovesco clip closure of lateral duodenal wall perforations.

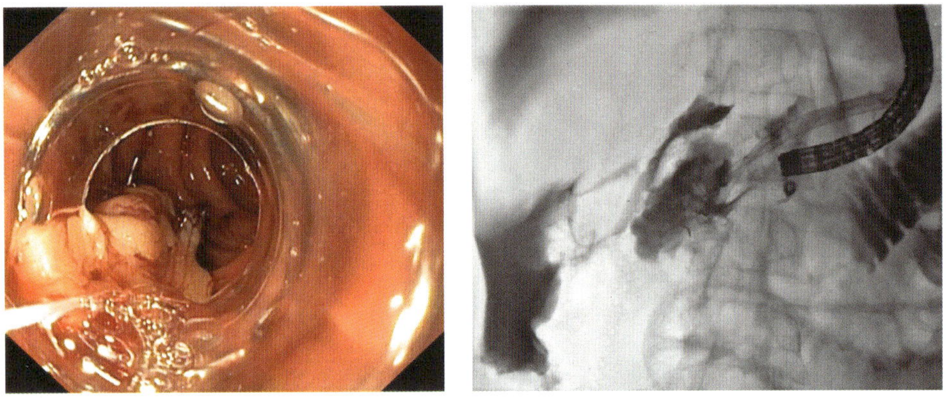

(a) (b)

Figure 2: A case with 40 mm perforation at duodenal wall. (a) Two Ovesco clips with omental patch were applied; (b) enterogram revealed persistent contrast leakage indicating an incomplete closure.

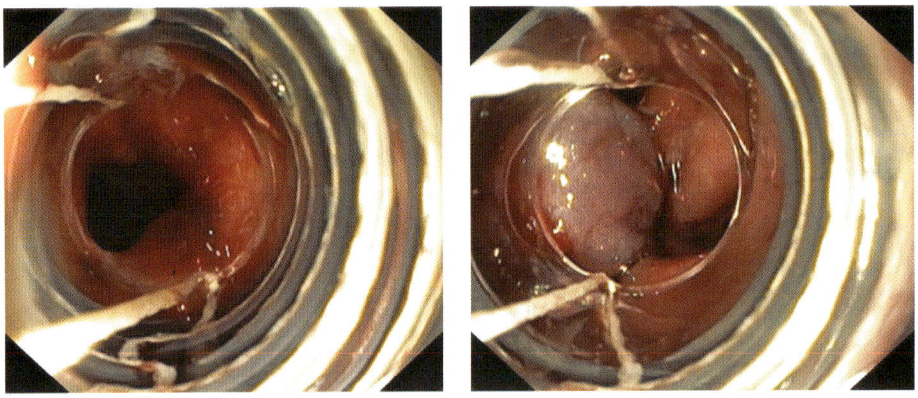

(a) (b)

Figure 3: Rescue band ligation after 2 Ovesco clips' application. (a) A residual perforation was detected; (b) successful closure with an additional band ligation.

of perforation in another patient. In the last two patients, after an endoscopic closure, the second ERCP was successfully repeated during subsequent admission. There was no mortality in this study.

4. Discussion

Ovesco clip has been commercially available in Thailand since 2012. The main indication in Thailand is for a closure of iatrogenic perforation. We collected data from 3 tertiary-care hospitals in Thailand; 2 hospitals are in Bangkok and 1 hospital is in Songkhla province. There were 6 iatrogenic perforations that underwent immediate endoscopic closure by using Ovesco clips. The technical and clinical success rates were 100% and 83.3%, respectively. The success rates per locations were 100% in colon and 80% in duodenum. There was no mortality in this study. The overall success rate and the success rate for colonic and duodenal closure are in line with previous reports, 87.8% [7], 76.9% [13, 14], and 88.2% [7], respectively.

Clinical failure in one patient was due to a large, 40 mm, perforation. In this patient, the 2 Ovesco clips were dislodged after band ligation. Consequently, surgical intervention was performed but only to remove the Ovesco clips. In retrospect, the perforation was already closed endoscopically. The patient can be safely discharged 1 day after surgery.

There was no report on the upper limit of perforation size closure in human [7, 13, 14]. In nonsurvival porcine model, the success rate for closure of colonic wall defect sizes of 24–27 mm and 29–55 mm was 83% and 29%, respectively [15]. In a prospective human study, the clinical success rate on Ovesco closure of 30 mm defect was reported as 97% [12]. Our study demonstrates that all perforations with the size range from 10 to 15 mm can be successfully closed by one Ovesco clip, and only the 40 mm perforation failed to be closed by one Ovesco clip. In our experience, the optimal upper limit of perforation size to be closed by one Ovesco clip should be smaller than 30 mm.

In 4 patients in which perforation developed before finishing therapeutic procedures, Ovesco clip closure allowed the continuation of the original therapeutic plan immediately after Ovesco clip closure in 1 patient (25%), in the next day in 1 patient (25%), and in the next admission in 2 patients (50%). In our series, the primary plan of endoscopic treatment was achieved without the need for readmission in 50% of patients.

In conclusion, Ovesco clip is a promising device for an endoscopic closure of iatrogenic perforation as it provides a high success rate and low complication rate. The limitations of this study are its retrospective descriptive design and small sample size, and all closures are performed by expert endoscopists. The data from a comparative study with long-term follow-up is needed before recommending the Ovesco clip as the primary device for perforation treatment.

Additional Points

Iatrogenic perforation traditionally requires surgery. Ovesco clip is a device that provides full thickness closure of gastrointestinal wall and has been increasingly used for a closure of iatrogenic perforation. It can be applied immediately in endoscopy suite and this in turn can prevent further spillage of gastrointestinal content into peritoneal space. It provides a high success rate especially in a lesion smaller than 30 mm and should be the preferred method for perforation closure.

Competing Interests

The authors have no competing interests.

Authors' Contributions

Phonthep Angsuwatcharakon, Piyapan Prueksapanich, Pradermchai Kongkam, Thawee Rattanachu-ek, Jaksin Sottisuporn, and Rungsun Rerknimitr substantially contributed to the conception and design; Phonthep Angsuwatcharakon drafted the paper; Rungsun Rerknimitr critically revised the important intellectual content; and Phonthep Angsuwatcharakon, Piyapan Prueksapanich, Pradermchai Kongkam, Thawee Rattanachu-ek, Jaksin Sottisuporn, and Rungsun Rerknimitr approved the final version before publishing.

References

[1] R. V. Putcha and J. S. Burdick, "Management of iatrogenic perforation," *Gastroenterology Clinics of North America*, vol. 32, no. 4, pp. 1289–1309, 2003.

[2] C. W. Iqbal, D. C. Cullinane, H. J. Schiller, M. D. Sawyer, S. P. Zietlow, and D. R. Farley, "Surgical management and outcomes of 165 colonoscopic perforations from a single institution," *Archives of Surgery*, vol. 143, no. 7, pp. 701–707, 2008.

[3] T. H. Luning, M. E. Keemers-Gels, W. B. Barendregt, A. C. I. T. L. Tan, and C. Rosman, "Colonoscopic perforations: a review of 30,366 patients," *Surgical Endoscopy*, vol. 21, no. 6, pp. 994–997, 2007.

[4] M. La Torre, F. Velluti, G. Giuliani, E. Di Giulio, V. Ziparo, and F. La Torre, "Promptness of diagnosis is the main prognostic factor after colonoscopic perforation," *Colorectal Disease*, vol. 14, no. 1, pp. e23–e26, 2012.

[5] F. Biancari, V. D'Andrea, R. Paone et al., "Current treatment and outcome of esophageal perforations in adults: systematic review and meta-analysis of 75 studies," *World Journal of Surgery*, vol. 37, no. 5, pp. 1051–1059, 2013.

[6] S. B. Cho, W. S. Lee, Y. E. Joo et al., "Therapeutic options for iatrogenic colon perforation: feasibility of endoscopic clip closure and predictors of the need for early surgery," *Surgical Endoscopy and Other Interventional Techniques*, vol. 26, no. 2, pp. 473–479, 2012.

[7] T. Verlaan, R. P. Voermans, M. I. van Berge Henegouwen, W. A. Bemelman, and P. Fockens, "Endoscopic closure of acute perforations of the GI tract: a systematic review of the literature," *Gastrointestinal Endoscopy*, vol. 82, no. 4, pp. 618–628, 2015.

[8] S. Banerjee, B. A. Barth, Y. M. Bhat et al., "Endoscopic closure devices," *Gastrointestinal Endoscopy*, vol. 76, no. 2, pp. 244–251, 2012.

[9] R. P. Voermans, F. Vergouwe, P. Breedveld, P. Fockens, and M. I. Van Berge Henegouwen, "Comparison of endoscopic closure modalities for standardized colonic perforations in a porcine colon model," *Endoscopy*, vol. 43, no. 3, pp. 217–222, 2011.

[10] A. Arezzo, T. Kratt, M. O. Schurr, and M. Morino, "Laparoscopic-assisted transgastric cholecystectomy and secure endoscopic closure of the transgastric defect in a survival porcine model," *Endoscopy*, vol. 41, no. 9, pp. 767–772, 2009.

[11] R. Mennigen, N. Senninger, and M. G. Laukoetter, "Novel treatment options for perforations of the upper gastrointestinal tract: endoscopic vacuum therapy and over-the-scope clips," *World Journal of Gastroenterology*, vol. 20, no. 24, pp. 7767–7776, 2014.

[12] R. P. Voermans, O. Le Moine, D. von Renteln et al., "Efficacy of endoscopic closure of acute perforations of the gastrointestinal tract," *Clinical Gastroenterology and Hepatology*, vol. 10, no. 6, pp. 603–608, 2012.

[13] A. Kirschniak, N. Subotova, D. Zieker, A. Königsrainer, and T. Kratt, "The Over-The-Scope Clip (OTSC) for the treatment of gastrointestinal bleeding, perforations, and fistulas," *Surgical Endoscopy and Other Interventional Techniques*, vol. 25, no. 9, pp. 2901–2905, 2011.

[14] C. Gubler and P. Bauerfeind, "Endoscopic closure of iatrogenic gastrointestinal tract perforations with the over-the-scope clip," *Digestion*, vol. 85, no. 4, pp. 302–307, 2012.

[15] D. von Renteln, A. Schmidt, M. C. Vassiliou, H.-U. Rudolph, and K. Caca, "Endoscopic full-thickness resection and defect closure in the colon," *Gastrointestinal Endoscopy*, vol. 71, no. 7, pp. 1267–1273, 2010.

2

Effectiveness and Safety of Endoscopic Treatment of Benign Biliary Strictures Using a New Fully Covered Self Expandable Metal Stent

Mihir S. Wagh, Disaya Chavalitdhamrong, Koorosh Moezardalan, Shailendra S. Chauhan, Anand R. Gupte, Michael J. Nosler, Chris E. Forsmark, and Peter V. Draganov

Division of Gastroenterology, Hepatology and Nutrition, University of Florida, 1600 SW Archer Road, Room HD 602, P.O. Box 100214, Gainesville, FL 32610, USA

Correspondence should be addressed to Mihir S. Wagh; mihir.wagh@medicine.ufl.edu

Academic Editor: Shai Friedland

Background. In patients with benign biliary strictures, the use of fully covered self-expandable metal stents (SEMS) has been proposed as an alternative to plastic stenting, but high quality prospective data are sparse. This study was performed to evaluate the long-term effectiveness and safety of a new fully covered SEMS for benign biliary strictures. *Methods.* All consecutive patients with benign biliary strictures were treated with placement of a fully covered SEMS (WallFlex) for 6 months. Short- and long-term stricture resolution, adverse events, and ease of stent removal were recorded. *Results.* 23 patients were enrolled. Stricture etiology was chronic pancreatitis (14), postorthotopic liver transplant (4), idiopathic (4), and biliary stones (1). All ERCPs were technically successful. All stents were successfully removed. Short-term stricture resolution was seen in 22/23 (96%) patients. Long-term success was 15/18 (83.3%). All 3 failures were patients with biliary strictures in the setting of chronic calcific pancreatitis. *Conclusions.* The use of the new SEMS for the treatment of benign biliary strictures led to short-term stricture resolution in the vast majority of patients. Over a long-term followup the success rate appears favorable compared to historical results achieved with multiple plastic stenting, particularly in patients with chronic pancreatitis. The study was registered with ClinicalTrials.gov (NCT01238900).

1. Introduction

Benign biliary strictures are common and challenging clinical problems. The two leading etiologies are chronic pancreatitis (CP) and postoperative complications, either related to bile duct injury at the time of cholecystectomy or anastomotic narrowing after orthotopic liver transplantation (OLT). The reported incidence of benign biliary strictures among CP patients ranges from 3 to 46% [1]. In post-OLT setting, biliary tract complications can occur in up to 30% of patients [2]. Furthermore, biliary strictures can occur in 0.5 to 0.9% of patients undergoing laparoscopic cholecystectomy [3, 4]. Other less frequent causes are primary sclerosing cholangitis, papillary stenosis, autoimmune pancreatitis, and bile duct stones [5]. Benign biliary strictures can present with a variety of clinical scenarios that range from mild elevation of liver enzymes to recurrent episodes of cholangitis to secondary biliary cirrhosis and end stage liver disease [6]. In order to prevent these serious complications, proper and early effective treatment of these strictures is essential.

Traditionally, benign biliary strictures had been treated surgically. Currently, endoscopic retrograde cholangiopancreatography (ERCP) with placement of multiple plastic stents has become the first line therapy. In the setting of postoperative biliary strictures, ERCP has shown a high rate of stricture resolution ranging from 75% to 89% [7–9]. The main drawbacks of the ERCP-based approach are the need for multiple procedures and a treatment period that usually lasts over a year. Furthermore, relatively high morbidity can occur due to stent occlusion [10], and endoscopic therapy for CP-related biliary stenosis has reported success rates of approximately only 25% [11].

In order to decrease the incidence of cholangitis and the need for multiple ERCPs, uncovered or partially covered self-expandable metal stents (SEMS) have been used. However, these stents have high rates of stent clogging caused by tissue ingrowth which could cause challenges with stent removal [10, 12]. Fully covered SEMS have been used with more favorable results; however, stent migration is a main concern [13, 14]. Only limited high quality data are available on the long-term efficacy and safety of fully covered SEMS in the treatment of benign biliary strictures [13, 15–22]. Therefore, we prospectively investigated the short- and long-term effectiveness and safety of a new fully covered SEMS in patients with benign biliary strictures.

2. Materials and Methods

This was a prospective cohort study. The study was approved by the Institutional Review Board (IRB) at the University of Florida. All patients signed informed consent. The study concept, hypothesis, and design were investigator initiated, and no financial support or free devices were received. The aim of this study was to evaluate the long-term effectiveness and safety of a new fully covered SEMS for benign biliary strictures.

2.1. Patients. Consecutive patients referred to the University of Florida for ERCP for benign biliary strictures were considered for study enrollment from July 2009 to December 2011. The inclusion criteria were strictures located at a minimum 2 cm downstream to the bifurcation and due to one of the following etiologies: CP, post-OLT, postcholecystectomy, postradiation or chemotherapy (for nonbiliary malignancies), bile duct stone related strictures, and idiopathic. Patients with prior endoscopic attempts with dilation and plastic stents were also included. The exclusion criteria were patients with bile duct strictures less than 2 cm from the bifurcation, autoimmune pancreatitis, primary sclerosing cholangitis, malignant strictures, age less than 18, and pregnancy.

2.2. Endoscopy Protocol. ERCP was performed by one of our four experienced therapeutic endoscopists (MSW, SSC, CEF, and PVD) using the TJF 160V duodenoscope (Olympus America, Center Valley, PA, USA). The stents used in this study were the fully covered WallFlex Biliary RX Stents (Boston Scientific Corporation, Natick, MA, USA) which are available in diameters of 8 or 10 mm and lengths of 40, 60, and 80 mm. Biliary sphincterotomy, if not done previously, was performed. Stricture dilation was not preformed prior to stent insertion. All stents were placed with the distal end extending into the duodenum. Per protocol, the intent was to keep the stent in place for 6-months. If the stricture had resolved at the 6-month follow-up ERCP, patients were classified as short-term success and then entered in the follow-up portion of the study. If at the time of the 6 month stent removal, the stricture was improved but still present, then a new fully covered SEMS (WallFlex) was placed. If the stricture had resolved at the time of the second stent removal, the patient was also classified as "short-term success." If the stricture was still present, the patient was classified as "short-term failure." A typical stenting sequence is shown on Figures 1, 2, and 3. Stents were removed by grasping the dedicated retrieval loop

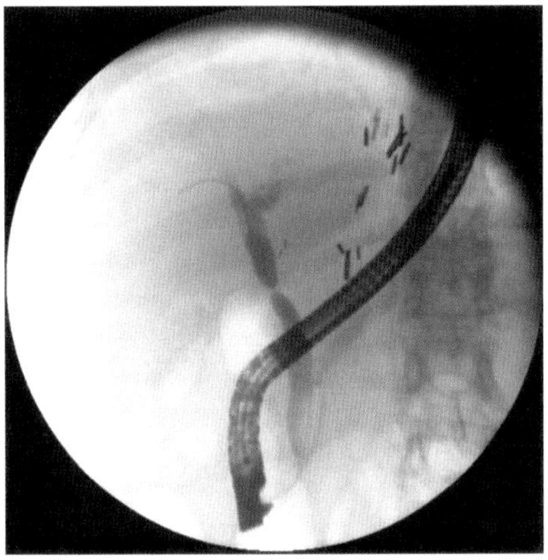

Figure 1: Cholangiogram of a patient with postliver transplant anastomotic stricture.

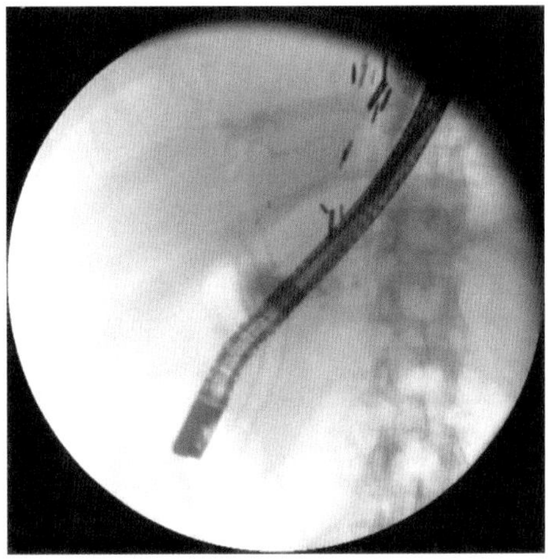

Figure 2: Fully expanded metal stent bridging the stricture.

at the proximal end of the stent using a rat-tooth forceps. If this was not feasible, the distal end of the stent was captured with a snare and then retrieved. Patients with post-OLT anastomotic biliary strictures received antibiotic prophylaxis prior to and up to 3 days after the stent placement to prevent cholangitis.

2.3. Outcomes. The primary outcome of this study was short- and long-term success rate in resolution of biliary strictures. Secondary outcomes were the frequency and severity of adverse events (including stent migration), duration and number of endoscopic treatment(s), and ease of stent removal.

2.4. Definitions. The procedure was considered technically successful if all of the following criteria were met: achieving deep bile duct cannulation, traversing the stricture with a wire, and deploying the SEMS across the stricture. For the follow-up ERCP, the procedure was considered technically successful if the SEMS could be extracted. The ease of stent

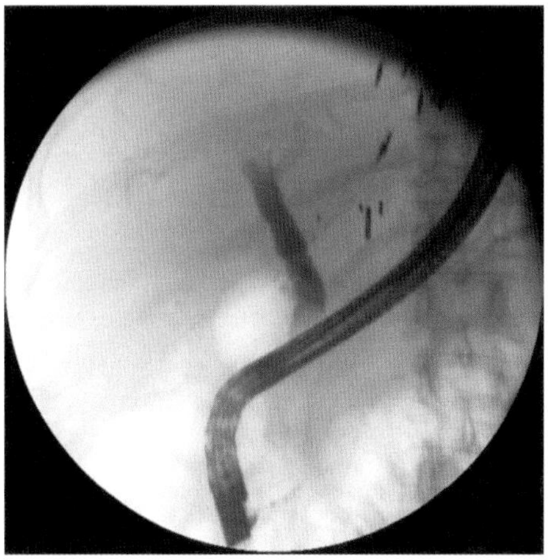

FIGURE 3: Resolution of the stricture.

TABLE 1: Patient characteristics.

Number	23
Age (years)	60 (51–70)
Male (% men)	10 (43%)
Etiology	
Chronic pancreatitis	14 (61%)
Orthotopic liver transplantation	4 (17%)
Idiopathic	4 (17%)
Gallstone related	1 (4%)
Prior common bile duct stenting	13 (56%)

Values listed as number (%) or median (IQR).

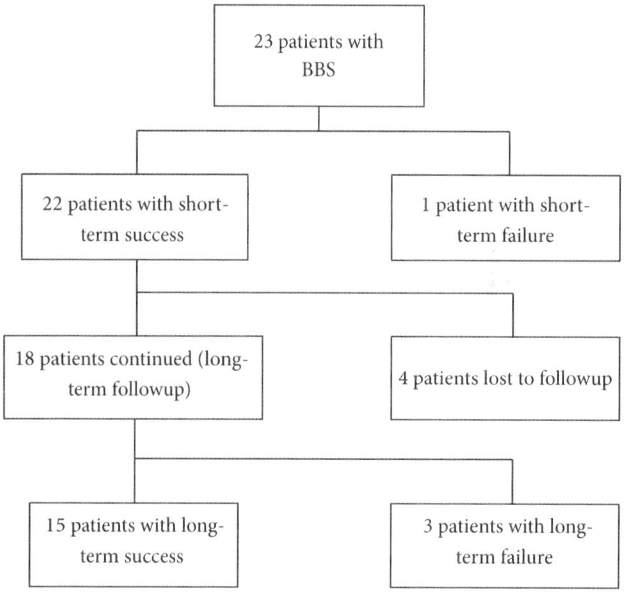

FIGURE 4: Flow diagram of the patients through the study.

extraction was graded on a 4-point scale (with ease, mild difficulty, significant difficulty, and failed). Short-term success was defined as resolution of the stricture as documented by rapid drainage of contrast out of the proximal biliary tree and easy passage of stone extraction balloon inflated to the size of the proximal bile duct. Long-term success was defined as no clinical evidence of recurrence of the biliary stricture during the follow-up period as documented by laboratory findings or imaging and no further need for further endoscopic or surgical interventions. The long-term follow-up was at least a 12-month period. The followup period started at the time of the metal stent removal. Adverse events were defined and graded using the 2010 American Society for Gastrointestinal Endoscopy consensus criteria [23].

2.5. Statistical Analysis. IBM SPSS version 19 was used for statistical analysis. The level of significance was set at $P < 0.05$ in statistical analyses. Per-protocol and intent-to-treat analysis was carried out.

3. Results

A total of 23 patients (10 male; mean age: 60.6; range: 24–81 years) were enrolled. Stricture etiologies were CP (14), OLT (4) (mean time after OLT was 2.7 months), idiopathic (4), and history of biliary stones (1). Patient characteristics are summarized in Table 1.

Of the 23 patients that completed the endoscopy protocol, 22 patients entered the followup phase (one patient had a persistent stricture and was therefore classified as short-term failure). Long-term follow-up was obtained in 18/22 (81.8%) of the patients. Therefore, 23 patients were available for the analysis of the technical success of the ERCPs and the short-term success rate of stricture resolution, and 18 patients were available for the analysis of the long-term success rate of stent therapy. Patient flow through the study is summarized on Figure 4.

All ERCP procedures were technically successful in all patients. The average number of ERCPs performed per patient was 2.4 (range 2–4). The average total stenting period per patient was 7.5 months (22 days to 17.6 months). Stent migration was seen in 9/23 (39.1%) patients (5 downstream, 4 upstream). In the cases of stent migration, all of the stent was still bridging the stricture except in two cases. In the first patient, the metal stent migrated out of the bile duct completely; however, the biliary stricture had resolved with no recurrence during followup. The second case was a patient with post-OLT anastomotic stricture at the upper third of the common bile duct. The stricture was located 70 mm proximal to the ampulla, and on the first ERCP a decision was made to deploy the longest size SEMS that was available (80 mm). The proximal end of the stent at the end of the deployment was 10 mm proximal to the stricture. On the followup ERCP, the proximal end of the stent was found below the stricture. Since stents longer than 80 mm are not manufactured, a decision was made to switch to plastic stents, and the patient was classified to be a short-term failure.

All stents were successfully removed in all patients. Stent removals were graded as "easy" except in 2 cases (8%) with upstream stent migration where the removal was graded as "with significant difficulty." Associated pathologies included

Table 2: Outcomes.

	Overall	Chronic pancreatitis	All others	P value
Short-term success	22/23 (96%)	14/14 (100%)	8/9 (89%)	0.39
Long-term success				
Per-protocol analysis	15/18 (83%)	8/11 (73%)	7/7 (100%)	0.21
Intention-to-treat analysis	15/22 (68%)	8/12 (67%)	7/10 (70%)	0.65

7 patients with common bile duct stones. Balloon extraction of the stones was successful in all cases.

The overall short-term treatment success rate for stricture resolution at the end of the stenting period was seen in 22/23 (95.6%) patients. The short-term success rate was 14/14 (100%) among the CP patients, 3/4 (75%) among the OLT patients, and 5/5 (100%) in remaining patients. The short-term failure was a patient with post-OLT anastomotic stricture as discussed in detail in the previous paragraph.

Long-term followup was available in 18/22 patients (81.8%). Patients were followed for a median follow-up period of 18.8 months (interquartile range of 14.1 to 21.3 months). The overall long-term success rate of stricture resolution was 15/18 (83.3%): in the CP group 8/11 (72.7%), in the OLT group 3/3 (100%), and the remaining patients 4/4 (100%) (Table 2). The failures included three patients with distal biliary strictures in the setting of CP with calcification. One patient underwent surgery with hepaticojejunostomy, and two patients needed further endoscopies with plastic stents.

The overall long-term treatment success on an intention to treat basis was 15/22 (68.2%): in the CP group 8/12 (66.7%), in the OLT group 3/3 (100%), and in the remaining patients 4/7 (57.1%) (Table 2). This analysis considered all patients lost to followup as long-term therapeutic failures, in a "worst-case" scenario analysis.

Adverse events included severe pain in one patient after placement of 10 mm wide stent. The stent had to be removed due to the pain; however, the patient subsequently did well with an 8 mm diameter stent, and the stricture was successfully treated with no recurrence during long-term followup. There was no incidence of post-ERCP pancreatitis or cholangitis. No other adverse events were noticed during followup period. Of note, in all 13 (56.5%) patients with gallbladder in situ, the SEMS was placed across the takeoff the cystic duct, and no acute cholecystitis was observed.

4. Discussion

Endoscopic treatment of benign biliary strictures has gained popularity as a less invasive approach compared to surgery. The preferred endoscopic strategy has been to sequentially dilate the stricture and insert incremental number of plastic stents during multiple consecutive endoscopic sessions [24–27]. Although good outcomes have been reported in patients with postoperative biliary strictures, the success rates in the setting of chronic pancreatitis have been disappointingly low [27, 28]. Furthermore, long-term success with plastic stents requires multiple endoscopic procedures which increase risks, costs, and patient burden [29].

Metal stents have been used in an attempt to improve the long-term success rate. The use of uncovered and partially covered SEMSs was abandoned due to the very high rate of tissue ingrowth, which leads to clogging of the stent and significant difficulty in stent removal [10, 12]. Recently, the use of various types of fully-covered metals has gained popularity, although concerns remain regarding safety and long-term outcomes [13, 16–22]. Our study expands on previously reported experiences with various fully covered SEMS and is the first one to report the prospective long-term outcomes with the use of the WallFlex Biliary RX Stent for benign biliary strictures. Summarized data from prior studies on other fully covered SEMS for benign biliary strictures with long-term followup are shown in Table 3.

Our data revealed that in patients with benign biliary strictures, placement and removal of fully-covered SEMS are technically highly successful (100%) and led to short-term stricture resolution in the vast majority of the patients (96%). Furthermore, long-term stricture resolution was achieved in 83% of the patients. Moreover, our long-term success rate in patients with CP-related strictures appeared significantly higher (73%) compared with prior experiences with plastic stents and other types of SEMS [13, 16]. Importantly, these successful outcomes were achieved with a very low number of ERCPs (mean of 2.4 procedures per patient). The vast majority of patients required only one ERCP for stricture resolution by SEMS placement (due to its radial expansion capability) and one ERCP for stent removal. This suggested the benefit of SEMS over plastic stents to overcome the problem of multiple plastic stent placements with repeated interventions.

We observed an overall very low incidence of adverse events. We noted only one episode of postprocedure pain due to continuous radial expansion force of the SEMS, and that was successfully treated by downgrading the stent size to a smaller diameter. There were no complications during stent placement or stent removal, and no stent dysfunction was noted. As we expected, stent migration was common (9/23; 39%), but it was without clinical consequences except in one case. All stents were successfully removed with ease. This could be explained by having loop for stent retrieval. The only two cases with significantly difficult removals occurred with upstream stent migration. After we encountered this problem with upstream migration, we modified our technique to leave 4 to 5 mm of the distal end of the stent protruding from the ampulla at the end of stent deployment.

We believe that our study provides preliminary evidence of the long-term clinical utility of fully-covered SEMS as a therapy for benign biliary strictures. Our study has several methodological strengths: (1) prospective design; (2) strict

TABLE 3: Prior prospective studies on fully covered SEMS for benign biliary strictures.

Study (year)	N	Type of stent	Stricture resolution success rate	Migration rate	Mean followup (months)
Traina et al. (2009) [17]	16	Niti-S Comvi	87.5%	38%	10.1
Mahajan et al. (2009) [13]	44	GORE VIABIL	83%	4.5%	3.8
Hu et al. (2011) [18]	13	A short stent with a retrieval suture	92.3%	None	12.1
Park et al. (2011) [19]	22	SEMS with anchoring flap	91%	None	3.6
	21	SEMS with flared end	88%	33%	4.2
Tarantino et al. (2012) [20]	39	Niti-S Comvi (after failure of conventional therapy)	71.8%	33.3%	22.1
	15	Niti-S Comvi (as first approach)	53.3%	46.7%	14.4
Poley et al. (2012) [16]	23	HANAROSTENT	61%	4%	15
Perri et al. (2012) [21]	7	Unflared end Niti-S	43%	100%	24
	10	Flared end Niti-S	90%	40%	24
Tarantino et al. (2012) [22]	62	Niti-S Comvi	90.3%	24.2%	15.9
Current study	23	Wallflex	96%	39.1%	18.8

and clinically meaningful predetermined definitions for procedure, short-term and long-term success; (3) predetermined treatment protocol; (4) included all patients presenting to our center which led to reducing the potential for selection bias; and (5) relatively long clinical follow-up period (mean of 18 months).

We also acknowledge the following limitations of this study: (1) relatively small number of patients. As a result, our study lacks the power to provide a meaningful comparison between various subgroups. (2) The patients included in this study were referred to a tertiary referral center. This reason raises the concerns about selection bias of more difficult cases. (3) Fifty-six percent of our patients had prior therapy for their benign biliary stricture with dilation and plastic stent placements; therefore they were not treatment naive. (4) We had a high prevalence of CP-related strictures which are known to be more difficult to treat. (5) Four patients were lost to followup. Although our "loss to followup" rate is within the methodologically expectable rate, we unfortunately could not obtain long-term followup in all patients. In order to account for this, we performed an intention-to-treat analysis which we considered all of the patients that were lost to followup to be failures of therapy. Therefore, this analysis should provide a "worst case scenario" interpretation of our data.

Overall, we achieved very good results, and the biliary stricture resolution rate in CP cases appeared to be superior to historical results achieved with plastic stenting. Furthermore, recurrence of the stricture in three patients happened in CP patients. This might be explained by the nature of the disease itself, not from the de novo stricture caused by SEMS. However, this should be interpreted with caution with the absence of a control group.

5. Conclusions

The use of fully-covered SEMSs for the treatment of benign biliary strictures leads to short-term stricture resolution in the vast majority of patients. Over a long-term follow-up period, the success rate appears favorable compared with historical results achieved with multiple plastic stenting, particularly in the patients with CP related strictures. Future randomized studies directly comparing plastic versus metal stents appear warranted. An optimal quality of fully-covered SEMS needs to be developed in order to make this stent a standard of care tool for patients suffering from benign biliary strictures with the best outcome and most cost effectiveness.

References

[1] A. A. Abdallah, J. E. J. Krige, and P. C. Bornman, "Biliary tract obstruction in chronic pancreatitis," *HPB*, vol. 9, no. 6, pp. 421–428, 2007.

[2] L. B. Johnson and F. H. Al-Kawas, "The bile duct—the achilles' heel of living donor liver transplantation," *American Journal of Gastroenterology*, vol. 99, no. 7, pp. 1296–1297, 2004.

[3] S. M. Strasberg, M. Hertl, and N. J. Soper, "An analysis of the problem of biliary injury during laparoscopic cholecystectomy," *Journal of the American College of Surgeons*, vol. 180, no. 1, pp. 101–125, 1995.

[4] G. Branum, C. Schmitt, J. Baillie et al., "Management of major biliary complications after laparoscopic cholecystectomy," *Annals of Surgery*, vol. 217, no. 5, pp. 532–541, 1993.

[5] P. G. A. Van Boeckel, F. P. Vleggaar, and P. D. Siersema, "Plastic or metal stents for benign extrahepatic biliary strictures: a systematic review," *BMC Gastroenterology*, vol. 9, article 96, 2009.

[6] A. L. Warshaw, R. H. Schapiro, J. T. Ferrucci, and J. J. Galdabini, "Persistent obstructive jaundice, cholangitis, and biliary cirrhosis due to common bile duct stenosis in chronic pancreatitis," *Gastroenterology*, vol. 70, no. 4, pp. 562–567, 1976.

[7] P. H. P. Davids, E. A. J. Rauws, P. P. L. O. Coene, G. N. J. Tytgat, and K. Huibregtse, "Endoscopic stenting for post-operative

biliary strictures," *Gastrointestinal Endoscopy*, vol. 38, no. 1, pp. 12–18, 1992.

[8] J. J. Bergman, L. Burgemeister, M. J. Bruno et al., "Long-term follow-up after biliary stent placement for postoperative bile duct stenosis," *Gastrointestinal Endoscopy*, vol. 54, no. 2, pp. 154–161, 2001.

[9] G. Morelli, A. Fazel, J. Judah, J. J. Pan, C. Forsmark, and P. Draganov, "Rapid-sequence endoscopic management of posttransplant anastomotic biliary strictures," *Gastrointestinal Endoscopy*, vol. 67, no. 6, pp. 879–885, 2008.

[10] A. M. van Berkel, D. L. Cahen, D. J. van Westerloo, E. A. J. Rauws, K. Huibregtse, and M. J. Bruno, "Self-expanding metal stents in benign biliary strictures due to chronic pancreatitis," *Endoscopy*, vol. 36, no. 5, pp. 381–384, 2004.

[11] D. L. Cahen, A. M. M. Van Berkel, D. Oskam et al., "Long-term results of endoscopic drainage of common bile duct strictures in chronic pancreatitis," *European Journal of Gastroenterology and Hepatology*, vol. 17, no. 1, pp. 103–108, 2005.

[12] B. Behm, A. Brock, B. W. Clarke et al., "Partially covered self-expandable metallic stents for benign biliary strictures due to chronic pancreatitis," *Endoscopy*, vol. 41, no. 6, pp. 547–551, 2009.

[13] A. Mahajan, H. Ho, B. Sauer et al., "Temporary placement of fully covered self-expandable metal stents in benign biliary strictures: midterm evaluation (with video)," *Gastrointestinal Endoscopy*, vol. 70, no. 2, pp. 303–309, 2009.

[14] M. Kahaleh, B. Behm, B. W. Clarke et al., "Temporary placement of covered self-expandable metal stents in benign biliary strictures: a new paradigm? (with video)," *Gastrointestinal Endoscopy*, vol. 67, no. 3, pp. 446–454, 2008.

[15] T. H. Baron, "Covered self-expandable metal stents for benign biliary tract diseases," *Current Opinion in Gastroenterology*, vol. 27, no. 3, pp. 262–267, 2011.

[16] J. W. Poley, D. L. Cahen, H. J. Metselaar et al., "A prospective group sequential study evaluating a new type of fully covered self-expandable metal stent for the treatment of benign biliary strictures (with video)," *Gastrointestinal Endoscopy*, vol. 75, no. 4, pp. 783–789, 2012.

[17] M. Traina, I. Tarantino, L. Barresi et al., "Efficacy and safety of fully covered self-expandable metallic stents in biliary complications after liver transplantation: a preliminary study," *Liver Transplantation*, vol. 15, no. 11, pp. 1493–1498, 2009.

[18] B. Hu, D. J. Gao, F. H. Yu, T. T. Wang, Y. M. Pan, and X. M. Yang, "Endoscopic stenting for post-transplant biliary stricture: usefulness of a novel removable covered metal stent," *Journal of Hepato-Biliary-Pancreatic Surgery*, vol. 18, no. 5, pp. 640–645, 2011.

[19] D. H. Park, S. S. Lee, T. H. Lee et al., "Anchoring flap versus flared end, fully covered self-expandable metal stents to prevent migration in patients with benign biliary strictures: a multicenter, prospective, comparative pilot study (with videos)," *Gastrointestinal Endoscopy*, vol. 73, no. 1, pp. 64–70, 2011.

[20] I. Tarantino, M. Traina, F. Mocciaro et al., "Fully covered metallic stents in biliary stenosis after orthotopic liver transplantation," *Endoscopy*, vol. 44, no. 3, pp. 246–250, 2012.

[21] V. Perri, I. Boškoski, A. Tringali et al., "Fully covered self-expandable metal stents in biliary strictures caused by chronic pancreatitis not responding to plastic stenting: a prospective study with 2 years of follow-up," *Gastrointestinal Endoscopy*, vol. 75, no. 6, pp. 1271–1277, 2012.

[22] I. Tarantino, B. Mangiavillano, R. Di Mitri et al., "Fully covered self-expandable metallic stents in benign biliary strictures: a multicenter study on efficacy and safety," *Endoscopy*, vol. 44, no. 10, pp. 923–927, 2012.

[23] P. B. Cotton, G. M. Eisen, L. Aabakken et al., "A lexicon for endoscopic adverse events: report of an ASGE workshop," *Gastrointestinal Endoscopy*, vol. 71, no. 3, pp. 446–454, 2010.

[24] C. Berkelhammer, P. Kortan, and G. B. Haber, "Endoscopic biliary prostheses as treatment for benign postoperative bile duct strictures," *Gastrointestinal Endoscopy*, vol. 35, no. 2, pp. 95–101, 1989.

[25] D. J. Geenen, J. E. Geenen, W. J. Hogan et al., "Endoscopic therapy for benign bile duct strictures," *Gastrointestinal Endoscopy*, vol. 35, no. 5, pp. 367–371, 1989.

[26] J. M. Dumonceau, J. Deviere, M. Delhaye et al., "Plastic and metal stents for postoperative benign bile duct strictures: the best and the worst," *Gastrointestinal Endoscopy*, vol. 47, no. 1, pp. 8–93, 1998.

[27] P. Draganov, B. Hoffman, W. Marsh, P. Cotton, and J. Cunningham, "Long-term outcome in patients with benign biliary strictures treated endoscopically with multiple stents," *Gastrointestinal Endoscopy*, vol. 55, no. 6, pp. 680–686, 2002.

[28] M. Barthet, J. P. Bernard, J. L. Duval, C. Affriat, and J. Sahel, "Biliary stenting in benign biliary stenosis complicating chronic calcifying pancreatitis," *Endoscopy*, vol. 26, no. 7, pp. 569–572, 1994.

[29] M. F. Catalano, J. D. Linder, S. George, E. Alcocer, and J. E. Geenen, "Treatment of symptomatic distal common bile duct stenosis secondary to chronic pancreatitis: comparison of single vs. multiple simultaneous stents," *Gastrointestinal Endoscopy*, vol. 60, no. 6, pp. 945–952, 2004.

3

Diagnostic Yield and Safety of Endoscopic Ultrasound Guided Fine Needle Aspiration of Central Mediastinal Lung Masses

Enrique Vazquez-Sequeiros,[1,2] Michael J. Levy,[3] Manuel Van Domselaar,[2] Fernando González-Panizo,[2] Jose Ramon Foruny-Olcina,[1,2] Daniel Boixeda-Miquel,[1] Diego Juzgado-Lucas,[2] and Agustin Albillos[1]

[1] *Gastroenterology Service, University Hospital Ramon y Cajal, 28801 Madrid, Spain*
[2] *Gastroenterology Service, University Hospital Quiron, Madrid, Spain*
[3] *Developmental Endoscopy Unit, Gastroenterology Division, Mayo Clinic, Rochester, MN, USA*

Correspondence should be addressed to Enrique Vazquez-Sequeiros; evazquezse@gmail.com

Academic Editor: Kazuo Inui

Background and Aims. EUS-FNA is an accurate and safe technique to biopsy mediastinal lymph nodes. However, there are few data pertaining to the role of EUS-FNA to biopsy central lung masses. The aim of the study was to assess the diagnostic yield and safety of EUS-FNA of indeterminate central mediastinal lung masses. *Methods.* Design: Retrospective review of a prospectively maintained database; noncomparative. Setting: Tertiary referral center. From 10/2004 to 12/2010, all patients with a lung mass located within proximity to the esophagus were referred for EUS-FNA. Main Outcome Measurement: EUS-FNA diagnostic accuracy and safety. *Results.* 73 consecutive patients were included. EUS allowed detection in 62 (85%) patients with lack of visualization prohibiting FNA in 11 patients. Among sampled lesions, one patient (1/62 = 1.6%) had a benign lung mass (hamartoma), while the remaining 61 patients (61/62 = 98.4%) had a malignant mass (primary lung cancer: 55/61 = 90%; lung metastasis: 6/61 = 10%). The sensitivity, specificity, and accuracy of EUS-FNA were 96.7%, 100%, and 96.7%, respectively. The sensitivity was 80.8% when considering nonvisualized masses. One patient developed a pneumothorax (1/62 = 1.6%). *Conclusions.* EUS-FNA appears to be an accurate and safe technique for tissue diagnosis of central mediastinal lung masses.

1. Background

Lung cancer represents the most common cause of cancer and cancer-related mortality [1]. Treatment strategy largely depends on the tumor stage, with tissue confirmation considered necessary to provide therapy. Pulmonologists and thoracic surgeons have classically relied on bronchoscopy (forceps biopsy of lumen tumor and/or blind transbronchial fine needle aspiration), computed tomography- (CT-) guided fine needle aspiration/biopsy (FNA), mediastinoscopy, or thoracoscopy for diagnosis [2].

The technique selected usually depends on local expertise and tumor and nodal location. The accuracy of each of these techniques is limited and each is associated with notable morbidity [2]. The sensitivity of bronchoscopically guided biopsy is poor, as it fails to reach a definitive diagnosis in 20 to 30% of patients [3]. CT-guided FNA provides a diagnostic accuracy of 77% to 95%, but is largely limited to sampling of masses larger than 2 cm in size and may result in pneumothorax in as many as 22%–62% of patients [4–6]. In addition, CT often cannot be performed in lesions abutting or located in close proximity to large mediastinal vessels [7]. While surgical techniques such as mediastinoscopy or thoracoscopy provide excellent diagnostic accuracy in this setting, both must be performed in the operating room under general anesthesia and have been associated with significant procedure-related mortality (as high as 0.4%) [8].

More recently, endoscopic ultrasound guided fine needle aspiration (EUS-FNA) has proven to be an accurate and safe technique to biopsy mediastinal lymph nodes to aid lung cancer staging [9–11]. In addition, limited data suggest that EUS-FNA may also allow imaging and biopsy lung masses and may complement or substitute for other biopsy techniques [12–14]. In recent years, pulmonologists and thoracic surgeons have also employed endobronchial ultrasound (EBUS) to examine and biopsy (EBUS-TBNA) lesions in the anterior mediastinum, with excellent results (accuracy > 80–90%) [11, 15]. Unfortunately, this modern technique is still beginning to spread in many countries and is not available in many institutions.

Aim. The aim of this study was to determine the diagnostic yield and safety of EUS-FNA in patients with a central mediastinal lung mass.

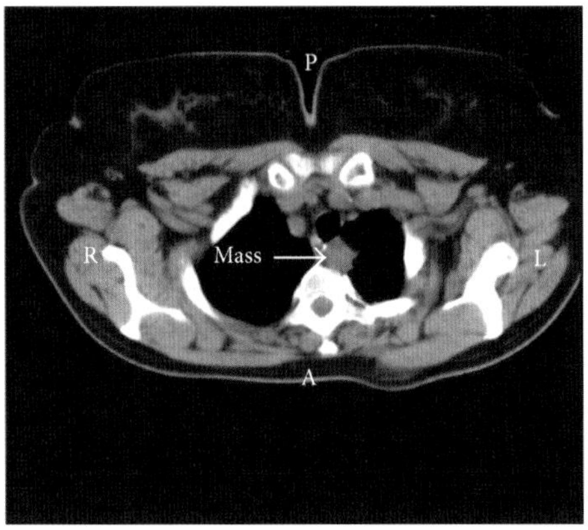

FIGURE 1: Chest CT scan showing a left upper-lobe lung mass adjacent to the esophagus.

2. Patient and Methods

2.1. Study Design. We conducted a retrospective review of a prospectively maintained database (at 2 tertiary referral centers) to identify consecutive patients with an indeterminate central lung mass who were referred for EUS-FNA. Central mediastinal lung masses were defined as those with the closest margin believe to be in sufficient proximity to the esophageal wall based on pre-EUS-CT or PET-CT to potentially permit transesophageal EUS-FNA. The study includes all consecutive patients evaluated since the first referral in November 2004 until January 2011. Of note, while prior biopsy efforts may have included bronchoscopy and/or CT-guided biopsy, endobronchial ultrasound (EBUS) and EBUS-guided FNA were not available in our institutions at the time of the study. Clinical followup was available for a minimum of 12 months in each patient. The study protocol was approved by the Institutional Review Board, and informed consent was obtained for all procedures.

In accordance with our standard of clinical practice, this study excludes patients with (1) serious comorbidities precluding EUS exam; (2) patient refusal to participate; (3) prior tissue diagnosis by other means; (4) other target lesions more easily accessible for biopsy (e.g., liver metastasis); (5) coagulation disorder precluding EUS-FNA (platelet count <50,000/μL and/or international normalized ratio INR > 1.5); or (6) prior radiation therapy for lung cancer.

Patient data (demographics, intervention, and followup) were prospectively collected and introduced in a predefined computer database for later review. A chest CT scan and/or a PET/CT scan demonstrating a lung mass adjacent to the esophagus, with no mediastinal lymphadenopathy and/or distant metastases, was obtained in all cases (Figure 1). Bronchoscopy was also performed in all patients.

2.2. EUS Exam and FNA. The EUS-FNA exam was performed on an outpatient basis by an endosonographer having performed more than 5000 EUS procedures using a curvilinear array echoendoscope (GF-UCT140-AL5, GF-UCT160-OL5 Olympus 5–10 MHz) and an Aloka (ProSound SSD-α5) or C-60 ultrasound processor. Conscious sedation was administered using a combination of midazolam, propofol, and fentanyl or meperidine. The EUS instrument was

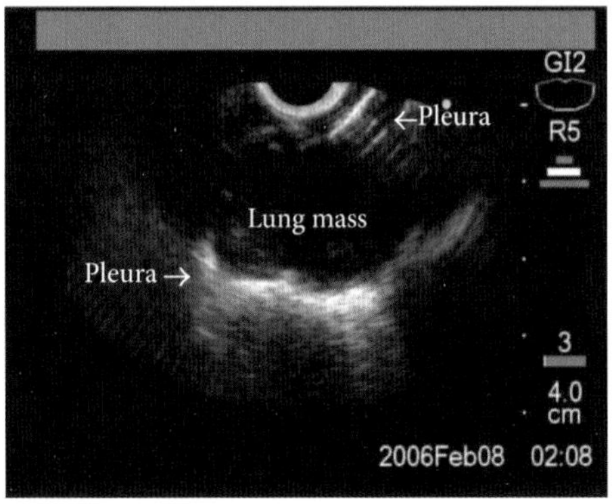

FIGURE 2: EUS exam of the same patient showing the hypoechogenic mass, 2 cm in size, located in the lung parenchyma.

advanced into the stomach with continuous imaging during withdrawal to exam the liver, left adrenal gland, perigastric region, and posterior mediastinum. A 22-gauge needle with stylet (Echo-Tip; Wilson Cook Medical Inc., Winston-Salem, North Carolina) was inserted in the mass under EUS guidance (Figures 2 and 3). In the preset study, we employed 25 gauge needles for biopsy. Per routine, after withdrawing the needle stylet, five cc of negative pressure was applied while 10 to and from movements were performed within the lesion. During subsequent needle passes, the amount of negative pressure was increased or decreased (range 0–10 cc) if the sample was grossly sparse or bloody appearing, respectively. When necessary, color Doppler US was used to avoid accidental puncture of intervening vascular structures.

The collected material was sprayed onto glass slides and evaluated by an on-site cytopathologist to assess adequacy. EUS-FNA aspirates were obtained until (1) a preliminary on site cytopathologic diagnosis of malignancy was given; or (2) a maximum of 3 passes had been performed, and adequate and representative material had been obtained by EUS-FNA means as assessed by the cytopathologist.

The definitive EUS-FNA cytologic diagnosis was based on formal review of all materials (Diff-Quik and Papanicolaou) with a positive test result mandating an interpretation of

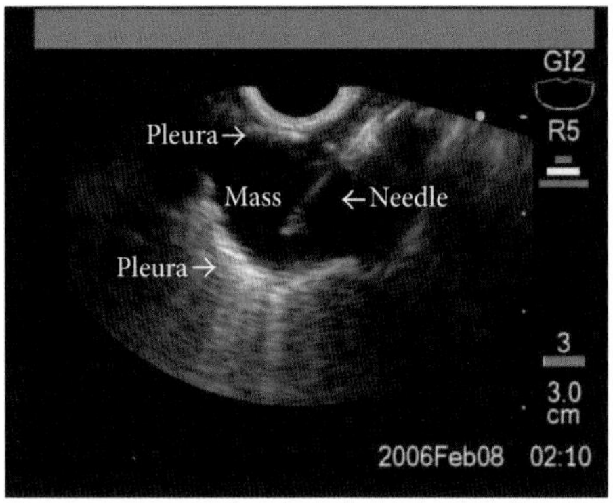

FIGURE 3: EUS-FNA of the lung mass identified was performed, disclosing a diagnosis of nonsmall-cell lung cancer.

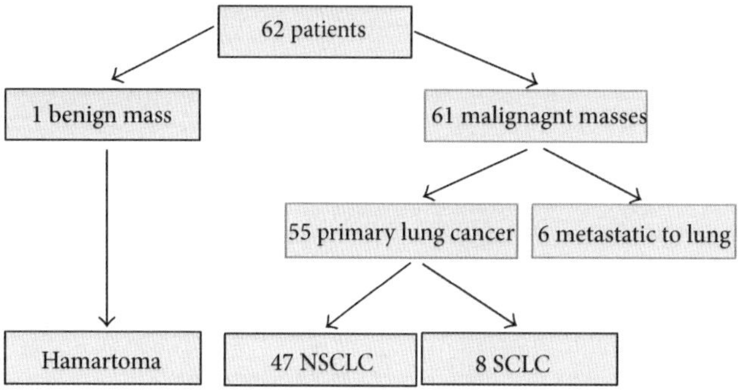

FIGURE 4: Final diagnosis of the 62 patients in whom EUS detection of the lung mass was possible. *Nonsmall-cell lung cancer (NSCLC); small-cell lung cancer (SCLC).

"positive for malignancy." All nonpositive interpretations (i.e., negative, atypical, and suspicious interpretations) were considered negative for malignancy.

As per routine clinical practice, patients were monitored after procedure for a minimum of 90 minutes during which development of complications was assessed. Patients were also evaluated for complications at standard clinical followup that is performed within 7 days after the procedure, during which a physical exam and chest X-ray were routinely obtained. Based on the patient status at initial followup, additional phone or in-person followup was conducted to identify any late complications.

2.3. Gold Standard for Lung Mass Diagnosis. The gold standard was based on strict cytohistologic correlation and a minimum 12-month followup [16]. A patient was considered to have malignancy if there was (1) cytologic and/or histologic evidence of malignancy based on material obtained via (a) EUS FNA, (b) surgical pathology (for those patients receiving surgical resection or mediastinoscopy or thoracoscopy), (c) percutaneous biopsy, or (d) autopsy; or (2) clinical course (≥12 months) suggesting malignancy based on presence of: (a) new radiographic abnormality including (i) regional or distant mass (hepatic, pulmonary, or bone), (ii) mass infiltrating large blood vessels, or (iii) malignant appearing lymphadenopathy with positive positron emission tomography imaging; or (b) cancer-related mortality. Designation of a lesion as benign required at least 12 months of followup and absence of any of the above criteria and/or follow-up imaging demonstrating complete resolution of the abnormality.

2.4. Statistical Analysis. A commercially available statistical software package (JMP 7.0.2 SAS Institute Inc., North Carolina, USA) was employed for statistical analysis. Descriptive analysis of data is presented in the paper as follows: (a) discrete variables, percentage and 95% confidence interval; (b) continuous variables, mean ± standard deviation (or median/interquartile range) and range [17]. The performance characteristics (sensitivity, specificity, and overall diagnostic accuracy) of EUS-FNA in this cohort of patients with a centrally located lung mass were calculated as previously described [17].

3. Results

From November 2004 to January 2011, 73 patients with a central mediastinal lung mass were referred for possible EUS-FNA. EUS allowed detection in 62 (85%) patients with lack of visualization prohibiting FNA in 11 patients. CT revealed that in 9 of the 11 patients the mass was located more than 1 cm distant to the cervical/upper esophagus potentially contributing to the failed EUS detection. In the other 2 patients, the lung mass was located in the mid esophagus, but >2 cm away from the esophageal wall, likely negatively impacting EUS detection.

For the 62 patients in whom EUS identification was possible, there was a male preponderance (male/female: 48/14 = 78%/22%), with a mean age of 68.0 ± 11.5 years (range 61–82). The lung masses were located in the vicinity of the cervical/upper esophagus (n = 19; each <1 cm from esophagus) or mid esophagus (n = 43 patients; each <2 cm from the esophagus). The lung masses measured a median long axis of 26 mm (range 12–65 mm), and the median number of EUS-FNA passes performed was 1 (range 1–3).

Based on the gold standard diagnosis, one of the visualized masses (1/62 = 1.6%; 95% CI: 0–9%) was ultimately diagnosed as a benign lesion (hamartoma), while the remaining 61 patients had a malignant mass (61/62 = 98.4%; 95% CI: 90–100%). Fifty-five malignant masses represented primary lung cancers (55/61 = 90%; 95% CI: 80–96%), while 6 were ultimately diagnosed as a lung metastasis (6/61 = 10%; 95% CI: 4–20%). Among the subgroup of primary lung cancers (n = 55), 47 were nonsmall-cell lung cancers (NSCLC), and 8 represented small-cell lung cancer (SCLC) (Figure 4).

An adequate EUS-FNA sample was obtained in all but one patient (61/62 = 98.4%; 95% CI: 93–100%), yielding the correct diagnosis in 60 patients (diagnostic accuracy: 60/62 = 96.7%; 95% CI: 88–99). The two false negative EUS-FNA results were obtained in patients with NSCLC, in which the EUS-FNA specimen contained only benign cells (n = 1) or no cytologic material was obtained (n = 1). The tumor sizes for these later two patients were 12 and 25 mm, respectively.

Therefore, the sensitivity of EUS-FNA among all 73 patients was 80.8% (59/73; 95% CI: 70–89%) compared to 96.7% (59/61 = 96.7%; 95% CI: 88–99%) for the cohort in whom EUS lung mass detection was possible.

One patient (1/62 = 1.6%; 95% CI: 0–9%) with a NSCLC developed a large tension pneumothorax within 24 hours of EUS-FNA-requiring chest tube placement and 24-hour intensive care unit observation. The patient fully recovered and was discharged from the hospital 7 days later. This complication was not recognized during the EUS-FNA procedure and was diagnosed due to patient dyspnea after release from the endoscopy unit. No other complications developed.

4. Discussion

The key to the evaluation and management of a lung mass is determining whether it represents a malignant or benign [18]. Standard techniques for obtaining a tissue diagnosis such as bronchoscopy or CT-guided biopsy yield a false negative rate of approximately 30% and risk pneumothorax [3–6]. More recently, introduced techniques such as EUS-FNA and EBUS-TBNA provide enhanced diagnostic sensitivity [9–16]. EUS-FNA is now routinely performed to evaluate indeterminate mediastinal structures and to enhance NSCLC staging largely through the targeted inspection of posterior mediastinal nodal stations (left lower paratracheal, aortopulmonary window, subcarinal, lower paraesophageal, and inferior pulmonary ligament) [19–30], providing a sensitivity and specificity of 81–97% and 83–100%, respectively [31]. EUS-FNA may be useful as the first diagnostic test in patients with suspected lung cancer or following negative bronchoscopy and computerized tomography [32]. EUS-FNA and EBUS-TBNA are now regarded as complementary staging modalities that combine to provide a diagnostic accuracy of 91% similar to surgical techniques [33–36]. Some suggest that these techniques may substitute for surgical diagnosis and staging of lung cancer patients [33–36].

Although EUS-FNA has been shown to be extremely useful for evaluation of mediastinal lymph nodes and masses in a minimally invasive manner, there are a paucity of data regarding the role of EUS-FNA to cytohistologically diagnose lung parenchyma masses. Varadarajulu et al. [12] conducted a retrospective study including 18 patients undergoing EUS-FNA of a lung mass abutting the esophageal wall. They reported a diagnostic yield of 100% without complications. Annema et al. [13] conducted a prospective and controlled study to assess the feasibility and diagnostic yield of EUS-FNA for diagnosis of centrally located lung tumors following a nondiagnostic bronchoscopy. EUS-FNA provided a diagnosis of malignancy in 31 of the 32 patients (97%) [13]. Hernandez et al. [14] described their retrospective experience in which EUS-FNA of centrally located primary lung cancers was diagnosed in all 17 patients evaluated.

Our data represent the largest study to date and support experience from other research groups. EUS-FNA provided the correct diagnosis in 96.7% of patients, and further diagnostic interventions (mediastinoscopy) were only required in two cases. Those 2 patients that could not be diagnosed by EUS-FNA corresponded to (1) one patient with a lung mass in which EUS-FNA obtained an inadequate/necrotic and nondiagnostic material; (2) one patient with a malignant lung mass (primary) and a false negative EUS-FNA result. Our findings also support the role of EUS-FNA in evaluating lung masses resulting from secondary metastasis.

A notable limitation of EUS-FNA is the impaired ability to identify and access lung tumors located distant (>2 cm) to the esophagus, which unfortunately comprise a majority of lung cancers. The impaired detection results from the acoustic impedance mismatch at the lung interface, which greatly limits ultrasound transmission. Our study is also limited by the lack of availability of EBUS and EBUS-TBNA in our centers during the study period. This may have resulted in some degree of referral bias that could theoretically impact our study findings.

To our knowledge, whether EUS-FNA or EBUS-TBNA may be better suited to perform biopsies of lung masses has not been investigated. Tournoy et al. demonstrated in a retrospective noncomparative study including 60 patients (82% with a prior nondiagnostic flexible bronchoscopy), that EBUS-TBNA reaches a sensitivity of 82% and a negative predictive value of 23% when biopsying centrally located lung masses [15]. Unfortunately, the present study was conducted at two institutions, in which EBUS-TBNA was not available at that time. Therefore, direct comparisons between both techniques could not be performed. We believe a combination of EUS-FNA and EBUS-TBNA will probably be the best approach for diagnosis of central mediastinal lung masses. Future studies designed for direct comparison of both techniques are definitively needed.

In summary, our data support the accuracy and general safety of EUS-FNA for evaluation of central mediastinal lung masses. Further research is needed to determine the role of EUS-FNA relative to EBUS-TBNA as the initial diagnostic test in patients with an indeterminate lung mass.

Abbreviations

CI:	Confidence interval
CT:	Computerized tomography
EUS-FNA:	Endoscopic ultrasound guided fine needle aspiration
NSCLC:	Nonsmall-cell lung cancer
SCLC:	Small cell lung cancer.

References

[1] A. J. Alberg and J. M. Samet, "Epidemiology of lung cancer," *Chest*, vol. 123, no. 1, supplement, pp. 21S–49S, 2003.

[2] F. C. Detterbeck, M. A. Jantz, M. Wallace, J. Vansteenkiste, and G. A. Silvestri, "Invasive mediastinal staging of lung cancer: ACCP evidence-based clinical practice guidelines (2nd edition)," *Chest*, vol. 132, no. 3, supplement, pp. 202S–220S, 2007.

[3] P. Mazzone, P. Jain, A. C. Arroliga, and R. A. Matthay, "Bronchoscopy and needle biopsy techniques for diagnosis and

staging of lung cancer," *Clinics in Chest Medicine*, vol. 23, no. 1, pp. 137–158, 2002.

[4] H. Li, P. M. Boiselle, J. A. O. Shepard, B. Trotman-Dickenson, and T. C. McLoud, "Diagnostic accuracy and safety of CT-guided percutaneous needle aspiration biopsy of the lung: comparison of small and large pulmonary nodules," *American Journal of Roentgenology*, vol. 167, no. 1, pp. 105–109, 1996.

[5] M. J. Wallace, S. Krishnamurthy, L. D. Broemeling et al., "CT-guided percutaneous fine-needle aspiration biopsy of small (≥1-cm) pulmonary lesions," *Radiology*, vol. 225, no. 3, pp. 823–828, 2002.

[6] E. A. Kazerooni, F. T. Lim, A. Mikhail, and F. J. Martinez, "Risk of pneumothorax in CT-guided transthoracic needle aspiration biopsy of the lung," *Radiology*, vol. 198, no. 2, pp. 371–375, 1996.

[7] Y. Ohno, H. Hatabu, D. Takenaka et al., "CT-guided transthoracic needle aspiration biopsy of small (≤ 20 mm) solitary pulmonary nodules," *American Journal of Roentgenology*, vol. 180, no. 6, pp. 1665–1669, 2003.

[8] K. Yasufuku and T. Fujisawa, "Staging and diagnosis of non-small cell lung cancer: invasive modalities," *Respirology*, vol. 12, no. 2, pp. 173–183, 2007.

[9] M. J. Wiersema, E. Vazquez-Sequeiros, and L. M. Wiersema, "Evaluation of mediastinal lymphadenopathy with endoscopic US-guided fine-needle aspiration biopsy," *Radiology*, vol. 219, no. 1, pp. 252–257, 2001.

[10] C. G. Micames, D. C. McCrory, D. A. Pavey, P. S. Jowell, and F. G. Gress, "Endoscopic ultrasound-guided fine-needle aspiration for non-small cell lung cancer staging: a systematic review and metaanalysis," *Chest*, vol. 131, no. 2, pp. 539–548, 2007.

[11] K. J. Tournoy, M. Carprieaux, E. Deschepper, J. P. van Meerbeeck, and M. Praet, "Are EUS-FNA and EBUS-TBNA specimens reliable for subtyping non-small cell lung cancer?" *Lung Cancer*, vol. 76, pp. 46–50, 2012.

[12] S. Varadarajulu, B. J. Hoffman, R. H. Hawes, and M. A. Eloubeidi, "EUS-guided FNA of lung masses adjacent to or abutting the esophagus after unrevealing CT-guided biopsy or bronchoscopy," *Gastrointestinal Endoscopy*, vol. 60, no. 2, pp. 293–297, 2004.

[13] J. T. Annema, M. Veseliç, and K. F. Rabe, "EUS-guided FNA of centrally located lung tumours following a non-diagnostic bronchoscopy," *Lung Cancer*, vol. 48, no. 3, pp. 357–361, 2005.

[14] A. Hernandez, M. Kahaleh, J. Olazagasti et al., "EUS-FNA as the initial diagnostic modality in centrally located primary lung cancers," *Journal of Clinical Gastroenterology*, vol. 41, no. 7, pp. 657–660, 2007.

[15] K. G. Tournoy, R. C. Rintoul, J. P. van Meerbeeck et al., "EBUS-TBNA for the diagnosis of central parenchymal lung lesions not visible at routine bronchoscopy," *Lung Cancer*, vol. 63, no. 1, pp. 45–49, 2009.

[16] F. G. Gress, T. J. Savides, A. Sandler et al., "Endoscopic ultrasonography, fine-needle aspiration biopsy guided by endoscopic ultrasonography, and computed tomography in the preoperative staging of non-small-cell lung cancer: a comparison study," *Annals of Internal Medicine*, vol. 127, no. 8 I, pp. 604–612, 1997.

[17] H. Motulsky, *Intuitive Biostatistics*, Oxford University Press, New York, NY, USA, 1995.

[18] J. L. Leef and J. S. Klein, "The solitary pulmonary nodule," *Radiologic Clinics of North America*, vol. 40, no. 1, pp. 123–143, 2002.

[19] M. J. Wiersema, P. Vilmann, M. Giovannini, K. J. Chang, and L. M. Wiersema, "Endosonography-guided fine-needle aspiration biopsy: diagnostic accuracy and complication assessment," *Gastroenterology*, vol. 112, no. 4, pp. 1087–1095, 1997.

[20] A. Affi, E. Vazquez-Sequeiros, I. D. Norton, J. E. Clain, and M. J. Wiersema, "Acute extraluminal hemorrhage associated with EUS-guided fine needle aspiration: frequency and clinical significance," *Gastrointestinal Endoscopy*, vol. 53, no. 2, pp. 221–225, 2001.

[21] M. B. Wallace, G. A. Silvestri, A. V. Sahai et al., "Endoscopic ultrasound-guided fine needle aspiration for staging patients with carcinoma of the lung," *Annals of Thoracic Surgery*, vol. 72, no. 6, pp. 1861–1867, 2001.

[22] A. Fritscher-Ravens, N. Soehendra, L. Schirrow et al., "Role of transesophageal endosonography-guided fine-needle aspiration in the diagnosis of lung cancer," *Chest*, vol. 117, no. 2, pp. 339–345, 2000.

[23] J. Laudanski, M. Kozlowski, J. Nikliński, and L. Chyczewski, "The preoperative study of mediastinal lymph nodes metastasis in lung cancer by endoscopic ultrasonography (EUS) and helical computed tomography (CT)," *Lung Cancer*, vol. 34, no. 2, pp. S123–S126, 2001.

[24] L. Aabakken, G. A. Silvestri, R. Hawes, C. E. Reed, V. Marsi, and B. Hoffman, "Cost-efficacy of endoscopic ultrasonography with fine-needle aspiration vs. mediastinotomy in patients with lung cancer and suspected mediastinal adenopathy," *Endoscopy*, vol. 31, no. 9, pp. 707–711, 1999.

[25] D. Kondo, M. Imaizumi, T. Abe, T. Naruke, and K. Suemasu, "Endoscopic ultrasound examination for mediastinal lymph node metastases of lung cancer," *Chest*, vol. 98, no. 3, pp. 586–593, 1990.

[26] D. L. Serna, H. E. Aryan, K. J. Chang, M. Brenner, L. M. Tran, and J. C. Chen, "An early comparison between endoscopic ultrasound-guided fine-needle aspiration and mediastinoscopy for diagnosis of mediastinal malignancy," *American Surgeon*, vol. 64, no. 10, pp. 1014–1018, 1998.

[27] K. J. Chang, R. A. Erickson, and P. Nguyen, "Endoscopic ultrasound (EUS) and EUS-guided fine-needle aspiration of the left adrenal gland," *Gastrointestinal Endoscopy*, vol. 44, no. 5, pp. 568–572, 1996.

[28] E. B. Stelow, S. M. Debol, M. W. Stanley, S. Mallery, R. Lai, and R. H. Bardales, "Sampling of the adrenal glands by endoscopic ultrasound-guided fine-needle aspiration," *Diagnostic Cytopathology*, vol. 33, no. 1, pp. 26–30, 2005.

[29] J. DeWitt, M. Alsatie, J. LeBlanc, L. McHenry, and S. Sherman, "Endoscopic ultrasound-guided fine-needle aspiration of left adrenal gland masses," *Endoscopy*, vol. 39, no. 1, pp. 65–71, 2007.

[30] N. C. Jhala, D. Jhala, M. A. Eloubeidi et al., "Endoscopic ultrasound-guided fine-needle aspiration biopsy of the adrenal glands: analysis of 24 patients," *Cancer*, vol. 102, no. 5, pp. 308–314, 2004.

[31] H. Kramer and H. J. M. Groen, "Current concepts in the mediastinal lymph node staging of nonsmall cell lung cancer," *Annals of Surgery*, vol. 238, no. 2, pp. 180–188, 2003.

[32] T. L. Ang, A. K. H. Tee, K. M. Fock, E. K. Teo, and T. S. Chua, "Endoscopic ultrasound-guided fine needle aspiration in the evaluation of suspected lung cancer," *Respiratory Medicine*, vol. 101, no. 6, pp. 1299–1304, 2007.

[33] N. Navani, J. M. Brown, M. Nankivell et al., "Suitability of endobronchial ultrasound-guided transbronchial needle aspiration specimens for subtyping and genotyping of non-small cell lung

cancer: a multicenter study of 774 patients," *American Journal of Respiratory and Critical Care Medicine*, vol. 185, no. 12, pp. 1316–1322, 2012.

[34] R. Ohnishi, I. Yasuda, T. Kato et al., "Combined endobronchial and endoscopic ultrasound guided fine needle aspiration for mediastinal nodal staging of lung cancer," *Endoscopy*, vol. 43, pp. 1082–1089, 2011.

[35] F. J. F. Herth, M. Krasnik, N. Kahn, R. Eberhardt, and A. Ernst, "Combined endoscopic-endobronchial ultrasound-guided fine-needle aspiration of mediastinal lymph nodes through a single bronchoscope in 150 patients with suspected lung cancer," *Chest*, vol. 138, no. 4, pp. 790–794, 2010.

[36] J. T. Annema, J. P. Van Meerbeeck, R. C. Rintoul et al., "Mediastinoscopy vs endosonography for mediastinal nodal staging of lung cancer: a randomized trial," *Journal of the American Medical Association*, vol. 304, no. 20, pp. 2245–2252, 2010.

4

The Current State of Diagnosis and Treatment for Early Gastric Cancer

Tomoyuki Yada,[1] Chizu Yokoi,[2] and Naomi Uemura[1]

[1] *Department of Gastroenterology, Kohnodai Hospital, National Center for Global Health and Medicine, 1-7-1 Kohnodai, Ichikawa, Chiba 272-8516, Japan*
[2] *Department of Gastroenterology, National Center for Global Health and Medicine, 1-21-1 Toyama, Shinjuku-ku, Tokyo 162-8655, Japan*

Correspondence should be addressed to Tomoyuki Yada; tomoyuki0618@yahoo.co.jp

Academic Editor: Tony C. K. Tham

The prognosis for gastric cancer depends on its stage; so, detection in the early stage of disease is important, when complete and curative removal is possible. Accurate diagnosis can be facilitated by a sound understanding of the basic findings of white light endoscopy of early gastric cancer, and diagnosis can be refined further by the combined use of other imaging modalities such as image-enhanced endoscopy including chromoendoscopy and endoscopic ultrasonography. Minimally invasive endoscopic treatment has come to be the preferred therapeutic approach for early gastric cancer. In addition to conventional endoscopic mucosal resection, a new technique known as endoscopic submucosal dissection (ESD) has spread rapidly worldwide. Indeed, strategies for ESD have been established, devices developed, its indications expanded, and its safety and long-term results extensively reported. Some unique combination therapies involving endoscopy and surgical treatment have also been reported. It is anticipated that the number of patients undergoing endoscopic therapy will continue to increase, and the ongoing developments in endoscopic treatment are expected not only to improve gastric cancer prognosis but also to maintain good quality of life after treatment.

1. Introduction

Despite both the incidence and mortality rates of gastric cancer showing decreasing trends, gastric cancer remains one of the most common causes of death by cancer worldwide [1, 2]. There are significant regional differences in gastric cancer onset, with East Asian countries, including Japan and Korea, known to have a particularly high incidence rate compared to the Western countries. In Japan, following the introduction of a mass screening program that utilizes double-contrast barium radiography for early the detection of gastric cancer and alongside developments in endoscopic equipment and improved diagnostic capability, gastric cancer is now being detected more often in the asymptomatic stages [3]. As a result, approximately 50% of the cases of gastric cancer currently treated in Japan are early stage disease [4]. In contrast, in Western countries, gastric cancer is often detected at an advanced stage and prognosis remains poor. Prognosis depends on the stage at which it is detected, and complete excision of the cancer is the only curative option. The excellent postoperative results for early gastric cancer, with a 5-year survival rate of over 90% in both Western countries and Japan, indicate just how important it is to detect the cancer at the earliest possible stage [5, 6]. Moreover, with the improved detection rate of early gastric cancer in Japan, more minimally invasive treatments have been investigated, and the use of endoscopic mucosal resection (EMR) has become widespread. This technique has the support of many endoscopists, including those in Western countries [7]. In addition, a new modality of endoscopic treatment, endoscopic submucosal dissection (ESD), has become commonly performed in facilities across Japan, helping to dramatically increase the number of early gastric cancer cases treated endoscopically [8]. This paper will give a basic summary of early gastric cancer, outline the current state of its diagnosis and treatment, and summarize the prospects for future management of the disease.

2. Classification of Early Gastric Cancer

Early gastric cancer is defined as remaining confined to the mucosa or submucosa, regardless of lymph node metastasis [9]. Japanese macroscopic classifications for gastric cancer are well known and divide early gastric cancer into three macroscopic types (0-I, 0-II, and 0-III) of which 0-II is then subclassified into 0-IIa, 0-IIb, and 0-IIc (Figures 1 and 2). The most common type of early gastric cancer is 0-IIc [10]. If two or more macroscopic types are mixed, the type that has spread further is recorded first. At an international workshop held in 2002, the Paris classification, which is based on the Japanese classification, was proposed and subsequently adopted as a simple and internationally unified classification for superficial gastrointestinal tumors [11].

Although cancer is pathologically diagnosed, the standards for pathological diagnosis are known to differ widely between Japan and Western countries [12]. In Western countries, cancer is diagnosed if the tumor has invaded the submucosa or muscularis mucosae and has at least invaded deeper than the lamina propria mucosae. In Japan, however, cancer is diagnosed based on cellular atypia or structural atypia, regardless of the extent of invasion. Although this discrepancy has lessened since the Vienna classification was proposed, lesions diagnosed as intramucosal carcinoma in Japan are still classified as high-grade adenoma/dysplasia (Vienna classification 4.1) in Western countries and often not diagnosed as cancer [13]. However, over 40% of lesions classified as equivalent to Vienna classification 3 or 4.1 on preoperative biopsy are diagnosed as cancer on the postendoscopic resection assessment, and it has been reported that a small number of cases are also accompanied by invasion into deeper regions of the submucosa [14, 15]. Therefore, when considering a complete cure, it is necessary to proceed carefully in cases with a histological diagnosis of neoplastic or dysplastic disease and, on case-by-case basis, to consider endoscopic resection.

Unlike advanced cancer which is easy to detect endoscopically, early gastric cancer often appears as subtle changes in the mucosal surface. To avoid missing the presence of cancer on endoscopy, the characteristics of early stage disease must be well understood and gastric observation must be thorough and detailed [16]. While diagnosis is based on conventional white light endoscopy findings, the use of dye-based image-enhanced endoscopy (chromoendoscopy), equipment-based image-enhanced endoscopy (narrow band imaging—NBI), and endoscopic ultrasonography (EUS) is contributing to improved diagnostic capabilities for early gastric cancer.

2.1. White Light Endoscopy. Accurate diagnosis of early gastric cancer relies on having a good grasp of the characteristics of early stage disease and learning effective methods of endoscopic observation. When conducting white light endoscopy, it is important to pay attention to points such as slight color changes in the mucosa (pale redness or fading of color), loss of visibility of underlying submucosal vessels, thinning of and interruptions in mucosal folds, and spontaneous bleeding. Each of these findings is often a subtle change, and the endoscopist must be sure to clean off mucus adherent to the gastric wall, suction excessive gastric juice, supply sufficient air, and thoroughly observe the entire area within the stomach. Furthermore, when a lesion is observed, although a diagnosis of invasion depth is required, the endoscopist makes a comprehensive diagnostic judgment considering mural thickness and hardness, color, fold concentration, depression depth, and protrusion length. Reduction of air volume within the stomach is effective for observing wall thickness and hardness. The accuracy of conventional endoscopy to discriminate between intramucosal carcinoma and submucosal carcinoma is reported to be 72%–84% [17–19]. Furthermore, although high-definition endoscopy was developed to improve image quality and diagnostic capability, it also allows for more accurate diagnosis of early gastric cancer than ultrathin endoscopy [20].

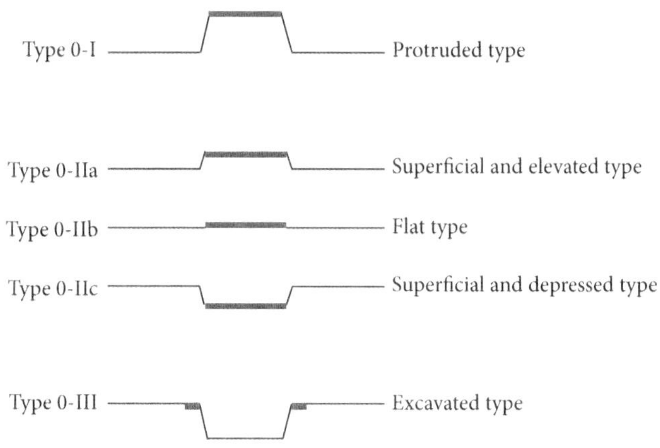

Figure 1: Macroscopic classification of early gastric cancer. (Type 0: superficial, flat tumor with or without minimal elevation or depression).

2.2. Dye-Based Image-Enhanced Endoscopy: Chromoendoscopy. When subtle mucosal changes such as those described earlier are observed, detailed chromoendoscopic observation has been shown to effectively aid diagnosis. Typically, 0.1% indigo carmine is sprayed directly via the forceps channel. Early gastric cancer is diagnosed through comparison with the surrounding mucosa; so, the dye must also be sprayed widely over the mucosa surrounding the lesion. This method highlights subtle differences in elevation of the mucosal surface and changes in the surface structure and color and helps to improve qualitative diagnosis and diagnosis of the extent of invasion [21, 22]. Spraying of indigo carmine can, however, actually make the lesion boundaries unclear when mucus is adherent to the stomach wall; therefore, it is important to wash the lesion meticulously prior to spraying [23]. In addition, it should be noted that indigo carmine spraying can actually make it more difficult to observe the lesion if it exhibits few color changes or small differences in elevation.

2.3. Equipment-Based Image-Enhanced Endoscopy: Narrow Band Imaging. NBI is a common type of equipment-based image-enhanced endoscopy that enhances the superficial surface structure and vascular architecture of the mucous layer by illuminating blue and green narrowband lights.

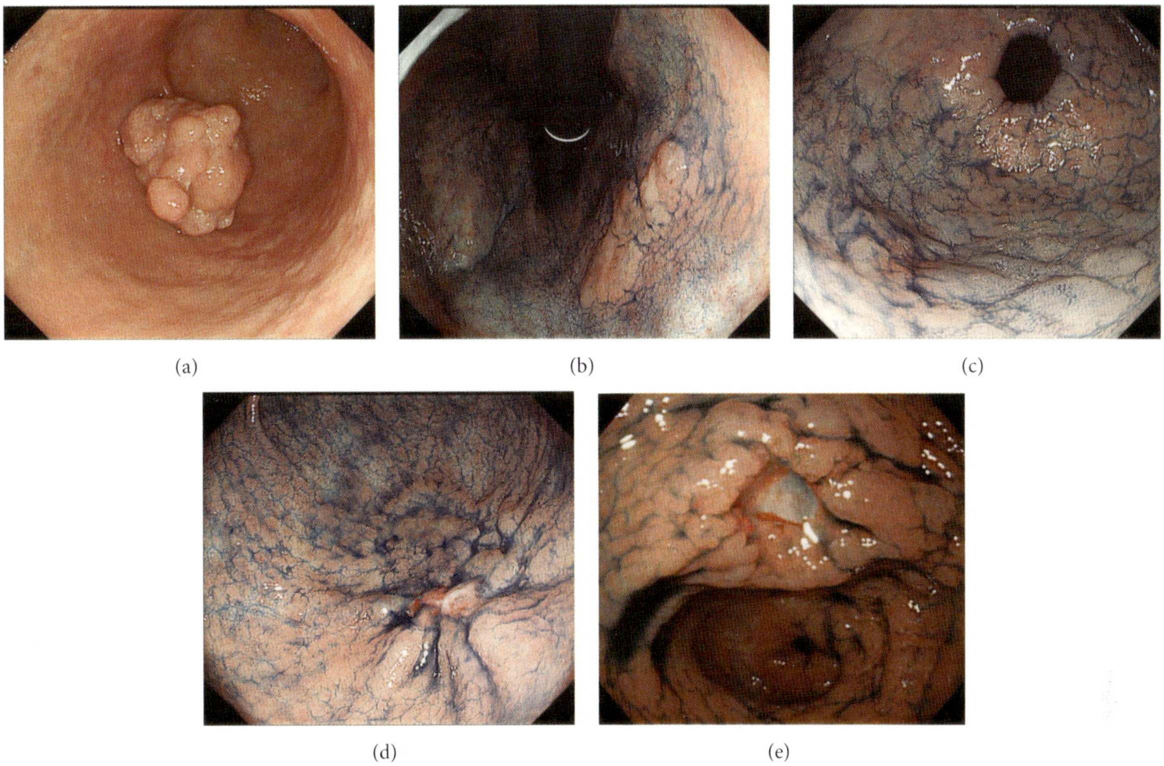

FIGURE 2: Macroscopic classification of early gastric cancer: (a) type 0-I (protruded type); (b) type 0-IIa (superficial and elevated type); (c) type 0-IIb (flat type); (d) type 0-IIc (superficial and depressed type); (e) type-III (excavated type).

Magnified endoscopy with NBI makes it possible to observe microvascular (MV) and microsurface (MS) patterns on the gastric mucosa in detail. Yao et al. combined changes in these patterns with the presence or absence of a demarcation line to establish a diagnostic system for gastric cancer called the VS classification system (Figure 3) [24]. This method has proven effective in actual clinical practice in two main areas.

The first area is differential diagnosis of small gastric cancer and gastritis. With conventional endoscopic observation, it has been difficult to discriminate between small gastric cancer and benign abnormalities (e.g., gastritis) accurately in many cases. A prospective randomized controlled trial that investigated differential diagnosis of small depressed gastric cancer and gastritis with depressed lesions of less than 1 cm proved that the accuracy with combined NBI magnification surpassed that with conventional white light endoscopy [25]. The trial revealed that when NBI magnification was conducted after conventional observation with white light, the diagnostic capabilities were excellent, with accuracy, sensitivity, and specificity all above 95%. The use of this method accurately distinguishes between cancer and gastritis, thereby reducing the number of unnecessary biopsies.

The second area is the utility of including NBI magnification for margin determination when conducting the detailed examination prior to endoscopic therapy. While securing lateral margins based on accurate diagnosis is crucial during endoscopic therapy, it is difficult to determine the margins for early gastric cancer with both conventional endoscopy and chromoendoscopy in approximately 20% of cases [26, 27]. Macroscopically flat types of lesions, such as type 0-IIb, are common in such cases; yet, combined NBI magnification can still help to improve margin determination capabilities [26, 28].

Observation using NBI appears, therefore, to have clear advantages for the diagnosis of early gastric cancer if the necessary knowledge and skills are acquired. Endoscopists must be aware as NBI is not an all-purpose method. For example, because of the large size of the gastric lumen, use of nonmagnified NBI darkens the screen, limiting its use to the type of magnification outlined earlier. This means that it is not suitable for identifying lesions within the stomach. Furthermore, while it is very useful for margin determination with differentiated cancers, it has only limited utility with undifferentiated cancers. Undifferentiated cancers are often localized to the height of the glandular neck within the lamina propria mucosae, and the tumor surface remains covered with normal crypt epithelium. In these situations, concomitant use of NBI magnification will not reveal the characteristic irregular MV and MS patterns of cancer. Accordingly, diagnosis of the extent of undifferentiated cancers requires at least four negative biopsies in the area surrounding the cancer (Figure 4) [24, 26].

2.4. Endoscopic Ultrasonography. With more endoscopic procedures being performed for early gastric cancer, it has become necessary to determine preoperative invasion depth more accurately [29]. As mentioned earlier, although conventional endoscopic observation has an accuracy of around

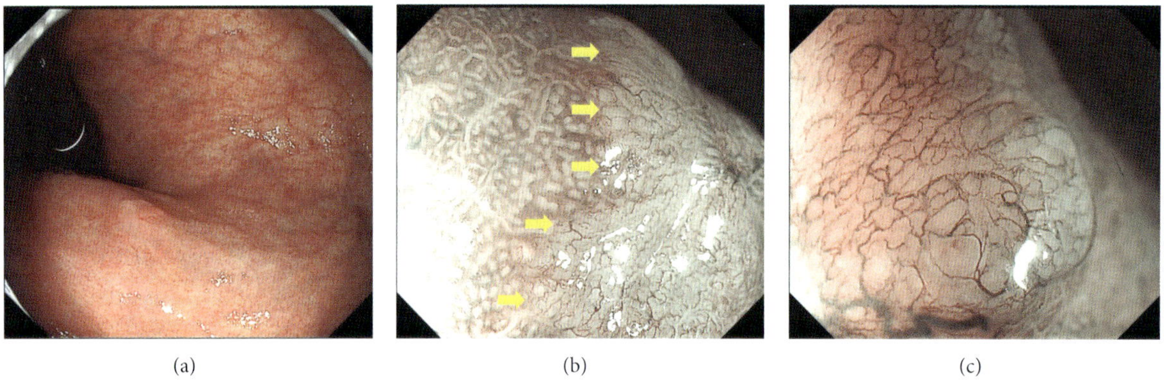

FIGURE 3: (a) A differentiated type 0-IIa lesion on the anterior wall of the middle gastric body. Magnifying endoscopy (ME) with narrow band imaging (NBI) shows (b) a clear demarcation line (arrows) at the border of the lesion with noncancerous mucosa to the left and cancerous mucosa to the right and (c) an irregular microvascular pattern plus the absence of a microsurface pattern in the cancerous mucosa.

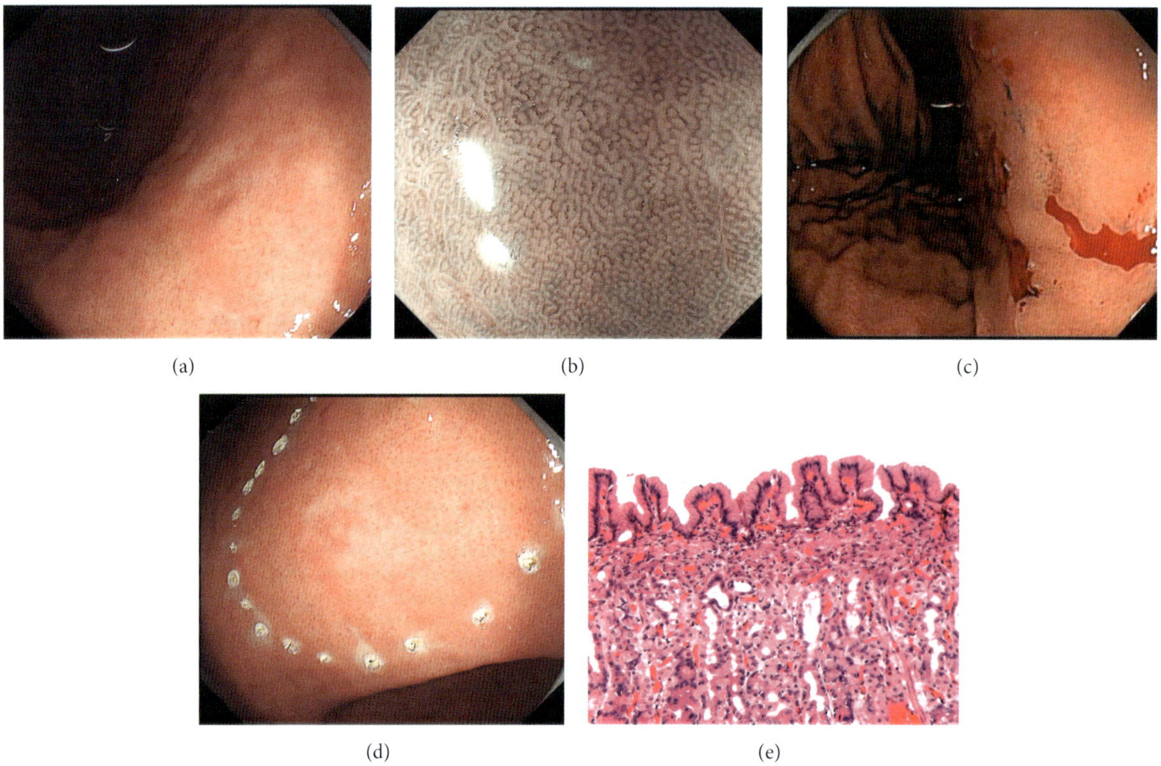

FIGURE 4: (a) An undifferentiated type 0-IIc lesion on the lesser curvature of the lower gastric body. (b) Magnifying endoscopy with narrow band imaging shows only a regular microvascular pattern plus a regular microsurface pattern in the cancerous mucosa with no identifiable demarcation line. (c) Multiple biopsies were taken from the mucosa surrounding the lesion to determine the horizontal extent of the cancer. (d) Marking dots were placed outside the scars of negative biopsies, and ESD was performed. (e) Histopathologically, the cancer extends to height of the glandular neck within the lamina propria mucosae and is covered with normal crypt epithelium.

80%, diagnosing invasion depth can be difficult in many cases. Furthermore, as such diagnosis with conventional endoscopic observation is subjective, EUS can be used to make a more objective diagnosis. Normally, the main objective of EUS for early gastric cancer is to determine whether the patient can undergo endoscopic therapy, and small diameter lesions are often targeted. Therefore, while the procedure is more often conducted using 20 MHz catheter-based miniprobes than with the 12 MHz catheter-based miniprobes, the latter are concomitantly used for large type 0-I lesions. The accuracy of depth diagnosis is reported to be 65%–86% and can reach 92% when normal endoscopic findings correspond to EUS findings [30–33]. However, these diagnostic capabilities drop for depressed lesions, undifferentiated cancers, cases accompanied by ulcers, cases of minute submucosal invasion, type 0-I lesions, and lesions located in the upper-third of the stomach. Accordingly, when it is difficult to diagnose lesion depth even with the combined use of EUS, endoscopic therapy can be conducted if there are no findings suggesting deep submucosal invasion, but doctors must judge whether or not to conduct curative resection on the basis of the pathological findings after endoscopic resection. Apart from the utility of EUS for diagnosing invasion depth, EUS can be used preoperatively to assess the submucosal vasculature in order to predict intraoperative bleeding during endoscopic therapy [34].

3. Endoscopic Therapy and Its Indications

In Japan, the 5-year postoperative survival rate for early gastric cancer excluding other causes of death is 99% for intramucosal carcinoma and 96% for submucosal carcinoma [35]. The frequency of lymph node metastasis in these patients is 3% for intramucosal carcinoma and 20% for submucosal carcinoma [36]. Given that favorable prognosis can be expected for early gastric cancer with the standard therapy of gastric resection accompanied by lymph node dissection, the indications for endoscopic therapy need to be strictly determined, as this therapy involves local excision and is not accompanied by lymph node dissection. Good indications for endoscopic therapy are, therefore, lesions where lymph node metastasis can be disregarded. In these cases, endoscopic therapy has significant advantages over surgery, as it is minimally invasive and preserves postoperative gastric function.

4. Endoscopic Diagnosis

Since endoscopic mucosal resection using the strip biopsy method (two-channel method) was first introduced for endoscopic therapy in 1984 [37], various methods of EMR have been developed, including endoscopic resection with a cap-fitted panendoscope (EMRC). They are widely used in Western countries as well as Japan [7]. Lesions with an extremely low likelihood of lymph node metastasis have been identified by clinicopathological investigations of multiple surgery cases, and indications for endoscopic therapy have been compiled by the Japan Gastric Cancer Association [38, 39]. In principle, these indications state that the likelihood of lymph node metastasis is extremely unlikely and that the tumor should be of a size and in a site that allows it to undergo en bloc resection. Specifically, the lesion must be (1) a differentiated elevated intramucosal cancer less than 2 cm in size or (2) a differentiated depressed intramucosal cancer less than 1 cm in size without ulcer findings. However, due to the nature of the excision technique, which uses a snare, EMR also has the disadvantage that only a small area can be excised at a time, and so for larger lesions, it has higher rates of piecemeal excision and local recurrence [5, 40].

In this context, ESD was developed to make accurate en bloc resection possible. Indeed, ESD enables en bloc resection of large lesions, lesions with accompanying ulcer scarring, and lesions recurring after EMR because it involves dissecting along the submucosal layer directly using a high-frequency knife (Figure 5) [5, 41–44]. Following its introduction, investigations into additional indications for ESD have been made. In 2000, Gotoda et al. analyzed 5265 cases of early gastric cancer treated by surgery and reported that there was an extremely low risk of lymph node metastasis in cases that were (1) differentiated intramucosal cancers without ulcer findings, irrespective of tumor size, (2) differentiated intramucosal cancers less than 3 cm in size with ulcer findings, and (3) differentiated minute invasive submucosal (less than 500 μm below the muscularis mucosa) cancers less than 3 cm in size [45]. Since then, the indications for ESD have been expanded to cover these lesions. With the accumulation of cases, there also appears to be an extremely low risk of lymph node metastasis for lesions that are undifferentiated intramucosal cancers less than 2 cm in size without ulcer findings, and these lesions are now indicated for ESD (Table 1) [46].

Although ESD is said to cause more complications than EMR, most instances of perforation or bleeding complications can be treated with endoscopy, and the risk for life-threatening complications is thought to be extremely low [47, 48]. Due to its widespread use for en bloc resection and low recurrence rate, a meta-analysis has shown ESD to be superior to EMR [49]. The continuing modification of endoscopic therapy devices and techniques and the spread of live demonstrations of ESD in Japan meant that many facilities are performing this technique nationwide and that the rate at which endoscopic therapy is being used for early gastric cancer is increasing dramatically [8]. There have also been reports, however, that conventional EMR and ESD produce the same results for lesions of less than 5 mm, and, rather than excising all lesions with ESD, EMR and ESD should be used properly weighing up the advantages and disadvantages [50]. Although ESD, like EMR, is now also conducted in Western countries, few cases of early gastric cancer are indicated for endoscopic therapy in the first place; so, it appears that it will take some time before it becomes widely used and for the techniques to become established [51, 52].

5. Postendoscopic Resection Management and Surveillance

Post-ESD management involves fasting on the day of the surgery in order to prevent delayed bleeding, resuming the intake of fluids from the following day and of food from the second day after surgery. Post-ESD ulcers require approximately 6–8 weeks to close completely, during which time antacids are administered [53]. Proton pump inhibitors (PPIs) are said to be more effective for preventing delayed bleeding than H2-receptor antagonists [54], and, recently, the combined use of mucosal protective antiulcer drugs with PPIs was reported to further promote ulcer healing [55, 56]. Long-term results for indicated lesions after EMR are favorable, with both the 5- and 10-year survival rates excluding death from other illnesses reported to be 99% [57]. It would appear then that if complete excision is achieved for an indicated lesion, the risk of local recurrence is extremely low, but it is desirable that patients undergo annual endoscopic surveillance to ensure early detection of metachronous cancer. Post-EMR/ESD metachronous cancer has a 3-year cumulative incidence rate of 5.9%, with a fairly high average time until initial detection of 3.1 ± 1.7 years [58].

With respect to the long-term ESD results for expanded indications, there is no difference in the 5-year survival rate

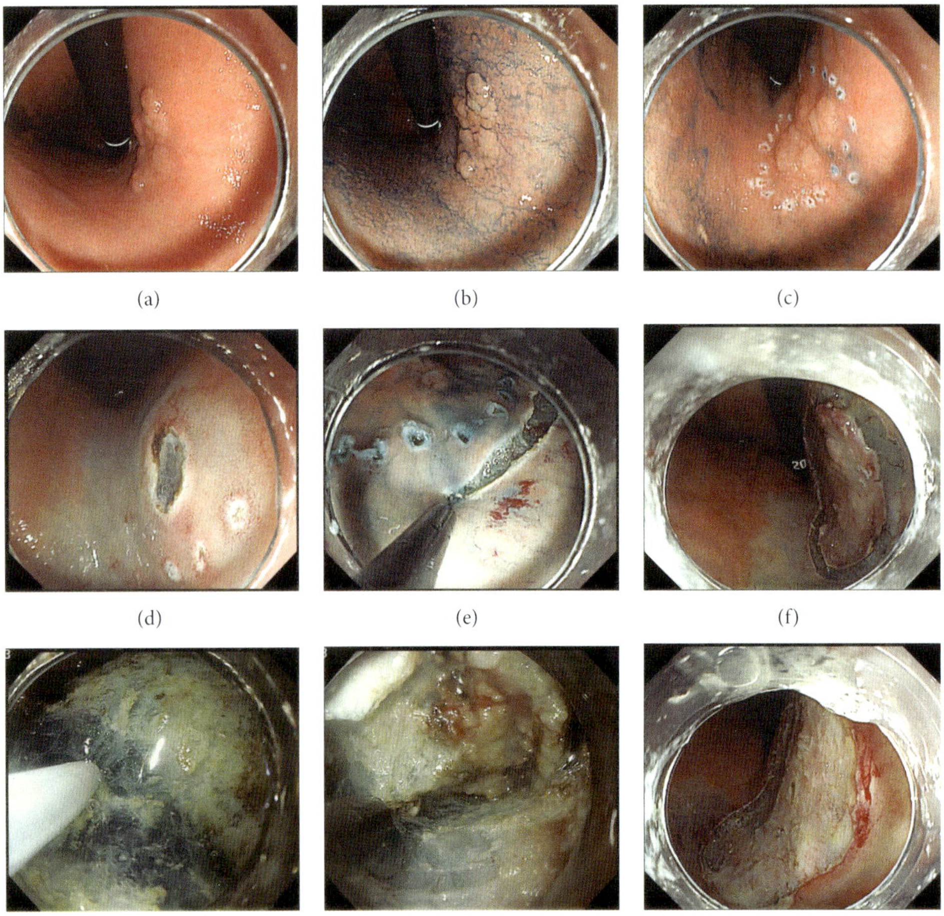

(a) (b) (c) (d) (e) (f) (g) (h) (i)

FIGURE 5: Procedure of endoscopic submucosal dissection. (a) Type 0-IIa lesion on the lesser curvature of the middle gastric body. (b) Chromoendoscopy with indigo carmine dye spraying. (c) Marking around the lesion. (d) Making small initial incision with a needle knife. (e) Mucosal cutting with an insulation-tipped diathermic knife-2 (IT knife-2). (f) Circumferential incision of the mucosa. (g) Additional submucosal injection of diluted epinephrine and indigo carmine. (h) Dissection of the submucosal layer with an IT knife-2. (i) The mucosal defect after resection of the lesion.

TABLE 1: Criteria for treatment of early gastric carcinoma.

	Mucosal carcinoma				Submucosal carcinoma	
	No ulcer		Ulcer		SM1	SM2
	≦20	>20	≦30	>30	≦30	Anysize
Differentiated carcinoma	EMR/ESD	ESD	ESD	Surgery	ESD	Surgery
Undifferentiated carcinoma	ESD	Surgery	Surgery	Surgery	Surgery	Surgery

of curative resection between the original and expanded indications [48, 59]. However, as there is currently insufficient evidence of the long-term results following curative resection under the expanded indications, these patients undergo annual endoscopic surveillance, in addition to half-yearly abdominal computed tomography or endoscopic ultrasonography, for at least 3 years in order to detect lymph node or distant metastasis.

When the pathological examination indicates noncurative resection, additional surgery including lymph node dissection is strongly recommended. The acceptability and safety of laparoscopy-assisted distal gastrectomy for early gastric cancer have been shown, and it is considered a first-line additional therapy after endoscopic resection in Japan [60–63]. Even in elderly patients aged 75 years or older, a noncurative resection group that underwent additional surgery had a higher survival rate than a noncurative resection group that underwent follow-up observation only. Thus, if patient activities of daily living and comorbidity allow, additional surgery can also be considered for elderly patients [64].

6. Prospects for the Future Management of the Disease

As the long-term ESD results under the expanded indications have yet to be established, the results of a prospective clinical trial by the Japan Clinical Oncology Group of its validity are eagerly awaited. If this study verifies the safety and effectiveness of ESD, the expanded indications may well become actual indications.

Although the number of early gastric cancer lesions that can be resected with endoscopic therapy is increasing, for nonindicated lesions, regular surgery remains the basic treatment. A large gap exists between these two treatment methods with regard to invasiveness, and minimally invasive surgical methods are being investigated to close this gap. One such method is ESD followed by laparoscopic lymph node dissection and histological evaluation [65]. Long-term results are now being reported, albeit only for a small number of cases, and this method may become an option for minimally invasive surgery in cases where lymph node metastasis cannot be confirmed or ruled out [66]. Furthermore, although the popularization of ESD has led to a clear decrease in lesions for which excision is technically difficult, lesions in the gastric fundus region or gastric corpus curvature or lesions with severe ulcer scarring can pose difficulties for ESD. These lesions have commonly been treated by radical surgery despite the extremely low likelihood of lymph node metastasis, but promising initial outcomes of laparoscopy-assisted full-thickness resection of the stomach, a minimally invasive surgical technique, have been published recently [67–70]. If sentinel node navigation is established for gastric cancer, it is likely that this minimally invasive surgical therapy will be developed even further.

7. Conclusion

Early detection and early treatment are vital, improving the prognosis of gastric cancer. As we have seen, endoscopic examination plays an important role in the early detection of gastric cancer, but in many cases, diagnostic accuracy is dependent on the skill of the endoscopist. First, it is important for endoscopists to conduct endoscopic observation carefully, fully aware that early gastric cancer is often indicated only by subtle changes on the mucosal surface. They must also acquire the necessary skills and knowledge to identify lesions on conventional white light endoscopy. In addition, the combined use of chromoendoscopy and image-enhanced endoscopy is expected to further improve diagnostic precision. Minimally invasive methods of treatment are currently the preferred treatment option for early gastric cancer, with the use of EMR, in particular, becoming widespread. At present, ESD is rapidly becoming favored in many countries including Japan as it shows an even greater potential for a complete cure. In the future, it is predicted that, with the development of technology and devices, endoscopic therapy will be performed more and more frequently, and that we will see more combinations of endoscopic therapy and surgery. A complete cure for early gastric cancer can be expected with radical surgery, but it is important to continue the development of minimally invasive endoscopic methods while also continually verifying their safety and complete curability.

References

[1] A. Jemal, R. Siegel, J. Xu, and E. Ward, "Cancer statistics, 2010," *CA Cancer Journal for Clinicians*, vol. 60, no. 5, pp. 277–300, 2010.

[2] J. Ferlay, H. R. Shin, F. Bray, D. Forman, C. Mathers, and D. M. Parkin, "Estimates of worldwide burden of cancer in 2008: GLOBOCAN 2008," *International Journal of Cancer*, vol. 127, no. 12, pp. 2893–2917, 2010.

[3] C. Hamashima, D. Shibuya, H. Yamazaki et al., "The Japanese guidelines for gastric cancer screening," *Japanese Journal of Clinical Oncology*, vol. 38, no. 4, pp. 259–267, 2008.

[4] K. Maruyama, M. Kaminishi, K. I. Hayashi et al., "Gastric cancer treated in 1991 in Japan: data analysis of nationwide registry," *Gastric Cancer*, vol. 9, no. 2, pp. 51–66, 2006.

[5] H. Ono, H. Kondo, T. Gotoda et al., "Endoscopic mucosal resection for treatment of early gastric cancer," *Gut*, vol. 48, no. 2, pp. 225–229, 2001.

[6] F. J. Oliveira, H. Ferrao, E. Furtado, H. Batista, and L. Conceicao, "Early gastric cancer: report of 58 cases," *Gastric Cancer*, vol. 1, no. 1, pp. 51–56, 1998.

[7] R. Soetikno, T. Kaltenbach, R. Yeh, and T. Gotoda, "Endoscopic mucosal resection for early cancers of the upper gastrointestinal tract," *Journal of Clinical Oncology*, vol. 23, no. 20, pp. 4490–4498, 2005.

[8] K. Hotta, T. Oyama, T. Akamatsu et al., "A comparison of outcomes of Endoscopic Submucosal Dissection (ESD) for early gastric neoplasms between high-volume and low-volume centers: multi-center retrospective questionnaire study conducted by the Nagano ESD Study Group," *Internal Medicine*, vol. 49, no. 4, pp. 253–259, 2010.

[9] Japanese Gastric Cancer Association, "Japanese classification of gastric carcinoma—2nd English edition," *Gastric Cancer*, vol. 1, no. 1, pp. 10–24, 1998.

[10] H. Katai and T. Sano, "Early gastric cancer: concepts, diagnosis, and management," *International Journal of Clinical Oncology*, vol. 10, no. 6, pp. 375–383, 2005.

[11] "The Paris endoscopic classification of superficial neoplastic lesions: esophagus, stomach, and colon: November 30 to December 1, 2002," *Gastrointestinal Endoscopy*, vol. 58, supplement 6, pp. S3–S43, 2003.

[12] R. J. Schlemper, M. Itabashi, Y. Kato et al., "Differences in diagnostic criteria for gastric carcinoma between Japanese and Western pathologists," *The Lancet*, vol. 349, no. 9067, pp. 1725–1729, 1997.

[13] R. J. Schlemper, R. H. Riddell, Y. Kato et al., "The Vienna classification of gastrointestinal epithelial neoplasia," *Gut*, vol. 47, no. 2, pp. 251–255, 2000.

[14] M. Kato, T. Nishida, S. Tsutsui et al., "Endoscopic submucosal dissection as a treatment for gastric noninvasive neoplasia: a multicenter study by Osaka University ESD Study Group," *Journal of Gastroenterology*, vol. 46, no. 3, pp. 325–331, 2011.

[15] K. Miwa, H. Doyama, R. Ito et al., "Can magnifying endoscopy with narrow band imaging be useful for low grade adenomas in preoperative biopsy specimens?" *Gastric Cancer*, vol. 15, no. 2, pp. 170–178, 2012.

[16] K. Sugano, K. Sato, and K. Yao, "New diagnostic approaches for early detection of gastric cancer," *Digestive Diseases*, vol. 22, no. 4, pp. 327–333, 2004.

[17] T. Sano, Y. Okuyama, O. Kobori, T. Shimizu, and Y. Morioka, "Early gastric cancer: endoscopic diagnosis of depth of invasion," *Digestive Diseases and Sciences*, vol. 35, no. 11, pp. 1340–1344, 1990.

[18] S. Abe, I. Oda, T. Shimazu et al., "Depth-predicting score for differentiated early gastric cancer," *Gastric Cancer*, vol. 14, no. 1, pp. 35–40, 2011.

[19] J. Choi, S. G. Kim, J. P. Im, J. S. Kim, H. C. Jung, and I. S. Song, "Endoscopic prediction of tumor invasion depth in early gastric cancer," *Gastrointestinal Endoscopy*, vol. 73, no. 5, pp. 917–927, 2011.

[20] H. Toyoizumi, M. Kaise, H. Arakawa et al., "Ultrathin endoscopy versus high-resolution endoscopy for diagnosing superficial gastric neoplasia," *Gastrointestinal Endoscopy*, vol. 70, no. 2, pp. 240–245, 2009.

[21] H. Tajiri, A. Ohtsu, N. Boku et al., "Routine endoscopy using electronic endoscopes for gastric cancer diagnosis: retrospective study of inconsistencies between endoscopic and biopsy diagnoses," *Cancer Detection and Prevention*, vol. 25, no. 2, pp. 166–173, 2001.

[22] Y. Kawahara, R. Takenaka, H. Okada et al., "Novel chromoendoscopic method using an acetic acid-indigocarmine mixture for diagnostic accuracy in delineating the margin of early gastric cancers," *Digestive Endoscopy*, vol. 21, no. 1, pp. 14–19, 2009.

[23] M. Dinis-Ribeiro, "Chromoendoscopy for early diagnosis of gastric cancer," *European Journal of Gastroenterology & Hepatology*, vol. 18, no. 8, pp. 831–838, 2006.

[24] K. Yao, G. K. Anagnostopoulos, and K. Ragunath, "Magnifying endoscopy for diagnosing and delineating early gastric cancer," *Endoscopy*, vol. 41, no. 5, pp. 462–467, 2009.

[25] Y. Ezoe, M. Muto, N. Uedo et al., "Magnifying narrowband imaging is more accurate than conventional white-light imaging in diagnosis of gastric mucosal cancer," *Gastroenterology*, vol. 141, no. 6, pp. 2017.e3–2025.e3, 2011.

[26] T. Nagahama, K. Yao, S. Maki et al., "Usefulness of magnifying endoscopy with narrow-band imaging for determining the horizontal extent of early gastric cancer when there is an unclear margin by chromoendoscopy (with video)," *Gastrointestinal Endoscopy*, vol. 74, no. 6, pp. 1259–1267, 2011.

[27] S. Yoshinaga, T. Gotoda, and I. Oda, "Clinical imaging of early gastric cancers—conventional endoscopy: including chromoendoscopy using indigo carmine," *Stomach Intestine*, vol. 44, pp. 650–662, 2009.

[28] S. Kiyotoki, J. Nishikawa, M. Satake et al., "Usefulness of magnifying endoscopy with narrow-band imaging for determining gastric tumor margin," *Journal of Gastroenterology and Hepatology*, vol. 25, no. 10, pp. 1636–1641, 2010.

[29] S. Yoshinaga, I. Oda, S. Nonaka, R. Kushima, and Y. Saito, "Endoscopic ultrasound using ultrasound probes for the diagnosis of early esophageal and gastric cancers," *World Journal of Gastrointestinal Endoscopy*, vol. 4, no. 6, pp. 218–226, 2012.

[30] H. Yanai, Y. Matsumoto, T. Harada et al., "Endoscopic ultrasonography and endoscopy for staging depth of invasion in early gastric cancer: a pilot study," *Gastrointestinal Endoscopy*, vol. 46, no. 3, pp. 212–216, 1997.

[31] K. Akahoshi, Y. Chijilwa, S. Hamada et al., "Pretreatment staging of endoscopically early gastric cancer with a 15 MHz ultrasound catheter probe," *Gastrointestinal Endoscopy*, vol. 48, no. 5, pp. 470–476, 1998.

[32] G. H. Kim, D. Y. Park, M. Kida et al., "Accuracy of high-frequency catheter-based endoscopic ultrasonography according to the indications for endoscopic treatment of early gastric cancer," *Journal of Gastroenterology and Hepatology*, vol. 25, no. 3, pp. 506–511, 2010.

[33] T. Tsuzukr, H. Okada, Y. Kawahara et al., "Usefulness and problems of endoscopic ultrasonography in prediction of the depth of tumor invasion in early gastric cancer," *Acta Medica Okayama*, vol. 65, no. 2, pp. 105–112, 2011.

[34] D. Kikuchi, T. Iizuka, S. Hoteya et al., "Usefulness of endoscopic ultrasound for the prediction of intraoperative bleeding of endoscopic submucosal dissection for gastric neoplasms," *Journal of Gastroenterology and Hepatology*, vol. 26, no. 1, pp. 68–72, 2011.

[35] M. Sasako, T. Kinoshita, and K. Maruyama, "Prognosis of early gastric cancer," *Stomach Intestine*, vol. 28, pp. 139–146, 1993.

[36] T. Sano, O. Kobori, and T. Muto, "Lymph node metastasis from early gastric cancer: endoscopic resection of tumour," *The British Journal of Surgery*, vol. 79, no. 3, pp. 241–244, 1992.

[37] M. Tada, M. Karita, H. Yanai, and T. Takemoto, "Endoscopic therapy of early gastric cancer by strip biopsy," *Japanese Journal of Cancer & Chemotherapy*, vol. 15, no. 4, part 2-3, pp. 1460–1465, 1988.

[38] S. Tsujitani, S. Oka, H. Saito et al., "Less invasive surgery for early gastric cancer based on the low probability of lymph node metastasis," *Surgery*, vol. 125, no. 2, pp. 148–154, 1999.

[39] Japanese Gastric Cancer Association, *Guidelines For the Treatment of Gastric Cancer*, Kanehara, Tokyo, Japan, 2001.

[40] M. Matsushita, K. Hajiro, K. Okazaki, and H. Takakuwa, "Endoscopic mucosal resection of gastric tumors located in the lesser curvature of the upper third of the stomach," *Gastrointestinal Endoscopy*, vol. 45, no. 6, pp. 512–515, 1997.

[41] H. Yamamoto, H. Kawata, K. Sunada et al., "Successful en-bloc resection of large superficial tumors in the stomach and colon using sodium hyaluronate and small-caliber-tip transparent hood," *Endoscopy*, vol. 35, no. 8, pp. 690–694, 2003.

[42] T. Oyama, A. Tomori, K. Hotta et al., "Endoscopic submucosal dissection of early esophageal cancer," *Clinical Gastroenterology and Hepatology*, vol. 3, no. 7, supplement 1, pp. S67–S70, 2005.

[43] N. Yahagi, M. Fujishiro, N. Kakushima et al., "Endoscopic submucosal dissection for early gastric cancer using the tip of an electrosurgical snare (thin type)," *Digestive Endoscopy*, vol. 16, no. 1, pp. 34–38, 2004.

[44] C. Yokoi, T. Gotoda, H. Hamanaka, and I. Oda, "Endoscopic submucosal dissection allows curative resection of locally recurrent early gastric cancer after prior endoscopic mucosal resection," *Gastrointestinal Endoscopy*, vol. 64, no. 2, pp. 212–218, 2006.

[45] T. Gotoda, A. Yanagisawa, M. Sasako et al., "Incidence of lymph node metastasis from early gastric cancer: estimation with a large number of cases at two large centers," *Gastric Cancer*, vol. 3, no. 4, pp. 219–225, 2000.

[46] T. Hirasawa, T. Gotoda, S. Miyata et al., "Incidence of lymph node metastasis and the feasibility of endoscopic resection for undifferentiated-type early gastric cancer," *Gastric Cancer*, vol. 12, no. 3, pp. 148–152, 2009.

[47] I. Oda, T. Gotoda, H. Hamanaka et al., "Endoscopic submucosal dissection for early gastric cancer: technical feasibility, operation time and complications from a large consecutive series," *Digestive Endoscopy*, vol. 17, no. 1, pp. 54–58, 2005.

[48] H. Isomoto, S. Shikuwa, N. Yamaguchi et al., "Endoscopic submucosal dissection for early gastric cancer: a large-scale feasibility study," *Gut*, vol. 58, no. 3, pp. 331–336, 2009.

[49] Y. M. Park, E. Cho, H. Y. Kang, and J. M. Kim, "The effectiveness and safety of endoscopic submucosal dissection compared with endoscopic mucosal resection for early gastric cancer: a systematic review and metaanalysis," *Surgical Endoscopy*, vol. 25, no. 8, pp. 2666–2677, 2011.

[50] S. Nakamoto, Y. Sakai, J. Kasanuki et al., "Indications for the use of endoscopic mucosal resection for early gastric cancer in Japan: a comparative study with endoscopic submucosal dissection," *Endoscopy*, vol. 41, no. 9, pp. 746–750, 2009.

[51] F. Catalano, A. Trecca, L. Rodella et al., "The modern treatment of early gastric cancer: our experience in an Italian cohort," *Surgical Endoscopy and Other Interventional Techniques*, vol. 23, no. 7, pp. 1581–1586, 2009.

[52] M. O. Othman and M. B. Wallace, "Endoscopic mucosal resection (EMR) and endoscopic submucosal dissection (ESD) in 2011, a Western perspective," *Clinics and Research in Hepatology and Gastroenterology*, vol. 35, no. 4, pp. 288–294, 2011.

[53] N. Kakushima, N. Yahagi, M. Fujishiro et al., "The healing process of gastric artificial ulcers after endoscopic submucosal dissection," *Digestive Endoscopy*, vol. 16, no. 4, pp. 327–331, 2004.

[54] N. Uedo, Y. Takeuchi, T. Yamada et al., "Effect of a proton pump inhibitor or an H2-receptor antagonist on prevention of bleeding from ulcer after endoscopic submucosal dissection of early gastric cancer: a prospective randomized controlled trial," *The American Journal of Gastroenterology*, vol. 102, no. 8, pp. 1610–1616, 2007.

[55] T. Kato, H. Araki, F. Onogi et al., "Clinical trial: rebamipide promotes gastric ulcer healing by proton pump inhibitor after endoscopic submucosal dissection-a randomized controlled study," *Journal of Gastroenterology*, vol. 45, no. 3, pp. 285–290, 2010.

[56] T. Inaba, S. Ishikawa, T. Toyokawa et al., "Basal protrusion of ulcers induced by Endoscopic Submucosal Dissection (ESD) during treatment with proton pump inhibitors, and the suppressive effects of polaprezinc," *Hepato-Gastroenterology*, vol. 57, no. 99-100, pp. 678–684, 2010.

[57] N. Uedo, H. Iishi, M. Tatsuta et al., "Longterm outcomes after endoscopic mucosal resection for early gastric cancer," *Gastric Cancer*, vol. 9, no. 2, pp. 88–92, 2006.

[58] T. Nakajima, I. Oda, T. Gotoda et al., "Metachronous gastric cancers after endoscopic resection: how effective is annual endoscopic surveillance?" *Gastric Cancer*, vol. 9, no. 2, pp. 93–98, 2006.

[59] T. Gotoda, M. Iwasaki, C. Kusano, S. Seewald, and I. Oda, "Endoscopie resection of early gastric cancer treated by guideline and expanded National Cancer Centre criteria," *The British Journal of Surgery*, vol. 97, no. 6, pp. 868–871, 2010.

[60] H. H. Kim, W. J. Hyung, G. S. Cho et al., "Morbidity and mortality of laparoscopic gastrectomy versus open gastrectomy for gastric cancer: an interim report-a phase III multicenter, prospective, randomized trial (KLASS trial)," *Annals of Surgery*, vol. 251, no. 3, pp. 417–420, 2010.

[61] H. Ohtani, Y. Tamamori, K. Noguchi et al., "A meta-analysis of randomized controlled trials that compared laparoscopy-assisted and open distal gastrectomy for early gastric cancer," *Journal of Gastrointestinal Surgery*, vol. 14, no. 6, pp. 958–964, 2010.

[62] X. Jiang, N. Hiki, H. Yoshiba et al., "Laparoscopy-assisted gastrectomy in patients with previous endoscopic resection for early gastric cancer," *The British Journal of Surgery*, vol. 98, no. 3, pp. 385–390, 2011.

[63] H. Tonouchi, Y. Mohri, M. Kobayashi, K. Tanaka, M. Ohi, and M. Kusunoki, "Laparoscopy-assisted distal gastrectomy with laparoscopic sentinel lymph node biopsy after endoscopic mucosal resection for early gastric cancer," *Surgical Endoscopy and Other Interventional Techniques*, vol. 21, no. 8, pp. 1289–1293, 2007.

[64] C. Kusano, M. Iwasaki, T. Kaltenbach, A. Conlin, I. Oda, and T. Gotoda, "Should elderly patients undergo additional surgery after non-curative endoscopic resection for early gastric cancer? long-term comparative outcomes," *The American Journal of Gastroenterology*, vol. 106, no. 6, pp. 1064–1069, 2011.

[65] N. Abe, T. Mori, H. Takeuchi et al., "Laparoscopic lymph node dissection after endoscopic submucosal dissection: a novel and minimally invasive approach to treating early-stage gastric cancer," *American Journal of Surgery*, vol. 190, no. 3, pp. 496–503, 2005.

[66] N. Abe, H. Takeuchi, A. Ohki et al., "Long-term outcomes of combination of endoscopic submucosal dissection and laparoscopic lymph node dissection without gastrectomy for early gastric cancer patients who have a potential risk of lymph node metastasis," *Gastrointestinal Endoscopy*, vol. 74, no. 4, pp. 792–797, 2011.

[67] N. Hiki, Y. Yamamoto, T. Fukunaga et al., "Laparoscopic and endoscopic cooperative surgery for gastrointestinal stromal tumor dissection," *Surgical Endoscopy and Other Interventional Techniques*, vol. 22, no. 7, pp. 1729–1735, 2008.

[68] S. Nunobe, N. Hiki, T. Gotoda et al., "Successful application of laparoscopic and endoscopic cooperative surgery (LECS) for a lateral-spreading mucosal gastric cancer," *Gastric Cancer*, vol. 15, no. 3, pp. 338–342, 2012.

[69] H. Inoue, H. Ikeda, T. Hosoya et al., "Endoscopic mucosal resection, endoscopic submucosal dissection, and beyond: full-layer resection for gastric cancer with nonexposure technique (CLEAN-NET)," *Surgical Oncology Clinics of North America*, vol. 21, no. 1, pp. 129–140, 2012.

[70] O. Goto, T. Mitsui, M. Fujishiro et al., "New method of endoscopic full-thickness resection: a pilot study of non-exposed endoscopic wall-inversion surgery in an ex vivo porcine model," *Gastric Cancer*, vol. 14, no. 2, pp. 183–187, 2011.

5

Narrow Band Imaging with Magnification Can Pick Up Esophageal Squamous Cell Carcinoma More Efficiently Than Lugol Chromoendoscopy in Patients after Chemoradiotherapy

Itsuko Asada-Hirayama,[1] Shinya Kodashima,[1] Mitsuhiro Fujishiro,[2] Satoshi Ono,[3] Keiko Niimi,[2] Satoshi Mochizuki,[1] Maki Konno-Shimizu,[1] Rie Mikami-Matsuda,[1] Chihiro Minatsuki,[1] Chiemi Nakayama,[1] Yu Takahashi,[1] Nobutake Yamamichi,[1] and Kazuhiko Koike[1]

[1] *Department of Gastroenterology, Graduate School of Medicine, The University of Tokyo, 7-3-1 Hongo, Bunkyo-ku, Tokyo 113-8655, Japan*
[2] *Department of Endoscopy and Endoscopic Surgery, Graduate School of Medicine, The University of Tokyo, 7-3-1 Hongo, Bunkyo-ku, Tokyo 113-8655, Japan*
[3] *Center for Epidemiology and Preventive Medicine, The University of Tokyo, 7-3-1 Hongo, Bunkyo-ku, Tokyo 113-8655, Japan*

Correspondence should be addressed to Shinya Kodashima; kodashima-tky@umin.ac.jp

Academic Editor: Kazuo Inui

Aim. Little is known about the usefulness of narrow band imaging (NBI) for surveillance of patients after chemoradiotherapy for esophageal neoplasia. Its usefulness in detecting esophageal squamous cell carcinoma (SCC) or high-grade intraepithelial neoplasia (HGIN) in these patients was retrospectively compared to Lugol chromoendoscopy. *Patients and Methods.* We assessed the diagnostic ability of NBI with magnification based on the biopsy specimens obtained from iodine-unstained lesions. Seventy-two iodine-unstained lesions were biopsied and consecutively enrolled for this study. The lesions were divided into NBI positive and NBI negative. Sensitivity, specificity, positive predictive value (PPV), negative predictive value (NPV), and accuracy of NBI with magnification and PPV of Lugol chromoendoscopy was calculated using histological assessment as a gold standard. *Results.* Forty-six endoscopic examinations using NBI with magnification followed by Lugol chromoendoscopy were performed to 28 patients. The prevalence of SCC and HGIN was 21.4%. Sensitivity, specificity, PPV, NPV, and accuracy of NBI were 100.0%, 98.5%, 85.7%, 100%, and 98.6%, respectively. On the contrary, PPV of Lugol chromoendoscopy were 8.3%. Compared to Lugol chromoendoscopy, NBI with magnification showed equal sensitivity and significantly higher PPV ($P < 0.0001$). *Conclusion.* NBI with magnification would be able to pick up esophageal neoplasia more efficiently than Lugol chromoendoscopy in patients after chemoradiotherapy.

1. Introduction

Posttreatment surveillance of esophageal squamous cell carcinoma (SCC) after chemoradiotherapy (CRT) is very important because early detection of local persistence or recurrence makes it possible to prevent delay in change of treatment. In addition, metachronous SCC of esophagus often develops in the patients with past history of esophageal SCC [1]. However, differential diagnosis between local persistence, recurrence, and metachronous SCC or normal posttherapeutic sequelae such as mucositis and fibrosis often becomes a problem after CRT [2]. Indeed, in our experience, many iodine-unstained areas which were proven to be nonneoplastic lesions by biopsy were frequently observed in patients after CRT for esophageal carcinoma.

Lugol chromoendoscopy is the gold standard for detecting esophageal SCC [3–6]. Lugol staining is based on a chemical reaction between iodine and the glycogen which is contained in normal epithelial cell microgranules in the stratum spinosum [7]. Dysplastic and cancerous cells are not stained by Lugol's solution because they do not contain glycogen due to their immaturity.

Recently, narrow band imaging (NBI) (Olympus Medical System Corporation, Tokyo, Japan) is reported to improve detection of esophageal neoplasia in patients at high risk for developing esophageal SCC [2, 8, 9]. It is an optical technique that enhances the diagnostic capability of endoscopes by using narrow-band spectrum optical filters. This filter is designed to correspond to the peak absorption spectrum of hemoglobin to enhance the visualization of mucosal and submucosal microvascular patterns [1].

To the best of our knowledge, there are few reports on the feasibility of using NBI endoscopy for the surveillance of esophagus in patients after CRT. In this study, usefulness of NBI with magnification in detecting esophageal SCC or high-grade intraepithelial neoplasia (HGIN) in patients after CRT for esophageal carcinoma was retrospectively assessed in comparison with chromoendoscopy using iodine solution.

2. Materials and Methods

2.1. Study Subjects. This is a retrospective study. We assessed the diagnostic ability of NBI with magnification based on the biopsy specimens obtained from iodine-unstained lesions. From January 2008 to March 2012, 90 lesions, which were unstained by spraying of Lugol's solution, were biopsied from the patients who had received CRT for esophageal SCC previously and gave written informed consent at the University of Tokyo, Tokyo, Japan; forty-six endoscopic examinations using conventional white light and NBI with magnification followed by Lugol chromoendoscopy were performed to 28 patients. Among the patients who underwent endoscopic examination and biopsy twice or more after CRT, the lesions which were judged to have been biopsied previous endoscopic examination on the basis of locations and shapes were excluded from the analysis. Consequently, 72 lesions were consecutively enrolled for this study.

2.2. Patient Characteristics. The locations of primary esophageal SCCs were diagnosed by endoscopic examination before CRT. Lymph node metastasis and distant metastasis were diagnosed by computed tomography (CT). The depth of the tumors was generally diagnosed comprehensively based on the findings of endoscopic examination and CT. As an exception, the depth of the tumors was determined based on the pathological assessment in the cases in which CRT was performed as an additional therapy after endoscopic submucosal dissection (ESD).

2.3. Endoscopic Procedure. All procedures were performed by using EVIS LUCERA SPECTRUM system (Olympus, Tokyo, Japan) and high-resolution upper gastrointestinal endoscopes, either GIF-Q240Z or GIF-H260Z (Olympus) by 4 endoscopists (S.K., S.O., K.N., and S.M.) with special endoscopic qualification.

First, the esophageal mucosa was carefully examined by white light and NBI without magnification in order to detect any abnormality of color or surface structure. Second, abnormal lesions found by white light or NBI were examined by NBI with magnification. We defined lesions which satisfied both following conditions by NBI with magnification as "NBI-positive"; (1) well-demarcated brownish area, and (2) abnormal changes of intraepithelial papillary capillary loop (IPCL) pattern, that were dilatation, tortuosity, and caliber change in a single IPCL, and variation in the shape of multiple IPCL [10] (Figure 1). We defined lesions which satisfied either or neither of them as "NBI-negative." The locations of "NBI-positive" lesions were strictly noted as a distance from the incisor teeth. Third, 10 to 20 mL of 3% Lugol's solution was applied on the esophageal mucosa using a spray catheter passed through the working channel of the endoscope by the same endoscopist who had performed NBI endoscopy. We defined well-demarcated unstained area of more than 5 mm of diameter as "Lugol positive" (Figure 2), and the locations were strictly noted. Lastly, biopsies from "Lugol-positive" lesions were performed, and 2.5% of sodium thiosulfate hydrate was sprayed over the esophageal mucosa to bleach the iodine.

2.4. Pathological Assessment. Biopsy specimens were obtained from each abnormal lesions using forceps. All specimens were soaked in formalin solution and routinely processed. Histological diagnoses were performed by experienced pathologists in our hospital. Histology was assessed according to the following four categories of the World Health Organization (WHO) classification and the Vienna classification [11, 12]: invasive SCC, HGIN, low -grade intraepithelial neoplasia (LGIN), and no tumor.

2.5. Statistical Analysis. Sensitivity, specificity, positive predictive value (PPV), negative predictive value (NPV), and accuracy of NBI with magnification in identifying esophageal SCC and HGIN from the lesions which were Lugol positive were calculated. To clarify how many lesions were SCC or HGIN among Lugol-positive lesions, PPV of Lugol chromoendoscopy was also calculated.

The continuous variables were expressed as medians and ranges. Pearson's χ^2 test was used to analyze categorical data. P value of less than 0.05 was considered significant. Statistical analysis was performed using JMP version 9.0.2 (SAS Institute Japan).

3. Results

A total of 46 endoscopic examinations using conventional white light and NBI with magnification followed by Lugol chromoendoscopy were performed to 28 patients. An average number of endoscopic examinations for each patient was 1.6 times. The median age of the 28 patients was 69 years (range: 56–86 years), and the median follow-up duration from CRT to endoscopic examination was 10 months (range: 3–42months). The location of the primary cancers was shown in Table 1.

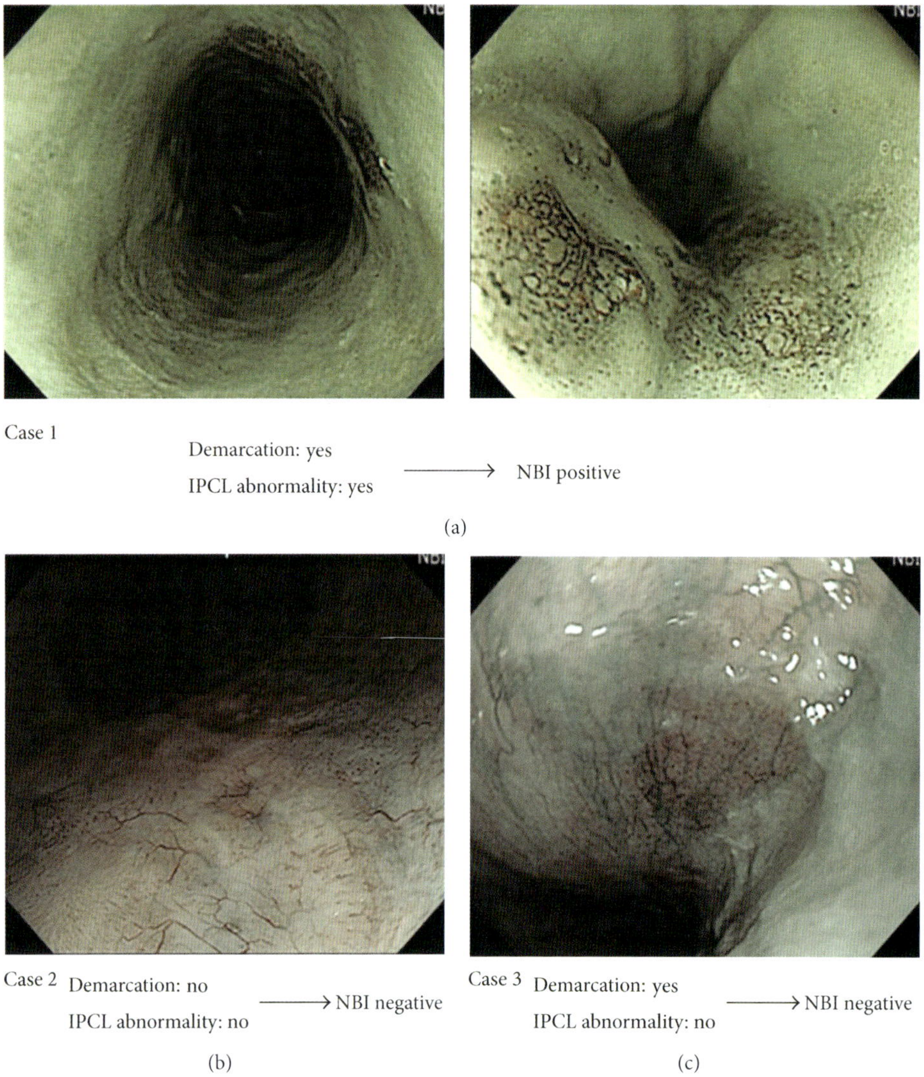

FIGURE 1: We defined lesions which satisfied both following conditions by NBI with magnification as "NBI-positive"; (1) well-demarcated brownish area, and (2) abnormal changes of intraepithelial papillary capillary loop (IPCL) pattern, that were dilatation, tortuosity, and caliber change in a single IPCL, and variation in the shape of multiple IPCL. We defined lesions which satisfied either or neither of them as "NBI negative." The abnormal blood vessels observed in Case 2 seemed to reflect neovascularization after chemoradiotherapy, so the lesion was judged to be negative for IPCL abnormality.

A total of 72 lesions biopsied form the Lugol-positive lesions were analyzed. The prevalence of SCC and HGIN was 21.4% (6/28). Seven superficial lesions in 7 patients were diagnosed as NBI positive using NBI endoscopy with magnification before iodine staining. All 7 lesions showed well-demarcated iodine-unstained areas by Lugol chromoendoscopy (Lugol positive). Among them, 4 lesions in 4 patients were histologically confirmed to be SCC, 2 lesions in 2 patients were HGIN, and 1 lesion was no tumor (Figure 3, Table 2). On the other hand, Lugol chromoendoscopy detected 65 iodine-unstained areas which were diagnosed as NBI negative. Among them, 5 lesions in 4 patients were diagnosed as LGIN, and 60 lesions in 20 patients were no tumor (Figure 3). The numbers of lesion detected by NBI with magnification versus Lugol chromoendoscopy were displayed in Table 3.

The sensitivity, specificity, PPV, NPV, and overall accuracy of NBI with magnification for the detection of esophageal SCC or HGIN using histological assessment as the gold standard were 100.0%, 98.5%, 85.7%, 100%, and 98.6%, respectively (Table 4). The PPV of Lugol chromoendoscopy was 8.3% (Table 4). No Lugol-negative lesions were biopsied in this study, so sensitivity, specificity, NPV, and accuracy of Lugol chromoendoscopy were indeterminate. Compared to Lugol chromoendoscopy, NBI with magnification was shown to have equal sensitivity and significantly higher PPV in detecting esophageal SCC or HGIN in patients after CRT ($P < 0.0001$).

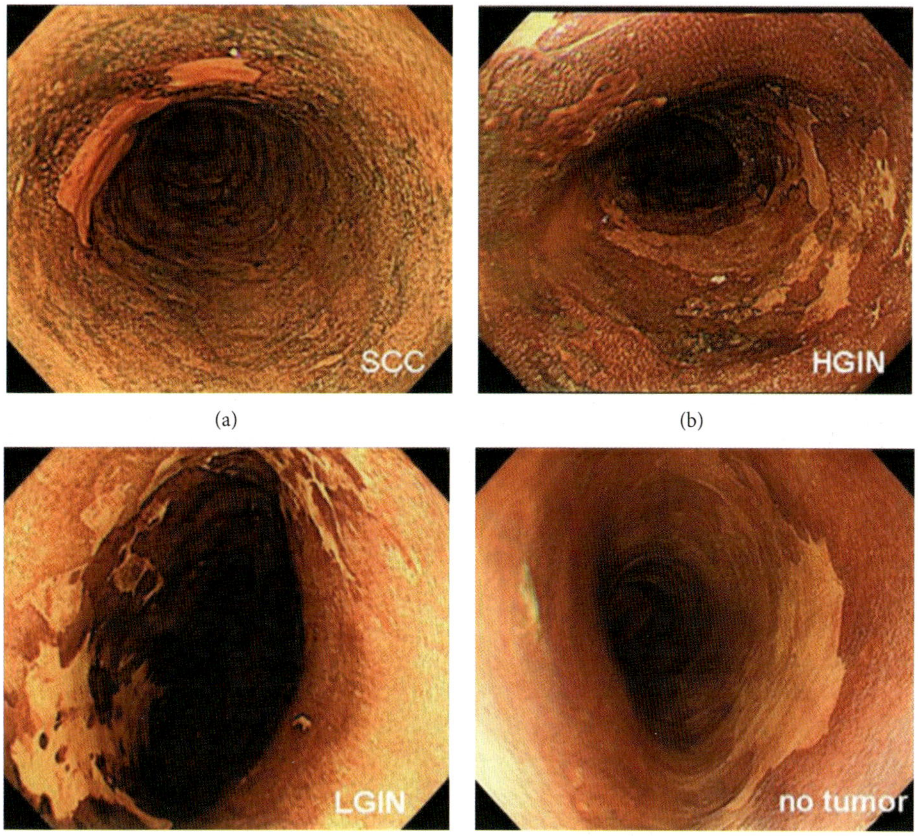

(c) (d)

FIGURE 2: We defined well-demarcated unstained area of more than 5 mm of diameter as "Lugol positive" and performed biopsy. The examples of Lugol-positive lesions were provided here.

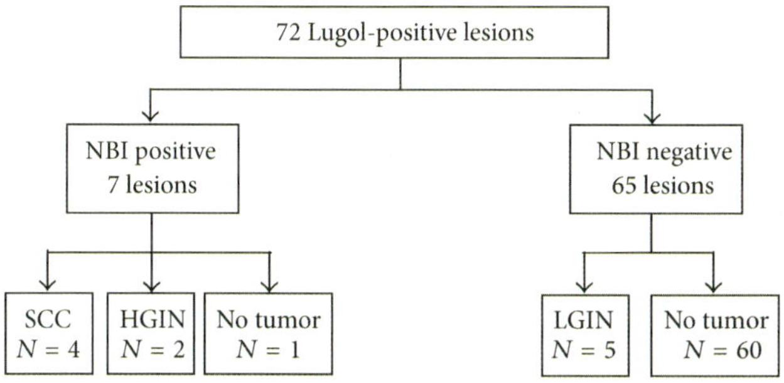

FIGURE 3: Seventy-two lesions biopsied from the Lugol-positive lesions were analyzed. The lesion observed as a well-demarcated brownish area with abnormal changes of intraepithelial papillary capillary loop (IPCL) pattern by NBI with magnification was defined as NBI positive. SCC squamous cell carcinoma; HGIN high-grade intraepithelial neoplasia; LGIN low-grade intraepithelial neoplasia; N = number of lesions.

4. Discussion

In this study, we assessed the diagnostic ability of NBI with magnification in detecting esophageal SCC or HGIN based on the biopsy specimens obtained from the lesions which were unstained by Lugol chromoendoscopy in the patients after CRT. There are many reports describing the superiority of Lugol chromoendoscopy to conventional endoscopy in detection of esophageal neoplasia in high-risk patients [1, 4]. However, the specificity of Lugol chromoendoscopy for the detection of esophageal SCC or HGIN was previously reported to be low, with values ranging from 40 to 95% [3, 4, 13–15]. At the same time, esophageal iodine staining can lead to a transient dysphagia related to an esophagospasm [16], esophagitis [17], and gastritis [18]. Moreover, Lugol chromoendoscopy requires taking some additional time to spray iodine solution and to wait until the whole mucosa is colored.

Recently, NBI is developed as one of the options to achieve optical chromoendoscopy. The benefits of NBI are its visualization of the superficial structure and image enhancement of vasculature within the mucosal layer. In particular, the recognition of changes in the IPCL pattern is useful for the detection of esophageal neoplasia [10]. Many studies reported the usefulness of NBI in detecting esophageal neoplasia in high-risk patients [1, 6, 8]. Furthermore, Chiu et al. reported that NBI with magnification had comparable sensitivity and superior specificity when comparing it to Lugol chromoendoscopy (sensitivity 92.3% versus 92.3%, specificity 91.7%

Table 1: Baseline characteristics of 28 patients and primary cancers.

Age, median (range), years	69 (56–86)
Sex (male, female)	25, 3
Location	
Ce	1
Ut	3
Mt	15
Lt	9
Ae	0
Depth	
M	1
SM	9
MP or more	18
LN metastasis	
Yes	16
No	12
Distant metastasis	
Yes	5
No	23
Chemotherapy	
CDDP + 5-FU	2
NPD + 5-FU	25
NPD + 5-FU → NPD + S-1	1
Radiation	
Median (range), Gy	50.4 (50–60)
Follow-up period	
Median (range), months	10 (3–42)

Table 2: Biopsy results displayed based on NBI with magnification results (number of lesions).

	SCC or HGIN	LGIN or no tumor	Total
NBI-positive	6	1	7
NBI-negative	0	65	65
Total	6	66	72

All 72 lesions were Lugol-positive. SCC: squamous cell carcinoma, HGIN: high-grade intraepithelial neoplasia, LGIN: low-grade intraepithelial neoplasia, NBI: narrow band imaging.

Table 3: Number of lesions detected by NBI with magnification versus Lugol chromoendoscopy.

	NBI with magnification n (%)	Lugol chromoendoscopy n (%)
SCC (4 lesions)	4 (100)	4 (100)
HGIN (2 lesions)	2 (100)	2 (100)
Other (66 lesions)	1 (1.5)	66 (100)

NBI: narrow band imaging, SCC: squamous cell carcinoma, HGIN: high-grade intraepithelial neoplasia.

versus 72.2%) [19]. Takenaka et al. also reported that NBI with magnification had comparable sensitivity (90.9% versus 100%, $P = 1$), superior specificity (95.4% versus 84.7%, $P < 0.001$), and superior accuracy (95.1% versus 85.9%, $P < 0.01$), compared with Lugol chromoendoscopy, in detecting esophageal SCC or HGIN in patients with head and neck cancer [20].

Table 4: (a) Diagnostic ability of the NBI with magnification in detecting esophageal SCC and HGIN. (b) Comparison of PPV of NBI with magnification and Lugol chromoendoscopy.

(a)

	Sensitivity	Specificity	PPV	NPV	Accuracy
NBI with magnification	100%	98.5%	85.7%	100%	98.6%

(b)

	NBI with magnification	Lugol chromoendoscopy	P value
PPV	85.7%	8.3%	$P < 0.0001$

NBI: narrow band imaging, SCC: squamous cell carcinoma, HGIN: high-grade intraepithelial neoplasia, PPV: positive predictive value, NPV: negative predictive value.

In this study, we focused on patients after CRT for esophageal carcinoma, among whom differential diagnosis between local persistence, recurrence, and metachronous SCC or normal post-therapeutic sequelae such as mucositis and fibrosis often becomes a problem. As a result, PPV of Lugol chromoendoscopy was only 8.3%. Compared to Lugol chromoendoscopy, NBI with magnification had equal sensitivity and significantly higher PPV (85.7% versus 8.3%) in detecting esophageal SCC or HGIN. This means that NBI with magnification would be able to pick up neoplastic lesions more efficiently than Lugol chromoendoscopy in these patients.

The prevalence of esophageal SCC and HGIN among the patients after CRT for esophageal carcinoma was 21.4% (6/28) in our study. The importance of regular surveillance for these patients was reconfirmed from this result. A surveillance endoscopy using NBI with magnification may improve acceptability of endoscopic procedures as compared with Lugol chromoendoscopy. Because the use of NBI would avoid all the side effects that can be observed with a Lugol's solution and would shorten the time of endoscopic procedure.

There were some limitations in this study. First, sensitivity, specificity, NPV, and accuracy of Lugol chromoendoscopy were indeterminate in this study because we assessed the diagnostic ability of NBI with magnification based on the biopsy specimens obtained from the lesions which were unstained by Lugol chromoendoscopy, that means no Lugol-negative lesions were biopsied in this study. However the results of our study suggested that NBI with magnification would be able to pick up esophageal neoplasia in patients after CRT more efficiently than Lugol chromoendoscopy. Second, patients who could not be examined using NBI with magnification because of stricture after CRT were excluded from the analysis because the aim of this study was to compare the diagnostic ability of "NBI with magnification" and "Lugol chromoendoscopy" Third, the diagnostic ability of NBI with magnification for esophageal neoplasia was not compared with that of conventional white light endoscopy. Muto et al. reported that the sensitivity and accuracy of NBI in detecting esophageal neoplasia were significantly higher than that of conventional white light endoscopy based on their multicenter randomized controlled trial [9]. Lastly, it seemed that both NBI with magnification and Lugol chromoendoscopy could not detect submucosal tumorlike SCCs [21] and recurrences [22] which were covered by normal epithelium and grew mainly in the submucosal layer of the esophagus because both methods diagnosed cancerous lesion based mainly on epithelial changes. Therefore other examinations should be considered to detect such lesions.

5. Conclusion

In conclusion, NBI with magnification has an equal sensitivity and significantly higher PPV in detecting esophageal neoplasia in patients after CRT compared to Lugol chromoendoscopy. So it would be able to pick up local persistence, recurrence, and metachronous SCC more efficiently with no side effects related to Lugol's solution. Although a large prospective study is desirable, NBI could replace Lugol chromoendoscopy as a surveillance tool for these patients.

References

[1] S. Lecleire, M. Antonietti, I. Iwanicki-Caron et al., "Lugol chromo-endoscopy versus Narrow Band Imaging for endoscopic screening of esophageal squamous-cell carcinoma in patients with a history of cured esophageal cancer: a feasibility study," *Diseases of the Esophagus*, vol. 24, no. 6, pp. 418–422, 2011.

[2] C. Piazza, D. Cocco, L. De Benedetto, F. D. Bon, P. Nicolai, and G. Peretti, "Role of narrow-band imaging and high-definition television in the surveillance of head and neck squamous cell cancer after chemo- and/or radiotherapy," *European Archives of Oto-Rhino-Laryngology*, vol. 267, no. 9, pp. 1423–1428, 2010.

[3] S. M. Dawsey, D. E. Fleischer, G.-Q. Wang et al., "Mucosal iodine staining improves endoscopic visualization of squamous dysplasia and squamous cell carcinoma of the esophagus in Linxian, China," *Cancer*, vol. 83, no. 2, pp. 220–231, 1998.

[4] H. Shiozaki, H. Tahara, K. Kobayashi et al., "Endoscopic screening of early esophageal cancer with the Lugal dye method in patients with head and neck cancers," *Cancer*, vol. 66, no. 10, pp. 2068–2071, 1990.

[5] Y. Shimizu, H. Tukagoshi, M. Fujita, M. Hosokawa, M. Kato, and M. Asaka, "Endoscopic screening for early esophageal cancer by iodine staining in patients with other current or prior primary cancers," *Gastrointestinal Endoscopy*, vol. 53, no. 1, pp. 1–5, 2001.

[6] E. Ide, F. Maluf-Filho, D. M. Chaves, S. E. Matuguma, and P. Sakai, "Narrow-band imaging without magnification for detecting early esophageal squamous cell carcinoma," *World Journal of Gastroenterology*, vol. 17, no. 39, pp. 4408–4413, 2011.

[7] H. Inoue, J. F. Rey, and C. Lightdale, "Lugol chromoendoscopy for esophageal squamous cell cancer," *Endoscopy*, vol. 33, no. 1, pp. 75–79, 2001.

[8] C. T. Lee, C. Y. Chang, Y. C. Lee et al., "Narrow-band imaging with magnifying endoscopy for the screening of esophageal cancer in patients with primary head and neck cancers," *Endoscopy*, vol. 42, no. 8, pp. 613–619, 2010.

[9] M. Muto, K. Minashi, T. Yano et al., "Early detection of superficial squamous cell carcinoma in the head and neck region and esophagus by narrow band imaging: a multicenter randomized controlled trial," *Journal of Clinical Oncology*, vol. 28, no. 9, pp. 1566–1572, 2010.

[10] T. Yoshida, H. Inoue, S. Usui, H. Satodate, N. Fukami, and S. E. Kudo, "Narrow-band imaging system with magnifying endoscopy for superficial esophageal lesions," *Gastrointestinal Endoscopy*, vol. 59, no. 2, pp. 288–295, 2004.

[11] R. J. Schlemper, R. H. Riddell, Y. Kato et al., "The vienna classification of gastrointestinal epithelial neoplasia," *Gut*, vol. 47, no. 2, pp. 251–255, 2000.

[12] S. R. Hamilton and L. A. Aaltonen, Eds., *World Health Organization Classification of Tumours. Pathology and Genetics of Tumours of the Digestive System*, IARC Press, Lyon, France, 2000.

[13] H. Ina, H. Shibuya, I. Ohashi, and M. Kitagawa, "The frequency of a concomitant early esophageal cancer in male patients with oral and oropharyngeal cancer: screening results using Lugol dye endoscopy," *Cancer*, vol. 73, no. 8, pp. 2038–2041, 1994.

[14] R. B. Fagundes, S. G. S. De Barros, A. C. K. Pütten et al., "Occult dysplasia is disclosed by Lugol chromoendoscopy in alcoholics at high risk for squamous cell carcinoma of the esophagus," *Endoscopy*, vol. 31, no. 4, pp. 281–285, 1999.

[15] M. Mori, Y. Adachi, T. Matsushima, H. Matsuda, H. Kuwano, and K. Sugimachi, "Lugol staining pattern and histology of esophageal lesions," *American Journal of Gastroenterology*, vol. 88, no. 5, pp. 701–705, 1993.

[16] T. Ponchon, "Endoscopic diagnosis of superficial neoplastic lesions of the digestive tract," *Gastroenterologie Clinique et Biologique*, vol. 24, no. 5, pp. B109–B122, 2000.

[17] F. P. B. Martins Thuler, G. A. De Paulo, and A. P. Ferrari, "Chemical esophagitis after chromoendoscopy with Lugol's solution for esophageal cancer: case report," *Gastrointestinal Endoscopy*, vol. 59, no. 7, pp. 925–926, 2004.

[18] A. Sreedharan, B. J. Rembacken, O. Rotimi, and B. J. Rembacken, "Acute toxic gastric mucosal damage induced by Lugol's iodine spray during chromoendoscopy," *Gut*, vol. 54, no. 6, pp. 886–887, 2005.

[19] P. W. Chiu, F. K. Cheung, and R. K. Tsang, "Narrow band imaging (NBI) against conventional Lugol staining for detection of superficial oesophageal neoplasia in high risk patients: a prospective comparative study," *Gastrointestinal Endoscopy*, vol. 65, p. AB332, 2007.

[20] R. Takenaka, Y. Kawahara, H. Okada et al., "Narrow-band imaging provides reliable screening for esophageal malignancy in patients with head and neck cancers," *American Journal of Gastroenterology*, vol. 104, no. 12, pp. 2942–2948, 2009.

[21] T. Kishino, Y. Yamaguchi, T. Yamagishi et al., "Submucosal tumor (SMT)—like esophageal squamous cell carcinoma with gastric metastasis," *Hepato-Gastroenterology*, vol. 47, no. 36, pp. 1581–1584, 2000.

[22] C. H. Tu, M. Muto, T. Horimatsu et al., "Submucosal tumor appearance is a useful endoscopic predictor of early primary-site recurrence after definitive chemoradiotherapy for esophageal squamous cell carcinoma," *Diseases of the Esophagus*, vol. 24, no. 4, pp. 274–278, 2011.

6

Endoscopic Papillary Large Balloon Dilation Reduces the Need for Mechanical Lithotripsy in Patients with Large Bile Duct Stones

Mohammad F. Madhoun,[1] Sachin Wani,[2] Sam Hong,[1] William M. Tierney,[1] and John T. Maple[1]

[1] *Division of Digestive Diseases and Nutrition, University of Oklahoma Health Sciences Center, 920 Stanton L. Young Boulevard, WP1345, Oklahoma City, OK 73104, USA*
[2] *Division of Gastroenterology and Hepatology, University of Colorado, Anschutz Medical Campus, and Veterans Affairs Medical Center, Aurora, Denver, CO, USA*

Correspondence should be addressed to John T. Maple; john-maple@ouhsc.edu

Academic Editor: Tony C.K. Tham

Background. Removal of large stones can be challenging and frequently requires the use of mechanical lithotripsy (ML). Endoscopic papillary large balloon dilation (EPLBD) following endoscopic sphincterotomy (ES) is a technique that appears to be safe and effective. However, data comparing ES + EPLBD with ES alone have not conclusively shown superiority of either technique. *Objective*. To assess comparative efficacies and rate of adverse events of these methods. *Method*. Studies were identified by searching nine medical databases for reports published between 1994 and 2013, using a reproducible search strategy. Only studies comparing ES and ES + EPLBD with regard to large bile duct stone extraction were included. Pooling was conducted by both fixed-effects and random-effects models. Risk ratio (RR) estimates with 95% confidence interval (CI) were calculated. *Results*. Seven studies (involving 902 patients) met the inclusion criteria; 3 of 7 studies were prospective trials. Of the 902 patients, 463 were in the ES + EPLBD group, whereas 439 underwent ES alone. There were no differences noted between the groups with regard to overall stone clearance (98% versus 95%, RR = 1.01 [0.97, 1.05]; $P = 0.60$) and stone clearance at the 1st session (87% versus 79%, RR = 1.11 [0.98, 1.25]; $P = 0.11$). ES + EPLBD was associated with a reduced need for ML compared to ES alone (15% versus 32%; RR = 0.49 [0.32, 0.74]; $P = 0.0008$) and was also associated with a reduction in the overall rate of adverse events (11% versus 18%; RR = 0.58 [0.41, 0.81]; $P = 0.001$). *Conclusions*. ES + EPLBD has similar efficacy to ES alone while significantly reducing the need for ML. Further, ES + EPLBD appears to be safe, with a lower rate of adverse events than traditional ES. ES + EPLBD should be considered as a first-line technique in the management of large bile duct stones.

1. Introduction

Endoscopic retrograde cholangiopancreatography (ERCP) with endoscopic sphincterotomy (ES) represents the standard of care for management of bile duct stones [1]. However, removal of stones > 10 mm in diameter can be challenging and often requires the use of mechanical lithotripsy (ML) [2, 3]. Dilation of the biliary orifice and distal common bile duct (CBD) after ES using 12- to 20 mm esophageal or pyloric-type balloons was first described in 2003 as an alternative technique to manage large bile duct stones [4]. The safety and efficacy of this technique, termed endoscopic papillary large balloon dilation (EPLBD), have been confirmed in a number of subsequent reports [5–7]. However, studies comparing ES + EPLBD versus ES alone have not conclusively shown the superiority of either technique.

The aims of this systematic review and meta-analysis were to compare ES + EPLBD with ES alone for (i) overall clearance of stone, (ii) clearance of stones at first session, (iii) need for ML, and (iv) rate of adverse events.

2. Methods

2.1. Study Identification. All published studies that compared ES alone versus ES + EPLBD in the management of large bile duct stones were reviewed. Studies were identified by searching nine medical databases including PubMed and Ovid MEDLINE for reports published between 1994 and August of 2013. A reproducible search strategy was employed which combined the terms: "sphincterotomy" OR "ES" and "balloon dilation" and "bile duct stone" OR "choledocholithiasis. " References from retrieved articles and abstracts presented at Digestive Diseases Week between 2003 and 2013 were also manually reviewed.

2.2. Study Eligibility. Two investigators (SW, SH) independently evaluated studies for inclusion in the systematic review, and any disagreements were adjudicated by the senior investigator (JM). Investigators were not blinded to journal titles, author names, or institutional affiliations. The studies (1) prospectively or retrospectively included comparative analyses between ES and ES + EPLBD, (2) reported (or provided data allowing calculation of) the overall clearance of bile duct stones, and (3) used a balloon diameter ≥ 12 mm for the ES + EPLBD arm.

2.3. Data Extraction. Two study investigators extracted these data independently for each study: (1) publication year, (2) country of origin, (3) study design, (4) patient demographics, (5) mean CBD diameter, (6) mean diameter of bile duct stone, (7) mean number of stones, (8) presence of periampullary diverticulum, (8) size of endoscopic sphincterotomy, (9) presence of distal common bile duct stricture, (10) use of precut sphincterotomy, (11) stone clearance at first session, (12) overall stone clearance, (13) need for mechanical lithotripsy, (14) need for extracorporeal shock wave lithotripsy, (15) mean number of sessions to achieve complete stone clearance, (16) total procedure time, (17) fluoroscopy time, and (18) rate of adverse events.

2.4. Outcomes for Analysis. The primary outcome of this systematic review and meta-analysis was to compare ES + EPLBD with ES alone for overall clearance of bile duct stones. Secondary outcomes included clearance of the stones at the first session, need for ML, and rate of adverse events.

2.5. Assessment of Study Quality. The Newcastle-Ottawa quality assessment scale was used to assess bias in studies included in this review [8]. This scale rates studies on three sources of bias based on eight criteria: (1) is the case definition adequate?; (2) representativeness of the cases; (3) selection of controls; (4) definition of controls; (5) comparability of cases and controls on the basis of the design or analysis (confounding); (6) ascertainment of exposure; (7) same method of ascertainment for cases and controls; (8) nonresponse rate. Each criterion is worth one star except confounding, which is worth two stars. The Cochrane Collaboration's Risk of Bias (a tool available in Review Manager 5) was used to assess bias in randomized trials meeting eligibility criteria [9]. This tool rates studies on four sources of bias based on six criteria: (1) adequate sequence generation to gauge selection bias; (2) allocation concealment to gauge selection bias; (3) blinding of participants, personnel, and outcome assessors to gauge performance and detection bias; (4) incomplete outcome data to gauge attrition bias; (5) selective reporting to gauge reporting bias; (6) a criterion for other forms of bias. Disagreement between the two extracting authors was resolved by consensus.

2.6. Data Synthesis and Statistical Analysis. The meta-analysis was performed using the Review Manager (RevMan) software, version 4.2.8 (The Nordic Cochrane Centre, Copenhagen, The Cochrane Collaboration) as a summary risk ratio (RR) with 95 percent confidence interval by using the Mantel-Haenszel fixed-effects method [10]. Estimates were also combined using the random-effects model by DerSimonian and Laird [11]. In the absence of significant heterogeneity ($P > 0.1$), the fixed-effects model results were presented. All pooled data were reported with the associated 95% confidence intervals. All statistical tests were 2 sided, and the significance level was set at 5%. Heterogeneity was assessed by both χ^2 and I^2 statistics [12, 13]. A P value <0.10 (or a large χ^2 statistic relative to degrees of freedom) was considered evidence of heterogeneity beyond chance. An I^2 value greater than 40% was considered substantial heterogeneity.

3. Results

3.1. Study Identifications and Selection. The literature search yielded 39 potentially pertinent studies for inclusion. Thirty-one of these studies were immediately excluded after initial review, most commonly because they presented a case series describing one technique or were review articles. One study met the inclusion criteria but was subsequently excluded as it described the overall rate of clearance among the ES + EPLBD group but not among the ES group [14]. Thus seven studies were included in the final analysis (Figure 1) [15–21]. Manual review of the references of retrieved manuscripts concerning ES + EPLBD versus ES alone did not yield any additional studies meeting inclusion criteria for this analysis.

3.2. Description of Variation in Study Methods. Of the seven studies meeting inclusion criteria for the meta-analysis (Table 1), three were prospective randomized studies [15, 17, 20] and four were retrospective studies [16, 18, 19, 21]. One study was published as an abstract [18] and the rest were complete papers [15–17, 19–21]. Four studies were conducted in Korea [15, 17–19], one in Japan [16], one in China [20], and one in Portugal [21]. All studies except one [18] provided detailed patient demographic information. The number of patients included in these studies ranged from 27 to 100. The range of balloon diameter used in the ES + EPLBD group was between 12 and 20 mm in the six studies that reported this variable. Four of these studies used balloons with a minimum diameter of 15 mm [16–18, 20], while two studies used balloons ≥ 12 mm [15, 21]. No study specified the exact distribution of balloon diameters used within the range

Table 1: Characteristics of included studies.

Study (year)	Country	Type of study	Number of patients ES/ES + EPLBD	Age (mean) ES/ES + EPLBD	Gender, M (%) ES/ES + EPLBD	Mean CBD diameter (mm ± SD) ES/ES + EPLBD	Large balloon dilation size (mm)	Mean size of the stone (mm ± SD) ES/ES + EPLBD	Size of ES ES/ES + EPLBD	Periampullary diverticulum (%) ES/ES + EPLBD
Heo (2007)	Korea	RCT	100/100	63/64	50/48	N/A	12–20	15 ± 0.7/16 ± 0.7	Full/Limited	45/49
Itoi (2009)	Japan	Retrospective	48/53	73/75	58/38	18 ± 4.3/17 ± 3.7	15–20	15 ± 3.2/15 ± 3.5	Full/Full	58/47
Kim HG (2009)	Korea	RCT	28/27	70/70	39/37	21 ± 5.7/21 ± 6.3	15–18	21 ± 5.2/21 ± 4.1	Full/Limited	36/33
Hong GY (2009)	Korea	Retrospective	65/70	N/A	N/A	N/A	15 or 20	N/A	N/A	49/57
Kim TH (2011)	Korea	Retrospective	77/72	69/69	49/54	19 ± 4.4/18 ± 3.3	N/A	N/A	Full/Limited	N/A
Teoh (2013)	China	RCT	78/73	73/72	51/44	N/A	15	N/A	Full/Limited	NA
Rosa (2013)	Portugal	Retrospective	43/68	73/71	35/34	16.4 ± 7.2/17.1 ± 3.4	12–18	16.0 ± 6.7/16.8 ± 4.4	N/A	N/A

RCT: randomized controlled trial; ES: endoscopic sphincterotomy; EPLBD: endoscopic papillary large balloon dilation; N/A: not available; CBD: common bile duct; SD: standard deviation.

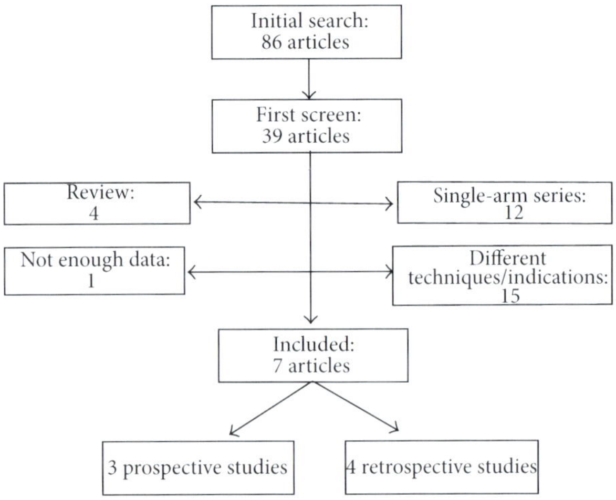

Figure 1: Flowchart of the studies included in the meta-analysis.

of permissible balloon sizes. A limited (submaximal) ES was implemented in conjunction with EPLBD in four studies [15, 17, 19, 20], full/maximal ES in one study [16], and two studies did not mention the extent of ES [18, 21]. All studies reported rates for overall stone clearance and the use of mechanical lithotripsy, and all except one [18] reported rates of clearance at the first session. Three studies reported total procedure time [16, 19, 20], and one study reported fluoroscopy time [16]. Five studies reported data regarding the size and/or number of biliary stones [15–17, 20, 21]. Among the three prospective randomized trials, randomization was conducted intraprocedurally after obtaining biliary access in two studies [15, 20] and prior to ERCP in one study [17].

3.3. Assessment of Study Quality. The assessment of bias in the retrospective studies indicated that three studies were of high methodological quality [16, 19, 21] and one of moderate methodological quality (Table 2) [18]. There appeared to be a consistent performance bias among all three randomized trials because of the fact that the nature of the study precludes blinding of the operator. Two studies were also limited by selection bias because of inadequate allocation concealment (Figure 2) [19, 20].

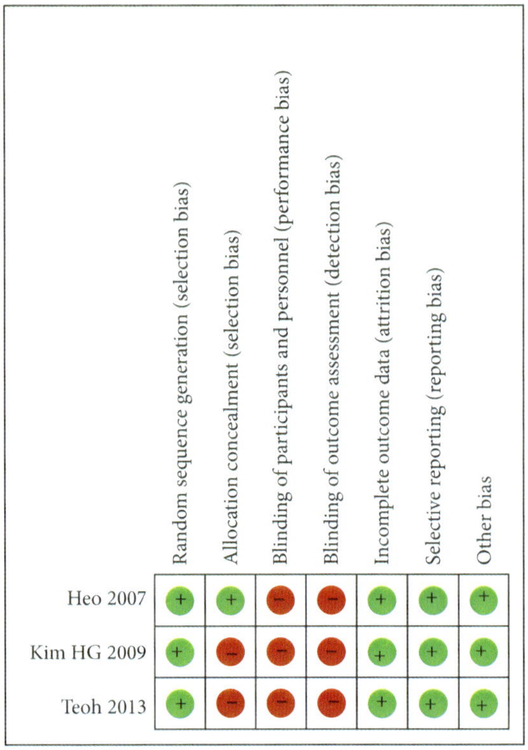

Figure 2: Risk of bias summary of randomized clinical trials.

Study or subgroup	ES + EPLBD Events	ES + EPLBD Total	ES Events	ES Total	Weight	Risk ratio M-H, random, 95% CI
Heo 2007	97	100	98	100	20.7%	0.99 [0.95, 1.03]
Hong 2009	70	70	65	65	0.0%	1.00 [0.97, 1.03]
Itoi 2009	53	53	47	48	19.0%	1.02 [0.97, 1.08]
Kim HG 2009	27	27	28	28	17.0%	1.00 [0.93, 1.07]
Kim TH 2011	70	72	73	77	17.6%	1.03 [0.96, 1.09]
Rosa 2013	65	68	30	43	5.2%	1.37 [1.12, 1.68]
Teoh 2013	71	73	78	78	20.4%	0.97 [0.93, 1.02]
Total (95% CI)		**393**		**374**	**100.0%**	**1.02 [0.97, 1.07]**
Total events	383		354			

Heterogeneity: $\tau^2 = 0.00$; $\chi^2 = 20.50$, df = 5 ($P = 0.001$); $I^2 = 76\%$

Test for overall effect: $Z = 0.04$ ($P = 0.52$)

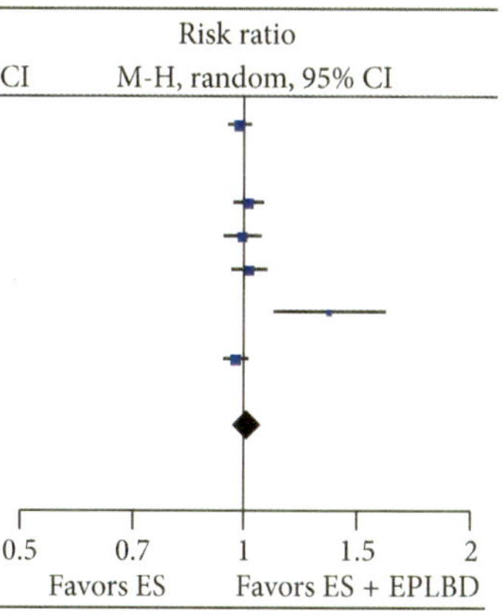

FIGURE 3: Forrest plot of the pooled risk ratio of overall clearance of duct stones and I^2 statistic for heterogeneity.

Study or subgroup	ES + EPLBD Events	ES + EPLBD Total	ES Events	ES Total	Weight	Risk ratio M-H, random, 95% CI
Heo 2007	83	100	87	100	20.4%	0.96 [0.85, 1.07]
Itoi 2009	51	53	41	48	19.7%	1.13 [0.99, 1.28]
Kim HG 2009	23	27	23	28	13.3%	1.04 [0.82, 1.31]
Kim TH 2011	63	72	57	77	17.7%	1.18 [1.01, 1.39]
Rosa 2013	56	68	19	43	8.3%	1.86 [1.31, 2.65]
Teoh 2013	65	73	69	78	20.6%	1.01 [0.90, 1.13]
Total (95% CI)		**393**		**374**	**100.0%**	**1.11 [0.98, 1.25]**
Total events	341		296			

Heterogeneity: $\tau^2 = 0.02$; $\chi^2 = 18.59$, df = 5 ($P = 0.002$); $I^2 = 73\%$

Test for overall effect: $Z = 1.59$ ($P = 0.11$)

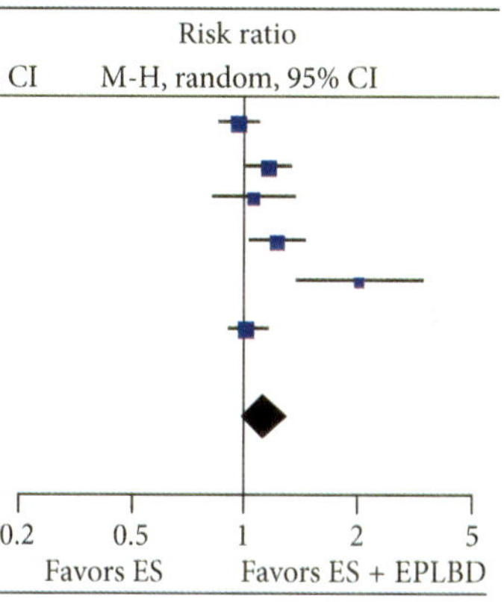

FIGURE 4: Forrest plot of the pooled risk ratio of clearance of stone at 1st session and I^2 statistic for heterogeneity.

TABLE 2: The Newcastle-Ottawa quality assessment in retrospective studies.

Study (year)	Selection	Comparability	Outcome/exposure
Itoi (2009)	* * **	**	**
Hong GY (2009)	* * *	N/A	**
Kim TH (2011)	* * **	**	**
Rosa (2013)	* * **	**	**

3.4. Data Synthesis. Seven studies involving 902 patients met the inclusion criteria. Of the 902 patients, 439 subjects were in the ES group, while 463 subjects underwent ES + EPLBD. The median stone diameter in the ES + EPLBD group was 16 mm compared to 15.3 mm in the ES group. The between-study variability (i.e., heterogeneity) beyond what could be expected by sampling error was substantially high for the pooled RR of overall clearance rate, clearance at 1st session, and the use of mechanical lithotripsy; hence, the random effects model was used. The I^2 of the pooled RR of the overall complication rate was 0%, which was not considered substantial heterogeneity as per *a priori* definition and thus the fixed effects model was used.

3.4.1. Overall Stone Clearance and Stone Clearance at 1st Session. The rate of overall stone clearance was not significantly different between the ES + EPLBD group and the ES group (98% versus 95%, RR = 1.01 [0.97, 1.05]; $P = 0.60$) (Figure 3). Similarly, the rate of stone clearance at the 1st session was not significantly different between the ES + EPLBD group and the ES group (87% versus 79%, RR = 1.11 [0.98, 1.25]; $P = 0.11$) (Figure 4).

3.4.2. Number of Sessions, Need for Mechanical Lithotripsy, and Procedure Duration. Among the four studies [17–19, 21] that reported the mean number of sessions needed for complete stone clearance, there was a nonsignificant trend toward fewer sessions needed among those who underwent ES + EPLBD versus ES (1.3 ± 0.3 versus 1.8 ± 0.7, $P = 0.245$). ES + EPLBD was associated with a reduced need for ML compared to ES alone (15% versus 32%; RR = 0.49 [0.32, 0.74]; $P = 0.0008$) (Figure 5). Total procedure time was numerically shorter in the ES + EPLBD group in each of the three studies that reported this variable [16, 17, 20], though this was statistically significant in only one study [16]. Total fluoroscopy time was significantly shorter in the ES + EPLBD group in the single study that reported this variable [16].

3.4.3. Adverse Events. ES + EPLBD was associated with a reduction in the overall rate of adverse events compared to ES alone (11% versus 18%; RR = 0.58 [0.41, 0.81]; $P = 0.001$)

Study or subgroup	ES + EPLBD Events	ES + EPLBD Total	ES Events	ES Total	Weight	Risk ratio M-H, random, 95% CI
Heo 2007	8	100	9	100	12.6%	0.89 [0.36, 2.21]
Hong 2009	13	70	47	65	0.0%	0.26 [0.15, 0.43]
Itoi 2009	3	53	12	48	8.0%	0.23 [0.07, 0.75]
Kim HG 2009	9	27	9	28	16.5%	1.04 [0.49, 2.21]
Kim TH 2011	6	72	15	77	13.0%	0.43 [0.18, 1.04]
Rosa 2013	10	68	16	43	18.7%	0.40 [0.20, 0.79]
Teoh 2013	21	73	36	78	31.2%	0.62 [0.40, 0.96]
Total (95% CI)		**393**		**374**	**100.0%**	**0.57 [0.40, 0.83]**
Total events	57		97			

Heterogeneity: $\tau^2 = 0.06$; $\chi^2 = 7.26$, df = 5 ($P = 0.20$); $I^2 = 31\%$
Test for overall effect: $Z = 2.97$ ($P = 0.003$)

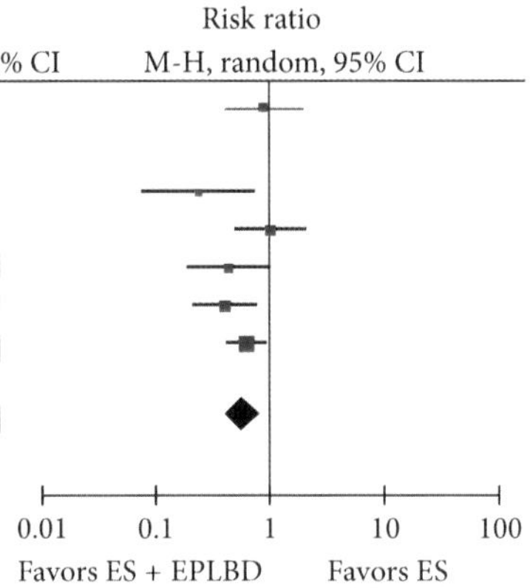

FIGURE 5: Forrest plot of the pooled risk ratio of the use of mechanical lithotripsy and I^2 statistic for heterogeneity.

Study or subgroup	ES + EPLBD Events	ES + EPLBD Total	ES Events	ES Total	Weight	Risk ratio M-H, fixed, 95% CI
Heo 2007	8	100	17	100	20.9%	0.47 [0.21, 1.04]
Hong 2009	8	70	19	65	24.3%	0.39 [0.18,0.83]
Itoi 2009	3	53	7	48	9.1%	0.39 [0.11,1.42]
Kim HG 2009	2	27	4	28	4.8%	0.52 [0.10,2.60]
Kim TH 2011	6	72	10	77	11.9%	0.64 [0.25,1.68]
Rosa 2013	10	68	5	43	7.5%	1.26 [0.46,3.45]
Teoh 2013	12	73	18	78	21.4%	0.71 [0.37,1.37]
Total (95% CI)		**463**		**439**	**100.0%**	**0.58 [0.41,0.81]**
Total events	49		80			

Heterogeneity: $\chi^2 = 4.45$, df = 6 ($P = 0.62$); $I^2 = 0\%$
Test for overall effect: $Z = 3.22$ ($P = 0.001$)

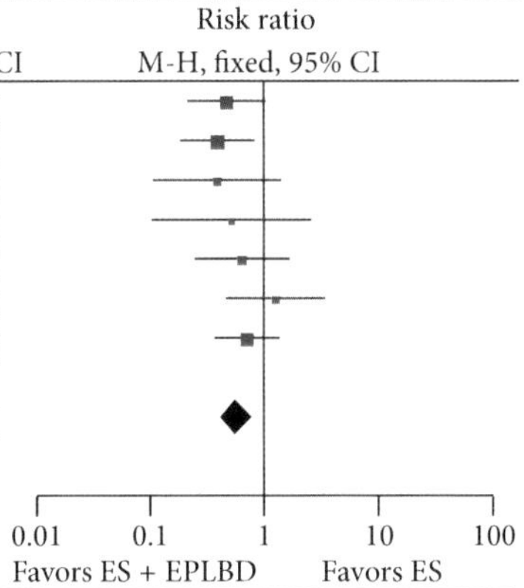

FIGURE 6: Forrest plot of the pooled risk ratio of the overall rate of adverse events and I^2 statistic for heterogeneity.

TABLE 3: Subgroup analysis of the complications rate.

	ES	ES + EPLBD	RR, (95% CI)	P value
All bleeding	38/439	20/463	0.5 (0.3, 0.8)	0.01
Pancreatitis	29/439	23/463	0.8 (0.4, 1.3)	0.29
Perforation	3/439	0/463	Not estimable	
Cholangitis	4/439	4/463	1.0 (0.24, 3.77)	0.94

(Figure 6). A subgroup analysis showed a significantly lower overall bleeding rate in the ES + EPLBD group (4% versus 9%; RR = 0.5 [0.3, 0.8]; $P = 0.003$). Bleeding could be further stratified into intraprocedural bleeding and clinically significant bleeding. The rate of intraprocedural bleeding was significantly higher in the ES alone group (8% versus 4%, $P = 0.008$), and while the rate of clinically significant bleeding was also numerically higher in the ES alone group, this trend did not attain statistical significance (0.9% versus 0.3%, $P = 0.19$). Individual studies generally required a 2-3 gram decrease in hemoglobin and/or overt melena for bleeding to be classified as "clinically significant." The rates of pancreatitis, perforation, and cholangitis were similar between the two groups (Table 3). No instances of perforation occurred in the 463 patients undergoing ES + EPLBD. Three perforations occurred in the ES arm: one retroperitoneal perforation of a diverticular wall during ES [19] and two suspected guidewire perforations [20]. All three perforations were managed conservatively. With regard to pancreatitis, a subanalysis demonstrated no difference in the rate of severe pancreatitis between patients undergoing ES versus ES + EPLBD (1.2% versus 0.7%, $P = 0.7$) [15, 17, 20, 21]. No life-threatening complications were reported across all patients in both groups.

3.4.4. Sensitivity Analyses. Sensitivity analyses were performed and most of the heterogeneity observed for the calculation of pooled overall clearance rate and clearance at 1st session could be attributed to a single study [21]. However, removing this study from the analysis did not alter the results. Similarly, no significant changes were seen across all outcomes when the study published only in abstract form was removed [18]. The retrospective and prospective studies were also analyzed separately. The pooled RR estimates for all primary and secondary outcomes when analyzed separately for only retrospective studies and for only prospective studies were concordant with pooled RR estimates for all of the studies combined (Table 4). A funnel plot of the overall clearance rate showed some asymmetry due to an unusually low rate of overall clearance (70%) in the ES-only arm in the study conducted by Rosa et al. (see Figure 7) [21].

TABLE 4: Sensitivity analysis of the primary and secondary outcomes stratified by the type of the studies.

	Relative risk (EPLBD + ES versus ES), (95% CI)		
	Retrospective studies	Randomized clinical trials	Combined
Overall clearance of bile duct stone	1.06 (0.95, 1.01)	0.98 (0.97, 1.01)	1.01 (0.97, 1.05)
Clearance of the stones at 1st session	1.29 (1.01, 1.46)	0.99 (0.91, 1.07)	1.11 (0.98, 1.25)
Need for ML	0.31 (0.22, 0.44)	0.73 (0.52, 1.03)	0.49 (0.32, 0.74)
Overall complication rate	0.57 (0.36, 0.91)	0.59 (0.36, 0.95)	0.58 (0.41, 0.81)

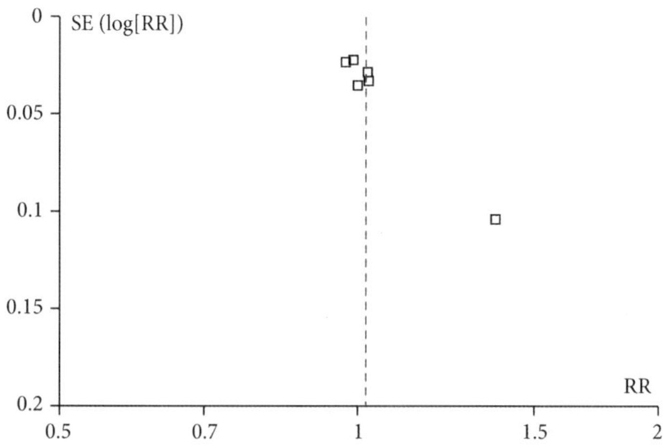

FIGURE 7: Funnel plot of the risk ratio of the overall clearance of bile duct stones.

4. Discussion

Approximately 85%–90% of bile duct stones can be removed with a balloon or basket following ES, with the most common reason for failure being large stone size [2, 22]. Historically, stones > 10 mm in diameter, and especially stones > 15 mm in diameter, have been associated with a lower success rate for endoscopic removal and a more frequent need for lithotripsy [3, 23]. Beyond stone size, factors such as small diameter of the distal CBD, ductal strictures distal to stones, and inadequate sphincterotomy, all may negatively impact the success rate of stone extraction at ERCP.

Despite the fact that the studies populating this meta-analysis were enriched with patients harboring large bile duct stones, we observed very high rates of success for overall duct clearance for both EPLBD after ES (98%) and for ES alone (95%). This likely reflects the expertise of the centers conducting these trials. Nonetheless, there was a trend observed towards more frequent clearance of the duct in one session with EPLBD after ES (87%) as compared with ES alone (79%, RR = 1.11 [0.98, 1.25]; $P = 0.11$). As such, it remains possible that rates of single session duct clearance may be enhanced with EPLBD after ES.

While mechanical lithotripsy is a valuable tool in the management of large or difficult stones, there are also potential issues associated with this technique including the challenge of cannulation with a through-the-scope lithotripter, difficulty with stone capture, need for repeated duct sweeping to remove stone fragments, and the potential need for stent placement if adequate duct clearance is not attained. EPLBD after ES holds potential advantages over ML in that many of these issues are avoided, as cannulation with the dilating balloon is not difficult, distal obstructive phenomena (e.g., duct strictures and inadequate sphincterotomies) are treated, and stones are removed *in toto*. As a result, stone clearance might be accomplished more quickly with this technique.

In this meta-analysis we found a significant reduction in the need for ML when EPLBD was employed after ES (15%) as compared with ES alone (32%). Limitations in data reporting preclude firm conclusions regarding time savings, but trends were noted for reductions in total procedure time and fluoroscopy time in the ES + EPLBD group when these variables were reported.

The use of EPLBD after ES was also associated with a reduction in the overall rate of adverse events as compared with ES alone. However, at least some of these differences appeared to be due to differences in intraprocedural bleeding events. Establishing a consistent threshold for reporting this endpoint is difficult, and for the endpoint of clinically significant bleeding, which may be more relevant, there was not a significant difference between the two groups. The rates for pancreatitis and cholangitis were similar between the two groups, and there were no perforations in the 463 patients who underwent ES + EPLBD. As such, it appears that ES + EPLBD is at least as safe as, and may be safer than, ES alone in patients undergoing ERCP for large bile duct stones.

A recently published meta-analysis [24] similarly aimed to compare ES alone versus ES + EPLBD. However, this meta-analysis is hindered by significant flaws with regard to study eligibility, inclusion criteria, and quality assessment that collectively detract from its overall validity. In this analysis, the authors erroneously included one study which was a randomized clinical trial of ES versus primary balloon sphincteroplasty (no preceding ES) using smaller balloons that did not exceed 12 mm in diameter [25]. The analysis also inappropriately included a randomized trial that compared ES + EPLBD versus ES + mechanical lithotripsy; in this study, no patients who underwent ES + EPLBD could receive ML, whereas all patients in the ES arm underwent ML also [26]. Another methodological concern involves the use of the Jadad score (an assessment tool only validated for assessing the quality of randomized clinical trials) to evaluate two retrospective studies [16, 19]. Finally, the authors reported that five studies in their analysis were "double blinded"—an impossibility given the nature of the interventions. These shortcomings grossly invalidate the findings of this analysis and the data we present represents the first methodologically robust meta-analysis comparing these two techniques.

The pooled results from this analysis are consistent with the trend from the majority of the included studies, which lacked adequate sample size to reach statistical significance independently. The results of this meta-analysis appear generalizable, given the variety of clinical settings, patient diversity, relatively uniform, readily available devices, and simple technique used to perform EPLBD after ES.

There are limitations in this study that merit mention. The inclusion of only English language studies could have potentially excluded some relevant trials. Significant heterogeneity noticed between the studies may be related to variations in study design, participant selection, use of different balloon sizes for dilation, the extent of the sphincterotomy, and operator skill level with mechanical lithotripsy. However, a sensitivity analysis that removed one study at a time demonstrated no effect on the overall conclusion of the pooled analysis. Combining retrospective and prospective studies can be problematic and is only advisable if the segregated results of pooled analyses of the retrospective and prospective studies are consistent, which is the case in our analysis.

In conclusion, the available literature demonstrates that ES + EPLBD has similar efficacy to ES alone for the removal of large bile duct stones while significantly reducing the need for ML. Further, ES + EPLBD appears to be safe, with a lower overall rate of complications in this pooled analysis relative to ES alone. ES + EPLBD should be considered a first-line technique in the management of large bile duct stones. Future prospective studies may allow for better comparisons between the two techniques with regard to total procedure time, fluoroscopy time, and costs.

References

[1] J. T. Maple, S. O. Ikenberry, M. A. Anderson et al., "The role of endoscopy in the management of choledocholithiasis," *Gastrointestinal Endoscopy*, vol. 74, no. 4, pp. 731–744, 2011.

[2] P. B. Cotton, "Non-operative removal of bile duct stones by duodenoscopic sphincterotomy," *The British Journal of Surgery*, vol. 67, no. 1, pp. 1–5, 1980.

[3] A. Lauri, R. C. Horton, B. R. Davidson, A. K. Burroughs, and J. S. Dooley, "Endoscopic extraction of bile duct stones: management related to stone size," *Gut*, vol. 34, no. 12, pp. 1718–1721, 1993.

[4] G. Ersoz, O. Tekesin, A. O. Ozutemiz, and F. Gunsar, "Biliary sphincterotomy plus dilation with a large balloon for bile duct stones that are difficult to extract," *Gastrointestinal Endoscopy*, vol. 57, no. 2, pp. 156–159, 2003.

[5] A. Minami, S. Hirose, T. Nomoto, and S. Hayakawa, "Small sphincterotomy combined with papillary dilation with large balloon permits retrieval of large stones without mechanical lithotripsy," *World Journal of Gastroenterology*, vol. 13, no. 15, pp. 2179–2182, 2007.

[6] A. Maydeo and S. Bhandari, "Balloon sphincteroplasty for removing difficult bile duct stones," *Endoscopy*, vol. 39, no. 11, pp. 958–961, 2007.

[7] P. V. Draganov, W. Evans, A. Fazel, and C. E. Forsmark, "Large size balloon dilation of the ampulla after biliary sphincterotomy can facilitate endoscopic extraction of difficult bile duct stones," *Journal of Clinical Gastroenterology*, vol. 43, no. 8, pp. 782–786, 2009.

[8] G. A. Wells, B. Shea, D. O'Connell et al., "The Newcastle-Ottawa Scale (NOS) for assessing the quality of nonrandomised studies in meta-analyses," http://www.ohri.ca/programs/clinical_epidemiology/oxford.asp.

[9] "Database C. Review Manager (RevMan)," http://ims.cochrane.org/revman.

[10] N. Mantel and W. Haenszel, "Statistical aspects of the analysis of data from retrospective studies of disease," *Journal of the National Cancer Institute*, vol. 22, no. 4, pp. 719–748, 1959.

[11] R. DerSimonian and N. Laird, "Meta-analysis in clinical trials," *Controlled Clinical Trials*, vol. 7, no. 3, pp. 177–188, 1986.

[12] J. P. Higgins and S. G. Thompson, "Quantifying heterogeneity in a meta-analysis," *Statistics in Medicine*, vol. 21, no. 11, pp. 1539–1558, 2002.

[13] T. B. Huedo-Medina, J. Sánchez-Meca, F. Marín-Martínez, and J. Botella, "Assessing heterogeneity in meta-analysis: Q statistic or I2 Index?" *Psychological Methods*, vol. 11, no. 2, pp. 193–206, 2006.

[14] J. García-Cano, L. T. Arana, C. J. Ayllón et al., "Biliary sphincterotomy dilation for the extraction of difficult common bile duct stones," *Revista Española de Enfermedades Digestivas*, vol. 101, no. 8, pp. 541–545, 2009.

[15] J. H. Heo, D. H. Kang, H. J. Jung et al., "Endoscopic sphincterotomy plus large-balloon dilation versus endoscopic sphincterotomy for removal of bile-duct stones," *Gastrointestinal Endoscopy*, vol. 66, no. 4, pp. 720–726, 2007.

[16] T. Itoi, F. Itokawa, A. Sofuni et al., "Endoscopic sphincterotomy combined with large balloon dilation can reduce the procedure time and fluoroscopy time for removal of large bile duct stones," *The American Journal of Gastroenterology*, vol. 104, pp. 560–565, 2009.

[17] H. G. Kim, Y. K. Cheon, Y. D. Cho et al., "Small sphincterotomy combined with endoscopic papillary large balloon dilation versus sphincterotomy," *World Journal of Gastroenterology*, vol. 15, no. 34, pp. 4298–4304, 2009.

[18] G. Y. Hong, S. W. Park, K. S. Seo, and H. Moon, "Endoscopic sphincterotomy plus large-balloon dilation versus endoscopic sphincterotomy for removal of large common bile duct stones," *Gastrointestinal Endoscopy*, vol. 69, Article ID AB148, 2009.

[19] T. H. Kim, H. J. Oh, J. Y. Lee, and Y. W. Sohn, "Can a small endoscopic sphincterotomy plus a large-balloon dilation reduce the use of mechanical lithotripsy in patients with large bile duct stones?" *Surgical Endoscopy*, vol. 25, no. 10, pp. 3330–3337, 2011.

[20] A. Y. Teoh, F. K. Cheung, B. Hu et al., "Randomized trial of endoscopic sphincterotomy with balloon dilation versus endoscopic sphincterotomy alone for removal of bile duct stones," *Gastroenterology*, vol. 144, no. 2, pp. 341–345.e1, 2013.

[21] B. Rosa, P. Moutinho-Ribeiro, A. Rebelo, A. Pinto-Correia, and J. Cotter, "Endoscopic papillary balloon dilation after sphincterotomy for difficult choledocholithiasis: a case-controlled study," *World Journal of Gastrointestinal Endoscopy*, vol. 5, no. 5, pp. 211–218, 2013.

[22] K. F. Binmoeller, M. Bruckner, F. Thonke, and N. Soehendra, "Treatment of difficult bile duct stones using mechanical, electrohydraulic and extracorporeal shock wave lithotripsy," *Endoscopy*, vol. 25, no. 3, pp. 201–206, 1993.

[23] J. J. Bergman, E. A. Rauws, P. Fockens et al., "Randomised trial of endoscopic balloon dilation versus endoscopic sphincterotomy for removal of bileduct stones," *The Lancet*, vol. 349, no. 9059, pp. 1124–1129, 1997.

[24] Y. Feng, H. Zhu, X. Chen et al., "Comparison of endoscopic papillary large balloon dilation and endoscopic sphincterotomy for retrieval of choledocholithiasis: a meta-analysis of randomized controlled trials," *Journal of Gastroenterology*, vol. 47, no. 6, pp. 655–663, 2012.

[25] C.-K. Lin, K.-H. Lai, H.-H. Chan et al., "Endoscopic balloon dilatation is a safe method in the management of common bile duct stones," *Digestive and Liver Disease*, vol. 36, no. 1, pp. 68–72, 2004.

[26] G. Stefanidis, N. Viazis, D. Pleskow et al., "Large balloon dilation vs. mechanical lithotripsy for the management of large bile duct stones: a prospective randomized study," *The American Journal of Gastroenterology*, vol. 106, pp. 278–285, 2011.

7

Endomicroscopy of the Pancreaticobiliary System

Shajan Peter, Ji Young Bang, Klaus Mönkemuller, Shyam Varardarajulu, and C. Mel Wilcox

Division of Gastroenterology and Hepatology, University of Alabama at Birmingham, Birmingham, AL 35294-0012, USA

Correspondence should be addressed to C. Mel Wilcox; melw@uab.edu

Academic Editor: Helmut Neumann

It is often difficult to accurately differentiate between benign and malignant pancreaticobiliary strictures, and some are interpreted as indeterminate despite ERCP, EUS, or radiological imaging techniques, thereby making it difficult for the clinician to make appropriate management decisions. Probe-based confocal laser endomicroscopy (pCLE) is an innovative imaging tool integrating real-time in vivo imaging of these difficult-to-interpret strictures in the pancreaticobiliary system during endoscopy. Recent studies of endomicroscopy have shown a promising role with improved accuracy in distinguishing these lesions, thus paving the way for future research addressing improving precise interpretation, training, and long long-term impact.

1. Introduction

Over the past few years, advanced imaging techniques have improved the diagnosis of pancreaticobiliary disorders. While there have been improvements in technology involving procedures such as endoscopic retrograde cholangiopancreaticography (ERCP), endoscopic ultrasound (EUS), computed tomography (CT) scan, magnetic resonance imaging (MRCP), and direct cholangioscopy/SpyGlass, there have also been major advancements in not only diagnosis but also in tissue procurement combined with therapeutic potential. However, in spite of such progress, it remains difficult to accurately differentiate between benign and malignant lesions such as strictures, which are vital for decision-making and appropriate management [1] (Figure 1). Often, conventional methods such as intraductal biopsy, cytological brushings, or FNA remain inconclusive or indeterminate resulting in low diagnostic accuracy [2] (Figure 5). These scenarios lead to further testing or intervention; delay diagnosis is important for a potential candidate requiring surgical resection or palliative therapy. Probe-based confocal laser endomicroscopy (pCLE) is one innovative tool that allows for real-time in vivo imaging of these difficult-to-interpret strictures in the pancreaticobiliary system.

Current diagnostic modalities (biopsy, brush cytology, or fine needle aspiration (FNA) through ERCP or EUS guided routes) have their limitations in accurate diagnosis of biliary strictures, and the sensitivity of tissue sampling varies between 20% and 60% [3–5]. The sensitivity increases when two sampling methods are utilized such as combining brush cytology with forceps yielding a sensitivity ranging from 54% to 70.4% and specificity from 97% to 100% [6]. Adding EUS-guided FNA to these methods increased the sensitivity marginally to 71% with specificity of 100%, though the EUS technique is the best method for diagnosing intrapancreatic lesions. In a recent study, standard ERCP-guided tissue sampling in indeterminate biliary strictures had 76% sensitivity and 88% accuracy, while these values were 57% and 78%, respectively, for cholangioscopic-directed (Spy Bite) biopsies [7]. These data show that given the best available techniques, the yield is still suboptimal. The site of stricture such as proximal versus distal, nature of sampling, superficial versus deep, and difficulty in focal targeting add to the existing challenges facing the diagnostic dilemma while evaluating indeterminate biliary strictures thereby underlying the dire need for improving overall accuracy.

Confocal laser endomicroscopy (CLE) has emerged as a new endoscopic imaging modality helping the endoscopist become an endopathologist by obtaining in vivo histological assessment. Thus it offers an additional or alternative method to tissue "sampling" in assessing strictures. There are two commercially available systems: (a) the endoscope-based CLE system where the confocal mechanism is incorporated in the tip of a conventional endoscope, integrated CLE (iCLE), and (b) the probe-based CLE (pCLE) system that can be passed through the biopsy channel of the endoscope. For real-time imaging of the biliary system owing to accessibility and delivery the latter system is currently being used [8].

The pCLE probe that is FDA approved specifically for pancreaticobiliary use is the CholangioFlex^{UHD} miniprobe (Mauna Kea Technologies, Paris, France) [9]. This probe consists of several fiber light bundles (>10000 optical fibers) with distal lens through which the laser beam is transmitted while being connected to a laser-scanning unit and light source. The diameter is smaller than a GastroFlex^{UHD} miniprobe, which is used for another upper gastrointestinal imaging. The specifications are listed in Table 1.

The CLE images are then sent to a laser scanning unit (LSU) that interprets the images and sends them to a processor. Data are collected at 12 frames per second. These images and acquired sequences are stored on computer systems, where they can be viewed and interpreted as real time or recorded and saved. They can be then reviewed, magnified, or exported. The specially designed software package (Cellvizio viewer) allows image correction and stabilization.

Table 1: Specifications of pCLE probe for pancreatico-biliary evaluation.

	Mini probe (CholangioFlex)
Laser wavelength	488 nm
Depth of imaging (μm)	40–60
Plane depth (μm)	0–50
Max field of view (mm)	325
Lateral resolution (μm)	3.5
Axial resolution (μm)	15
Imaging rate (frames/s)	12
External diameter (mm)	0.94

Table 2: Type of catheters for pCLE access.

Catheter device	Manufacturer
Cotton Graduated Dilatation Catheter	Cook Medical
OASIS One Action Stent Introduction System	Cook Medical
Memory Dormia Basket	Cook Medical
Howell Biliary Introducer	Cook Medical
Geenen Graduated Dilatation Catheter	Cook Medical
Swing Tip ERCP Cannula	Olympus Medical

2. Contrast Agents

Exogenous fluorescent agents are needed for detection of cellular details while performing a CLE test. Intravenous fluorescein sodium is commonly used at 10% concentration, which then helps in highlighting vessels, intercellular spaces, vascular pattern, lamina propria, and overall cellular architecture. It does not stain nuclei. Thus, disruption of cellular architecture or vasculature or leaky blood vessels are indicative of disease. When used mostly by ophthalmologists fluorescent agents have shown a high safety profile, and adverse events are few [10]. One must caution the patient that they may experience transient yellowing of the skin, eyes, and urine that could persist for a few hours. Typically an injection of 2.5 to 5.0 mL of fluorescein is sufficient for visualization of epithelial cells, and the effect lasts for 30 minutes.

3. Technique

The pCLE probe is inserted through the working channel of an ERCP scope or through various catheter devices (Table 2). It is advanced until the radiopaque tip is visible under fluoroscopic vision or cholangioscopic visualization. It is then positioned in direct contact with the mucosa of the biliary tract or site of interest. It might be preferred to go from an area of normal mucosa to abnormality. After injecting fluorescein intravenously, using the foot pedals provided or from the computer screen activates the laser, and real-time endomicroscopy is performed. Given the narrowing of lumen specially while imaging biliary duct strictures, the main challenge is positioning the probe to maintain it perpendicular to the mucosa rather than parallel. The video sequences and images can be captured or recorded. Tissue sampling such as for cytology or biopsies are preferably done after image acquisition by pCLE as they could result in art factual errors. Access of the pCLE probe can also be achieved through the SpyGlass system (Boston Scientific, Natick, Massachusetts, USA), Olympus cholangioscopes (Olympus Corp, Tokyo, Japan), and Storz prototype cholangioscope (Karl Storz GmbH, Tuttlingen, Germany) [17].

4. Interpretation

Features that differentiate benign mucosa from malignant mucosa include loss of the reticular pattern of epithelial bands <20 μm, irregular epithelial lining, gland-like structures, tortuous dilated vessels with abnormal branching, and clumps of black areas showing focal decreased areas of fluorescein or fluorescein leakage (Figures 2, 3, and 4). Putting all these observations together, the Miami classification has been adopted for classification of biliary and pancreatic lesions especially for indeterminate strictures [18]. Using specific criteria such as thick white bands (>20 μm), or thick dark bands (>40 μm) or dark clumps and epithelial structures, resulted in sensitivity of 97%, specificity (33%), PPV (80%), and NPV, (80%) compared with 45%, 100%, 100%, and 69%, respectively, for standard cytopathology. The interobserver variability was moderate for most criteria. In retrospective analysis, combining two or more criteria increased the sensitivity as compared to single criteria interpretation.

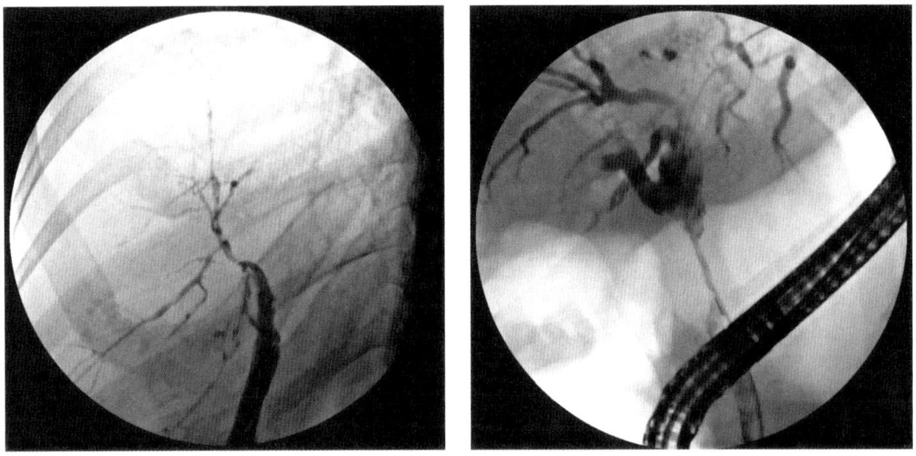

(a) (b)

Figure 1: ERCP images of biliary strictures.

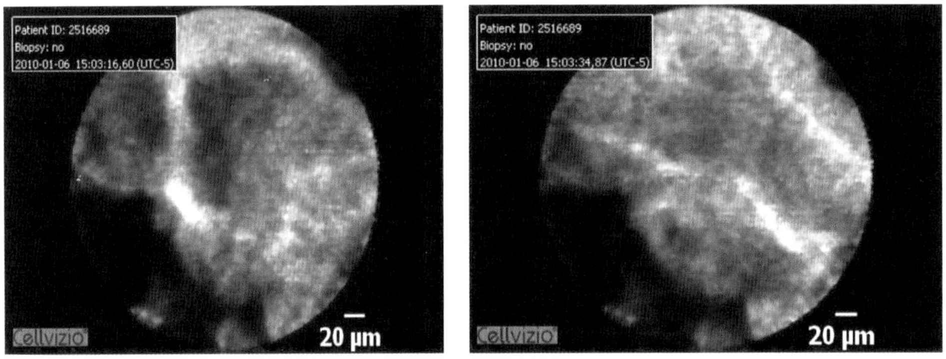

(a) (b)

Figure 2: Normal appearing bile duct with fine, reticular pattern.

5. Studies

Few studies have evaluated the role of pCLE in evaluating pancreaticobiliary strictures (Table 3). Shieh et al. used the GastroFlex miniprobe for CBD evaluation and noted that cellular architecture was better visualized using this probe as compared to the CholangioFlex probe with no major side effects [13]. Giovannini et al. used the Cholangioflex probe in 37 patients who had ERCP for bile duct stones or stenosis and interpreted images in 33 [15]. Their study predicted an accuracy of 86%, sensitivity of 83%, and specificity of 75% compared to routine biopsies with respective values of 53%, 65%, and 53%. Meining et al. conducted a multicenter study in 89 patients with indeterminate biliary strictures using the CholangioFlex probe with a one-month followup after the procedure [19]. They were able to predict malignancy in 40 patients that was subsequently confirmed on followup. pCLE had a sensitivity of 98%, specificity of 67%, and accuracy of 81% as compared to 45%, 100%, and 75%, respectively, for index pathology. Accuracy for combination of ERCP and pCLE was also significantly higher compared with ERCP and tissue acquisition (90% versus 73%). Also of interest, there was no improvement in pCLE diagnostic accuracy during the course of the study suggesting a short learning curve. Loeser et al. evaluated a smaller sample of 14 patients with indeterminate strictures of bile ducts using both the Cholangioflex and occasionally the GastroFlex probes [14]. They pointed to a normal reticular network pattern in benign lesions and comparison was made to multiphoton reconstructions of intact rat bile ducts [16]. The similarly observed reticular pattern corresponded to lymphatic structures, and presumably distortion of this pattern could be occurring in malignancy. Other criteria such as dilated blood vessels were not specific as they were observed in both benign and malignant strictures such that the negative predictive value suggests ruling out a malignancy.

6. Limitations and Promising Role

These studies shed light on the emerging role of pCLE for evaluation of indeterminate biliary strictures although limited by small sample size and specific population subsets. The diagnostic criteria are still evolving, and the exact anatomic correlates that result in the observed "abnormal" features remain undefined. One might speculate that white bands

TABLE 3: Relevant studies for pCLE of the biliary system [11].

Study (year)	Number of patients	Number malignant	Specificity	Sensitivity	Accuracy
Meining et al. [12] (2008)	14	6	88	83	86
Shieh et al. [13] (2012)	11	NA	NA	NA	NA
Loeser et al. [14] (2011)	14	6	NA	NA	NA
Giovannini et al. [15] (2011)	37	23	75	83	86
Meining et al. [19] (2011)	89	40	67	98	81

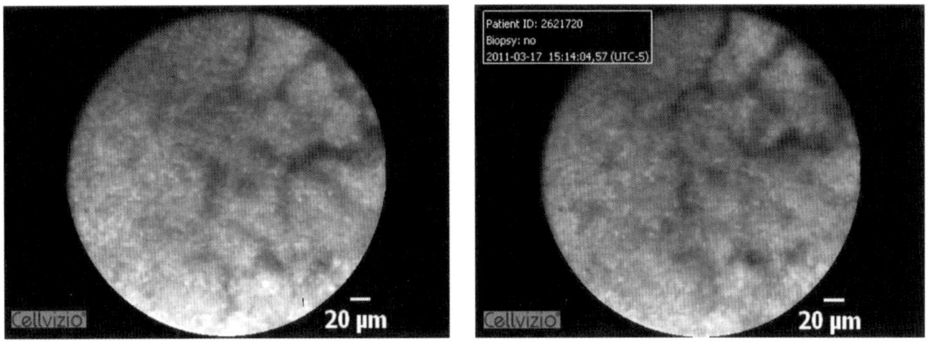

(a) (b)

FIGURE 3: Normal appearing bile duct and reticular pattern.

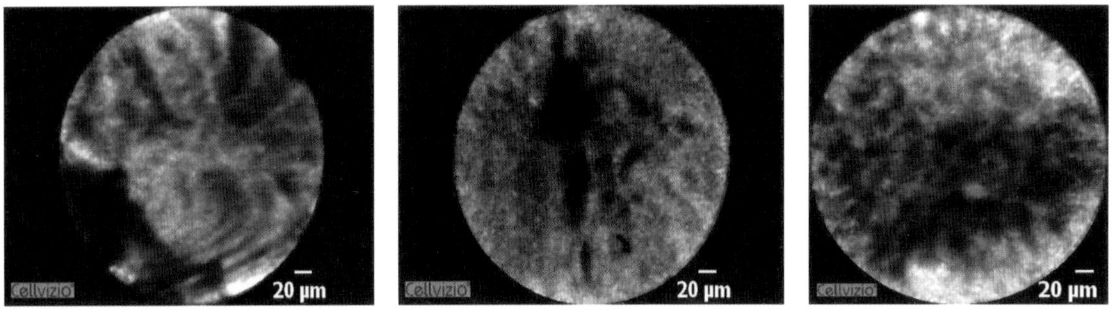

(a) (b) (c)

FIGURE 4: Biliary malignancy showing features of dark irregular structures, thick bands >20 μm, tortuous dilated blood vessels, and areas of dark clumps.

reflect blood vessels and increased neovascularization. Black bands could resemble lymphatic vessels, and the "clumps-" like structures correspond to tissue proliferation patterns, or these could mirror a paraneoplastic phenomenon. Observations such as the mucosal band and clump thickness are visual estimates and therefore subject to interpreter error. Also it is yet not clear which of these findings are specific to biliary versus pancreatic malignancies. In many of these studies, the endoscopists were aware of the clinical history and ERCP/CT or MRI findings while interpreting the imaging resulting in an interpreter bias. In a recent multicenter study, twenty-five deidentified pCLE video clips of indeterminate biliary strictures were sent to 6 observers at 5 institutions. Using the Miami Classification for standard image interpretation, they concluded that overall interobserver agreement with Kappa scores was poor to fair [20]. Further, the choice of optimal access delivery catheter versus cholangioscopic is still not clear and needs to be investigated, as well as the difference between using a larger diameter probe (Gastroflex) from the miniprobe (Cholangioflex) keeping in mind the respective spatial resolution and image quality. These factors may be important while manipulating and targeting those challenging malignant lesions in the bile duct especially when growth occurs longitudinally along the wall rather than an intraluminal ingrowth manner. The cost effectiveness of pCLE is yet to be determined as it is not clear whether this tool is sufficient enough to replace histology. Nevertheless, it could prevent repeated endoscopic evaluations with attempt at biopsies in indeterminate cases. The possibilities of use during laparoscopy or laparotomy identifying disease-free margins are other potential areas where pCLE might play an expanding role.

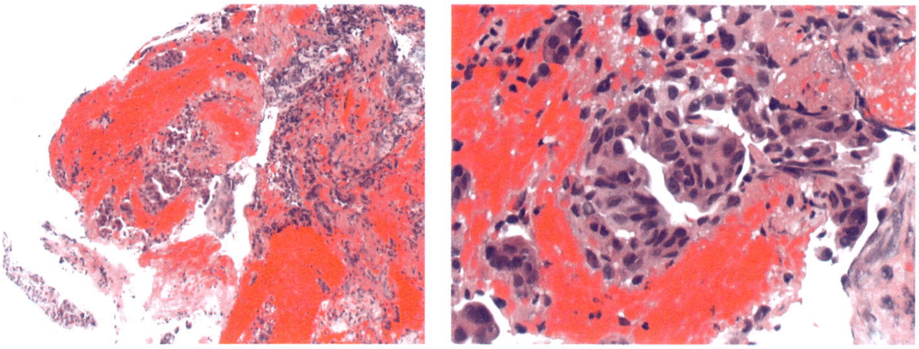

(a) (b)

Figure 5: Cytopathology images of malignant biliary strictures (a) 10x resolution and (b) 40x resolution.

7. Future

Clearly, further studies are needed before pCLE is adopted as an integral technique for evaluation of pancreaticobiliary disease. Future studies should focus on prospective validating while defining one or more specific criteria for pancreaticobiliary disorders ranging from normal to inflammatory, early neoplastic, to disease specific such as cholangiocarcinomas, gallbladder malignancies, infiltrative pancreatic cancers, and primary-sclerosing-cholangitis-(PSC-) related tumors. Modification of probes for better image stability and resolution will be technical innovative challenge. Use of EUS-guided FNA needles is being studied and could potentially help to reach territories such as pancreatic cysts. Molecular imaging using fluorescent-tagged peptides developed from bacteriophage libraries selective to biliary tissues focuses on newer areas of research [21]. These peptides could then be detected by CLE and differentiate between benign and dysplastic/neoplastic tissues.

8. Conclusions

The newer endoscopic imaging modality of CLE has kindled an interest in the field of advanced imaging offering real-time histopathologic evaluation of the pancreaticobiliary system. It has strengthened and extended the arm of the gastroenterologist from a therapeutic endoscopist to an endopathologist. The novel use of this technique is particularly of significance in differentiating indeterminate biliary strictures as treatment depends on an accurate and prompt diagnosis. More studies will ultimately determine its precise role in the immediate or long-term impact as well in combination with available modalities in the treatment of pancreaticobiliary disorders.

References

[1] D. Uhlmann, M. Wiedmann, F. Schmidt et al., "Management and outcome in patients with Klatskin-mimicking lesions of the biliary tree," *Journal of Gastrointestinal Surgery*, vol. 10, no. 8, pp. 1144–1150, 2006.

[2] J. J. Bennett and R. H. Green, "Malignant masquerade: dilemmas in diagnosing biliary obstruction," *Surgical Oncology Clinics of North America*, vol. 18, no. 2, pp. 207–214, 2009.

[3] T. Ponchon, P. Gagnon, F. Berger et al., "Value of endobiliary brush cytology and biopsies for the diagnosis of malignant bile duct stenosis: results of a prospective study," *Gastrointestinal Endoscopy*, vol. 42, no. 6, pp. 565–572, 1995.

[4] R. Schoefl, M. Haefner, F. Wrba et al., "Forceps biopsy and brush cytology during endoscopic retrograde cholangiopancreatography for the diagnosis of biliary stenoses," *Scandinavian Journal of Gastroenterology*, vol. 32, no. 4, pp. 363–368, 1997.

[5] T. Rösch, K. Hofrichter, E. Frimberger et al., "ERCP or EUS for tissue diagnosis of biliary strictures? A prospective comparative study," *Gastrointestinal Endoscopy*, vol. 60, no. 3, pp. 390–396, 2004.

[6] A. Weber, R. M. Schmid, and C. Prinz, "Diagnostic approaches for cholangiocarcinoma," *World Journal of Gastroenterology*, vol. 14, no. 26, pp. 4131–4136, 2008.

[7] D. J. Hartman, A. Slivka, D. A. Giusto, and A. M. Krasinskas, "Tissue yield and diagnostic efficacy of fluoroscopic and cholangioscopic techniques to assess indeterminate biliary strictures," *Clinical Gastroenterology and Hepatology*, vol. 10, no. 9, pp. 1042–1046, 2012.

[8] A. Meining, D. Saur, M. Bajbouj et al., "In vivo histopathology for detection of gastrointestinal neoplasia with a portable, confocal miniprobe: an examiner blinded analysis," *Clinical Gastroenterology and Hepatology*, vol. 5, no. 11, pp. 1261–1267, 2007.

[9] V. Becker, T. Vercauteren, C. H. von Weyhern, C. Prinz, R. M. Schmid, and A. Meining, "High-resolution miniprobe-based confocal microscopy in combination with video mosaicing (with video)," *Gastrointestinal Endoscopy*, vol. 66, no. 5, pp. 1001–1007, 2007.

[10] M. B. Wallace, A. Meining, M. I. Canto et al., "The safety of intravenous fluorescein for confocal laser endomicroscopy in the gastrointestinal tract," *Alimentary Pharmacology and Therapeutics*, vol. 31, no. 5, pp. 548–552, 2010.

[11] I. Smith, P. E. Kline, M. Gaidhane, and M. Kahaleh, "A review on the use of confocal laser endomicroscopy in the bile duct," *Gastroenterology Research and Practice*, vol. 2012, Article ID 454717, 5 pages, 2012.

[12] A. Meining, E. Frimberger, V. Becker et al., "Detection of cholangiocarcinoma in vivo using miniprobe-based confocal fluorescence microscopy," *Clinical Gastroenterology and Hepatology*, vol. 6, no. 9, pp. 1057–1060, 2008.

[13] F. K. Shieh, H. Drumm, M. H. Nathanson, and P. A. Jamidar, "High-definition confocal endomicroscopy of the common bile duct," *Journal of Clinical Gastroenterology*, vol. 46, no. 5, pp. 401–406, 2012.

[14] C. S. Loeser, M. E. Robert, A. Mennone, M. H. Nathanson, and P. Jamidar, "Confocal endomicroscopic examination of malignant biliary strictures and histologic correlation with lymphatics," *Journal of Clinical Gastroenterology*, vol. 45, no. 3, pp. 246–252, 2011.

[15] M. Giovannini, E. Bories, G. Monges, C. Pesenti, F. Caillol, and J. R. Delpero, "Results of a phase I-II study on intraductal confocal microscopy (IDCM) in patients with common bile duct (CBD) stenosis," *Surgical Endoscopy*, vol. 25, no. 7, pp. 2247–2253, 2011.

[16] M. O. Othman and M. B. Wallace, "Confocal laser endomicroscopy: is it prime time?" *Journal of Clinical Gastroenterology*, vol. 45, no. 3, pp. 205–206, 2011.

[17] M. Wallace, G. Y. Lauwers, Y. Chen et al., "Miami classification for probe-based confocal laser endomicroscopy," *Endoscopy*, vol. 43, no. 10, pp. 882–891, 2011.

[18] A. Meining, R. J. Shah, A. Slivka et al., "Classification of probe-based confocal laser endomicroscopy findings in pancreaticobiliary strictures," *Endoscopy*, vol. 44, no. 3, pp. 251–257, 2012.

[19] A. Meining, Y. K. Chen, D. Pleskow et al., "Direct visualization of indeterminate pancreaticobiliary strictures with probe-based confocal laser endomicroscopy: a multicenter experience," *Gastrointestinal Endoscopy*, vol. 74, no. 5, pp. 961–968, 2011.

[20] J. P. Talreja, A. Sethi, P. A. Jamidar et al., "Interpretation of probe-based confocal laser endomicroscopy of indeterminate biliary strictures: is there any interobserver agreement?" *Digestive Diseases and Sciences*, vol. 57, no. 12, pp. 3299–3302, 2012.

[21] P. L. Hsiung, J. Hardy, S. Friedland et al., "Detection of colonic dysplasia in vivo using a targeted heptapeptide and confocal microendoscopy," *Nature Medicine*, vol. 14, no. 5, pp. 454–458, 2008.

8

Endoscopic Ultrasound-Guided Celiac Plexus Neurolysis in Pancreatic Cancer: A Prospective Pilot Study of Safety Using 10 mL versus 20 mL Alcohol

Julia K. LeBlanc,[1] Susan Rawl,[2] Michelle Juan,[1] Cynthia Johnson,[3] Kurt Kroenke,[4,5,6] Lee McHenry,[1] Stuart Sherman,[1] Kathy McGreevy,[1] Mohammad Al-Haddad,[1] and John DeWitt[1]

[1] *Division of Gastroenterology and Hepatology, Indiana University Medical Center, 550 North University Boulevard, UH 4100, Indianapolis, IN 46202, USA*
[2] *Department of Adult Health, School of Nursing, Indiana University, Indianapolis, IN 46202, USA*
[3] *Department of Biostatistics, School of Medicine, Indiana University, 410 W. Tenth Sreet, Suite 3000, Indianapolis, IN 46202-3012, USA*
[4] *School of Medicine, Indiana University, Indianapolis, IN 46202-3082, USA*
[5] *Regenstrief Institute, Indianapolis, IN, USA*
[6] *Houston VA Health Services Research & Development Center of Excellence, Indianapolis, IN, USA*

Correspondence should be addressed to Julia K. LeBlanc, juleblan@iupui.edu

Academic Editor: Charles Melbern Wilcox

Background. The dose of alcohol used in EUS-CPN is not standardized. The objective was to compare the safety of 20 mL alcohol versus 10 mL alcohol during EUS-CPN for patients with pancreatic cancer-related pain. *Methods.* 20 patients were selected to receive 10 mL or 20 mL of alcohol during EUS-CPN. Followup was done at baseline, 24 hours, and weekly. Health-related quality of life (HRQoL) was assessed at baseline, week 2, week 4, and every 4 weeks thereafter until pain returned. *Results.* There were no major complications in both groups. Minor self-limited adverse effects were seen in 6 (30%) subjects and included lightheadedness in 1 (5%), transient diarrhea in 2 (10%), and transient nausea and vomiting in 3. Pain relief was similar in both groups: 80% in the 10 mL group and 100% in the 20 mL group ($P = 0.21$). The mean (± SD) duration of pain relief in the 10 mL and 20 mL groups was 7.9 ± 10.8 and 8.4 ± 9.2 weeks, respectively. 30% of patients in each group had complete pain relief. *Conclusions.* EUS-CPN using 20 mL of alcohol is safe. Similar clinical outcomes were seen in both groups. Further investigations to confirm these findings are warranted.

1. Introduction

One of the main concerns of patients with pancreatic cancer is pain [1]. For patients with pancreatic cancer, pain has a negative impact on quality of life (HRQoL) [2]. Pain will be present in a third of patients at the time of diagnosis, 30% to 50% undergoing treatment, and up to 90% with advanced disease [3–10]. After surgery for pancreatic cancer from 60% to 84% of patients reported moderate-to-severe pain [11]. While opioids are commonly used to relieve pain, their adverse side effects such as sedation, constipation, nausea, and vomiting have a negative impact on quality of life [3]. Celiac plexus neurolysis is not associated with these adverse effects and may improve survival among unresectable pancreatic cancer patients [5]. Although endoscopic ultrasound-guided celiac plexus neurolysis (EUS-CPN) does not have the side effects of opioids, it is not free of risks [12, 13]. Acute spinal cord infarction has been reported after EUS-CPN [13].

The amount of alcohol used in EUS-CPN ranges from 2 to 20 mL of alcohol [14–18]. There are no randomized studies that compare the safety of varying amounts of alcohol in celiac plexus neurolysis. We hypothesized that 20 mL of alcohol was safe in EUS-CPN. Onset of HRQoL and survival were also examined.

2. Methods

This study was approved by the Institutional Review Board at Indiana University Medical Center. Consecutive patients with known or suspected unresectable pancreatic cancer and pain were enrolled. Written informed consent to participate in this study was obtained from all patients enrolled. Patients were excluded if they had the following: previous CPN (endoscopic or percutaneous), an implanted pain relieving device, or an arterial abdominal aneurysm. Patients were selected to receive 20 mL of 0.75% bupivacaine followed by 10 mL or 20 mL of alcohol for EUS-CPN. Opioid use was not a prerequisite for entry into this study. Pain relief was defined as a pain score less than or equal to 4, or at least a 30% decrease in the pain score compared to baseline pain without an increase in pain medication usage.

2.1. EUS-CPN Procedure. EUS-CPN is defined as injection of a neurolytic agent into the celiac plexus area or directly into celiac ganglia. After providing informed consent, subjects were sedated with intravenous fentanyl, midazolam, and/or Propofol. A 22-gauge hollow Echotip Ultra needle (Cook Medical, Winston-Salem, NC, USA) was passed through the working channel of the echoendoscope, through the posterior wall of the stomach and directly into the celiac ganglia (Figures 1(a) and 1(b)) when visualized or anterior to the celiac trunk. A 5 mL sterile saline-filled syringe was loaded onto the needle and was used to "test" the position of the needle tip. Through the needle 20 mL of 0.75% bupivacaine was injected followed by 10 mL or 20 mL of 98% alcohol. If celiac ganglia were visualized, they were directly injected until the ganglia borders were blurred. When celiac ganglia were not sonographically identified, the needle was targeted to the origin of the celiac artery takeoff within 2 to 3 mm. The medication is administered in the same sequential fashion. After the EUS-CPN procedure, each patient was observed for at least one hour in the recovery room. Each patient received 1000 mL of intravenous fluids and antibiotics. Oral antibiotics were prescribed for three days. Prior to discharge each patient was assessed by the physician.

2.2. Followup. Baseline pain medication use and pain scores were documented for each patient. Each patient was called at 24 hours and weekly by a blinded research coordinator. Followup continued until the patient reported a return of their pain to baseline or died. Patients rated pain using a numeric rating scale (NRS) that ranges from 0 to 10 where 0 is "no pain" and 10 is "worst pain." During each phone interview, patients were also asked to quantify their use of pain medications. During each phone interview, the subject's pain was assessed using the brief pain inventory (BPI). The BPI is a three question survey that rates intensity of pain (severity) and interference of pain with mood, physical activity, work, social activity, relations with others, sleep, and enjoyment of life [19, 20]. Two HRQoL instruments, EORTC QLQ-30 and EORTC PAN-26, were administered during phone interviews at baseline, week 2, week 4, and every 4 weeks thereafter until the subject reported a return of their pain to baseline or died. The date of death was documented for each subject.

Table 1: Patient characteristics.

	10 mL alcohol	20 mL alcohol	P value
Gender			0.65
Male	5	4	
Female	5	6	
Mean (SD) age	66 (14)	63 (10)	0.5
Race			0.3
Caucasian	9	10	
African American	1	0	
Location in pancreas			0.41
Head	3	4	
Uncinate		1	
Body	4	1	
Tail	0	1	
Multiple	3	3	
Immediate complications			0.11
None	8	4	
Lightheadedness	1		
Diarrhea	1	5	
Nausea/vomiting	0	1	
Ganglia injection	5	5	1
Adjuvant radiation	4	2	0.61
Adjuvant chemotherapy	6	7	0.87
ED visit prior EUS-CPN*	4	5	0.81

*Subjects who visited the emergency department for pain control prior to study entry.

2.3. Statistical Methods. The frequency of complications was calculated. Complete response was defined as a pain score of zero without an increase in pain medication usage. Kaplan-Meier estimates of duration of pain relief were calculated. Health-related quality of life (HRQoL) scores were summarized for each patient. Patients who died while still experiencing pain relief are censored from our calculation of pain-free survival. Patients who did not achieve pain relief within the first four weeks of followup are assigned zero for duration of pain relief and were not be censored. The overall survival is calculated from the time of EUS-CPN.

3. Results

Patient characteristics are demonstrated in Table 1. The characteristics of pain relief in each group are demonstrated in Table 2. Among patients who received adjuvant chemotherapy and/or radiation, the median (range) duration of pain relief was 2.6 (0–32) weeks. Among patients who did not receive adjuvant chemotherapy and/or radiation the median (range) duration of pain relief was 2 (0–32) weeks. Pain scores are shown in Table 3. Four of 20 (20%) subjects (2 in each group) had pain relief that lasted over 16 weeks. Characteristics of complete responders (patients who had complete pain relief) are shown in Table 4. There were no

TABLE 2: Characteristics of pain relief.

	10 mL alcohol	20 mL alcohol	*P* value
Total subjects	10	10	
Number of subjects who had ganglia injected	5	5	1
Pain relief	8 (80%)	10 (100%)	0.21
Median (range) *onset* of pain relief (days)	1 (1–14)	1 (1–14)	
Mean (SD) *onset* of pain relief (days)	4.3 (6.0)	4.2 (5.5)	0.81
Median (range) *duration* of pain relief (weeks)	3.0 (0–32)	3.5 (2–30)	
Mean (SD) *duration* of pain relief (weeks)	7.9 (10.8)	8.4 (9.2)	0.9

SD: standard deviation.

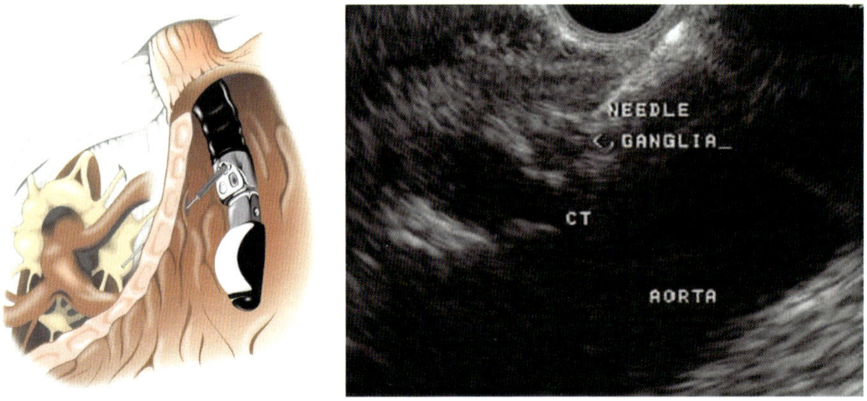

(a) (b)

FIGURE 1: (a) EUS-CPN with direct injection into the celiac ganglia. (b) EUS image of direct celiac ganglia injection.

deaths during the phone interview followup period of this study. Among the 10 patients who had direct injection of celiac ganglia, the median (range) duration of pain relief was 3 (0–32) and 3 (2–30) weeks for the 10 mL and 20 mL groups, respectively, ($P = 0.69$). In patients who *did not* have direct injection of celiac ganglia, the median (range) duration of pain relief 3 (2–8) and 1 (1–14) for the 10 mL and 20 mL alcohol groups, respectively, ($P = 0.19$). A Kaplan Meier survival curve is shown in Figure 2.

3.1. Quality of Life. HRQoL at the week 4 of followup is shown in Table 5. Scores directly correlated with pain relief on multiple measures. Minor adverse effects seen in the 10 mL group included transient diarrhea in 1 and lightheadedness in 1. Minor adverse effects seen in the 20 mL group included transient diarrhea in 5 and nausea and vomiting in 1.

3.2. Complications. There were minor self-limited postprocedure adverse effects in 6 subjects including lightheadedness in 1 (5%), transient diarrhea in 2 (10%), and transient nausea and vomiting in 3 (15%). Only subject in the 20 mL group required an emergency room visit for pain control at week 2. There were no complications of bleeding or paralysis.

4. Discussion

There were no major complications seen with the 20 mL of 98% alcohol group compared to the 10 mL group. During the EUS-CPN procedure all patients received a combination of fentanyl, versed, and propofol for sedation which likely explains the absence of pain in the recovery room. We found that EUS-CPN with 20 mL of alcohol compared to 10 mL of alcohol was safe. However, we also noted that clinical outcomes of the two groups were similar with respect to overall pain relief (100% in 20 mL group versus 80% in 10 mL group), weekly pain scores, onset of pain relief, duration of pain relief, and proportion of complete responders. This suggests that 20 mL alcohol during EUS-CPN may not provide significant pain relief despite its safety. A statistically significant difference is not observed between the two groups, however, as our study was a pilot study. A larger prospective study is warranted to confirm our findings.

We also noted an equal number of complete responders in each group. Two thirds of these complete responders in each group had direct injection of celiac ganglia. This suggests that direct visualization and injection of celiac ganglia may improve the accuracy of EUS-CPN. The overall efficacy, however, of EUS-CPN is likely explained by the diffuse spread of alcohol in the celiac region which likely explains this result.

With respect to pancreatic pain, digestive symptoms, nausea, and vomiting, relatively better HRQoL scores were seen in the 20 mL group. This finding has not previously been reported, and a larger prospective study is necessary for confirmation. There is a subtle trend in improved survival in the 20 mL group. Survival in general may be related to pain relief and may reflect the patient's ability to perform daily activities of living and have better nutrition. A larger

TABLE 3: Pain scores over time.

Time	10 mL alcohol				20 mL alcohol			
	N	Mean	SD	% relief*	*N*	Mean	SD	% relief*
Baseline	10	5.9	2.81		10	5.5	3.06	
24 hours	10	2.9	1.79	80%	9	3.6	3.5	67%
Week 1	8	3.75	3.28	50%	10	3.6	2.5	60%
Week 2	8	3.88	2.9	63%	8	3.13	3.27	75%
Week 3	8	3.13	2.85	75%	8	1.88	2.17	88%
Week 4	4	2	1.83	100%	5	2.2	2.17	100%
Week 5	4	2.75	0.5	100%	3	2	1.73	100%
Week 6	3	1	1.73	100%	2	2	2.83	100%

NRS: numeric rating scale (0–10), SD: standard deviation, *pain relief as defined by a 30% reduction in pain scores without an increase in pain medication consumption.

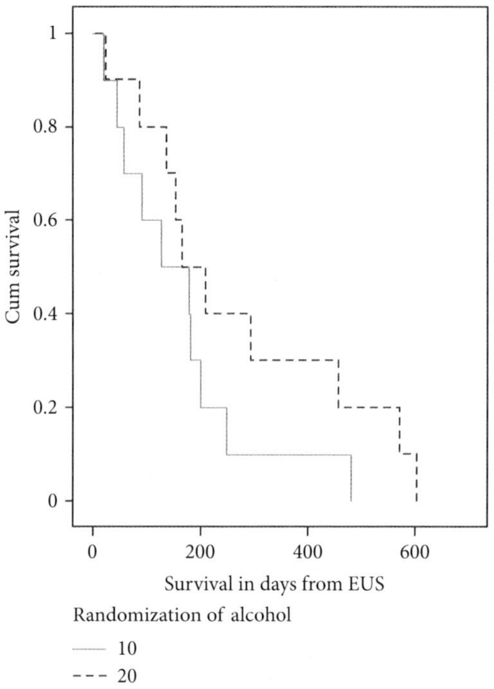

FIGURE 2: Survival in subjects by randomization. The survival curve shows the length of survival in days from the EUS-CPN procedure. The slashed line represents subjects in the 20 mL alcohol group, and the straight line represents subjects in the 10 mL alcohol group.

prospective study, however, is necessary to confirm these observations.

It has been reported that patients with pancreatic cancer have lower pain scores and pain medication consumption up to 16 weeks after EUS-CPN [15, 21]. In 2006 the precise identification and injection of celiac ganglia during EUS-CPN were reported in 16 of 22 (73%) patients [22]. In 2008 efficacy and safety of directly injected celiac ganglia during EUS-CPN were reported in 17 patients with unresectable pancreatic cancer and pain [16]. At 2 and 4 weeks, 94% of subjects reported pain relief as "complete," or "partial" [16]. Likewise, percutaneous and intraoperative celiac plexus neurolysis (CPN) have been performed with varying concentrations (50% to 100%) and amounts (15 to 50 mL)

TABLE 4: Characteristics of complete responders*.

Characteristics	10 mL alcohol	20 mL alcohol
N	3	3
Mean age (SD)	51 (10)	66 (10)
Number of subjects with ganglia injected	2	2
Median (range) *onset* of pain relief (days)	1 (1–14)	1 (1–14)
Median (range) *duration* of pain relief (weeks)	23 (3–32)	8 (3–30)
Median (range) *duration* of complete response (weeks)	17 (1–22)	11 (3–21)

*Complete responders were subjects who had pain scores of zero.

of alcohol [23–27] with efficacy ranging from 70% to 90% [23]. The variable response rates may be attributed to lack of targeted injection into ganglia [5, 23, 26, 28–30]. In a recent meta-analysis of percutaneous CPN, pain relief was rated as good to excellent in 89% after 2 weeks, partial to complete in 90% at 3 months, and partial to complete in 70–90% at the time of death [23].

In our study minor self-limited postprocedure adverse effects were seen in a third of subjects including transient lightheadedness, diarrhea, nausea, and vomiting. Our experience is similar to previous reports of adverse effects including diarrhea (17%), postural hypotension (1%), and postprocedure-related abdominal pain (9%) [14, 31]. In a report by Levy and colleagues, 7 of 17 patients (36%) experienced pain exacerbation in the recovery room which lasted 2.2 days [16]. Procedure-related transient abdominal pain was noted in 9% of subjects who did not have direct injection of celiac ganglia [14]. There have been 2 reports of major complications occurring after EUS-CPB using steroids for chronic pancreatitis including death after an arterial pseudoaneurysm hemorrhage [32], and a peripancreatic abscess developed 5 days after EUS-CPB treated with intravenous antibiotics [33]. A recent report of acute spinal cord infarction following EUS-CPN was attributed to 24 mL of a 1 : 5 mixture of bupivacaine 0.25% with epinephrine and alcohol (5 mL into a celiac ganglia, and 19 mL into the celiac trunk area) [13]. In this patient with pancreatic adenocarcinoma of

Table 5: Quality of life scores at 4 weeks.

	10 mL alcohol			20 mL alcohol		
	N	mean	SD	N	mean	SD
Higher score is better						
Physical functioning	4	63.3	11.5	4	43.3	42.3
Role functioning	4	58.3	21.5	4	29.2	47.9
Emotional functioning	4	62.5	28.5	4	56.3	41.6
Cognitive functioning	4	50	23.6	4	45.8	45.9
Social functioning	4	62.5	21	4	58.3	41.9
Global health status/QoL	4	54.2	16	4	47.9	23.9
Lower score is better						
Fatigue	4	50	14.3	4	66.7	24
Nausea/vomiting	4	33.3	27.2	4	25	21.5
Pain	4	33.3	0	4	58.3	28.9
Dyspnea	4	16.7	33.3	4	50	43
Insomnia	4	16.7	19.2	4	25	50
Appetite loss	4	50	19.2	4	66.7	38.5
Constipation	4	16.7	19.2	4	33.3	27.2
Diarrhea	4	16.7	19.2	4	25	31.9
Financial problems	4	33.3	27.2	4	50	57.7
Higher score is better						
PANCPAIN	4	54.2	21	4	60.4	26.7
DIGSYPTOMS	4	50	19.2	4	70.8	28.5
ALTBOWELHAB	4	79.2	16	4	58.3	39.7
HEPATIC	4	80.6	5.6	4	75	19
BODYIMAGE	4	70.8	21	4	41.7	50
SATHEALTHCARE	4	83.3	19.2	4	87.5	16
SEXUALITY	4	54.2	31.5	4	50	57.7
Overall	4	62.5	9	4	59.9	17.1

SD: standard deviation, dyspnea: shortness of breath, PANCPAIN: pancreatic pain, DIGSYPTOMS: digestive symptoms, ALTBOWLHAB: altered bowel habits, HEPATIC: hepatic/liver abnormalities, BODYIMAGE: body image, SATHEALTHCA: satisfaction with health care, SEXUALITY: sexual function.

the head, the procedure resulted in paraplegia. This incident lends to support that targeted injection of the celiac ganglia is preferred, as the spinal artery can be injured during EUS-CPN.

Lillemoe and colleagues demonstrated improved survival after intraoperative CPN (20 mL of 50% alcohol) in a double-blinded randomized placebocontrolled study of 139 subjects with unresectable pancreatic cancer [5]. A survival benefit was not seen, however, with percutaneous CPN (20 mL 100% alcohol) in patients with unresectable pancreatic cancer [26].

The main limitation of our study is the size. In our pilot study we have demonstrated preliminary evidence that EUS-CPN 20 mL 98% alcohol appears safe. Injection of ganglia appears to improve accuracy of EUS-CPN and possibly the duration of pain relief. A larger prospective trial is warranted to confirm our findings and further understandhow to examine the potential predictors of adjuvant therapy (chemotherapy, radiation, or both) and direct ganglia injection (versus injection into the celiac region) on the clinical outcomes of pain relief, quality of life, and survival.

References

[1] J. Coleman, S. J. Olsen, P. K. Sauter et al., "The effect of a frequently asked questions module on a pancreatic cancer web site patient/family chat room," *Cancer Nursing*, vol. 28, no. 6, pp. 460–468, 2006.

[2] J. Müller-Nordhorn, S. Roll, M. Böhmig et al., "Health-related quality of life in patients with pancreatic cancer," *Digestion*, vol. 74, no. 2, pp. 118–125, 2007.

[3] A. Caraceni and R. K. Portenoy, "Pain management in patients with pancreatic carcinoma," *Cancer*, vol. 78, pp. 639–653, 1996.

[4] R. de Oliveira, M. P. dos Reis, and W. A. Prado, "The effects of early or late neurolytic sympathetic plexus block on the management of abdominal or pelvic cancer pain," *Pain*, vol. 110, no. 1-2, pp. 400–408, 2004.

[5] K. D. Lillemoe, J. L. Cameron, H. S. Kaufman, C. J. Yeo, H. A. Pitt, and P. K. Sauter, "Chemical splanchnicectomy in patients with unresectable pancreatic cancer: a prospective randomized trial," *Annals of Surgery*, vol. 217, no. 5, pp. 447–457, 1993.

[6] L. C. Goudas, R. Bloch, M. Gialeli-Goudas, J. Lau, and D. B. Carr, "The epidemiology of cancer pain," *Cancer Investigation*, vol. 23, no. 2, pp. 182–190, 2005.

[7] M. H. Levy, "Drug therapy: pharmacologic treatment of cancer pain," *The New England Journal of Medicine*, vol. 335, no. 15, pp. 1124–1132, 1996.

[8] R. K. Portenoy and P. Lesage, "Management of cancer pain," *The Lancet*, vol. 353, no. 9165, pp. 1695–1700, 1999.

[9] H. P. Greenwald, J. J. Bonica, and M. Bergner, "The prevalence of pain in four cancers," *Cancer*, vol. 60, no. 10, pp. 2563–2569, 1987.

[10] R. L. Krech and D. Walsh, "Symptoms of pancreatic cancer," *Journal of Pain and Symptom Management*, vol. 6, no. 6, pp. 360–367, 1991.

[11] S. M. Singh, W. P. Longmire Jr., and H. A. Reber, "Surgical palliation for pancreatic cancer. The UCLA experience," *Annals of Surgery*, vol. 212, no. 2, pp. 132–139, 1990.

[12] U. S. Loeve and M. B. Mortensen, "Lethal necrosis and perforation of the stomach and the aorta after multiple EUS-guided celiac plexus neurolysis procedures in a patient with chronic pancreatitis," *Gastrointestinal Endoscopy*. In press.

[13] M. K. Mittal, A. A. Rabinstein, and E. F. Wijdicks, "Pearls & oy-sters: acute spinal cord infarction following endoscopic ultrasound-guided celiac plexus neurolysis," *Neurology*, vol. 78, no. 9, pp. e57–e59, 2012.

[14] N. T. Gunaratnam, A. V. Sarma, I. D. Norton, and M. J. Wiersema, "A prospective study of EUS-guided celiac plexus neurolysis for pancreatic cancer pain," *Gastrointestinal Endoscopy*, vol. 54, no. 3, pp. 316–324, 2001.

[15] M. J. Wiersema and L. M. Wiersema, "Endosonography-guided celiac plexus neurolysis," *Gastrointestinal Endoscopy*, vol. 44, no. 6, pp. 656–662, 1996.

[16] M. J. Levy, M. D. Topazian, M. J. Wiersema et al., "Initial evaluation of the efficacy and safety of endoscopic ultrasound-guided direct ganglia neurolysis and block," *American Journal of Gastroenterology*, vol. 103, no. 1, pp. 98–103, 2008.

[17] A. V. Sahai, V. Lemelin, E. Lam, and S. C. Paquin, "Central versus bilateral endoscopic ultrasound-guided celiac plexus block or neurolysis: a comparative study of short-term effectiveness," *American Journal of Gastroenterology*, vol. 104, no. 2, pp. 326–329, 2009.

[18] H. Sakamoto, M. Kitano, K. Kamata et al., "EUS-guided broad plexus neurolysis over the superior mesenteric artery using a 25-gauge needle," *American Journal of Gastroenterology*, vol. 105, no. 12, pp. 2599–2606, 2010.

[19] C. S. Cleeland, R. Gonin, A. K. Hatfield et al., "Pain and its treatment in outpatients with metastatic cancer," *The New England Journal of Medicine*, vol. 330, no. 9, pp. 592–596, 1994.

[20] K. Kroenke, M. Bair, T. Damush et al., "Stepped care for affective disorders and musculoskeletal pain (SCAMP) study. Design and practical implications of an intervention for comorbid pain and depression," *General Hospital Psychiatry*, vol. 29, no. 6, pp. 506–517, 2007.

[21] N. Harada, M. J. Wiersema, and L. M. Wiersema, "Endosonography-guided celiac plexus neurolysis," *Gastrointestinal Endoscopy Clinics of North America*, vol. 7, no. 2, pp. 237–245, 1997.

[22] H. Gerke, R. G. Silva Jr., D. Shamoun, C. J. Johnson, and C. S. Jensen, "EUS characteristics of celiac ganglia with cytologic and histologic confirmation," *Gastrointestinal Endoscopy*, vol. 64, no. 1, pp. 35–39, 2006.

[23] E. Eisenberg, D. B. Carr, and T. C. Chalmers, "Neurolytic celiac plexus block for treatment of cancer pain: a meta-analysis," *Anesthesia and Analgesia*, vol. 80, no. 2, pp. 290–295, 1995.

[24] X. Garcia-Eroles, V. Mayoral, A. Montero, J. Serra, and J. Porta, "Celiac plexus block: a new technique using the left lateral approach," *Clinical Journal of Pain*, vol. 23, no. 7, pp. 635–637, 2007.

[25] P. J. Wang, M. Y. Shang, Z. Qian, C. W. Shao, J. H. Wang, and X. H. Zhao, "CT-guided percutaneous neurolytic celiac plexus block technique," *Abdominal Imaging*, vol. 31, no. 6, pp. 710–718, 2006.

[26] G. Y. Wong, D. R. Schroeder, P. E. Carns et al., "Effect of neurolytic celiac plexus block on pain relief, quality of life, and survival in patients with unresectable pancreatic cancer: a randomized controlled trial," *The Journal of the American Medical Association*, vol. 291, no. 9, pp. 1092–1099, 2004.

[27] M. Caratozzolo, M. M. Lirici, M. Consalvo, F. Marzano, E. Fumarola, and L. Angelini, "Ultrasound-guided alcoholization of celiac plexus for pain control in oncology," *Surgical Endoscopy*, vol. 11, no. 3, pp. 239–244, 1997.

[28] S. Mercadante, "Celiac plexus block versus analgesics in pancreatic cancer pain," *Pain*, vol. 52, no. 2, pp. 187–192, 1993.

[29] E. Polati, G. Finco, L. Gottin, C. Bassi, P. Pederzoli, and S. Ischia, "Prospective randomized double-blind trial of neurolytic coeliac plexus block in patients with pancreatic cancer," *British Journal of Surgery*, vol. 85, no. 2, pp. 199–201, 1998.

[30] R. Squier, J. S. Morrow, and R. Roman, "Pain therapy for pancreatic carcinoma with neurolytic celiac plexus block," *Connecticut Medicine*, vol. 53, no. 5, pp. 269–271, 1989.

[31] M. J. Levy and M. J. Wiersema, "EUS-guided celiac plexus neurolysis and celiac plexus block," *Gastrointestinal Endoscopy*, vol. 57, no. 7, pp. 923–930, 2003.

[32] F. Gress, D. Ciaccia, J. Kiel, S. Sherman, and G. Lehman, "Endoscopic ultrasound (EUS) guided celiac plexus block (CB) for management of pain due to chronic pancreatitis (CP): a large single center experience," *Gastrointestinal Endoscopy*, vol. 45, no. 4, Article ID AB173, 1997.

[33] F. Gress, C. Schmitt, S. Sherman, D. Ciaccia, S. Ikenberry, and G. Lehman, "Endoscopic ultrasound-guided celiac plexus block for managing abdominal pain associated with chronic pancreatitis: a prospective single center experience," *American Journal of Gastroenterology*, vol. 96, no. 2, pp. 409–416, 2001.

9

Peroral Endoscopic Myotomy for the Treatment of Achalasia

Dennis Yang and Mihir S. Wagh

Division of Gastroenterology, University of Florida, 1600 SW Archer Road, Room HD 602, Gainesville, FL 32610, USA

Correspondence should be addressed to Mihir S. Wagh; mihir.wagh@medicine.ufl.edu

Academic Editor: Daniel M. Herron

Achalasia is a motility disorder of the esophagus, characterized by aperistalsis of the esophageal body and incomplete relaxation of the lower esophageal sphincter (LES). Treatment of achalasia is currently aimed at decreasing the resting pressure in the LES. Peroral endoscopic myotomy (POEM) is an emerging novel endoscopic procedure for the treatment of achalasia with initial data suggesting an acceptable safety profile, excellent short-term symptom resolution, low incidence of postprocedural gastroesophageal reflux (GER), and improvement in manometric outcomes. Further prospective randomized trials are required to evaluate the long-term effectiveness of this promising technique compared to other treatment modalities for achalasia. In this review we outline the technical aspects of POEM, summarize the available data on safety and outcomes, and suggest future directions for further advancement of this minimally invasive approach for the treatment of achalasia.

1. Introduction

Achalasia is a motility disorder of the esophagus, characterized by aperistalsis of the esophageal body and incomplete relaxation of the lower esophageal sphincter (LES). In some cases, the underlying pathophysiology has been attributed to the selective loss of inhibitory ganglion cell function in the myenteric plexus [1]. Typical clinical symptoms include dysphagia for solids and liquids, food regurgitation, and retrosternal chest pain. The diagnosis of achalasia is based on clinical, endoscopic, and radiographic findings, with esophageal manometry considered the gold standard [2, 3]. Treatment of achalasia is currently aimed at decreasing the resting pressure in the LES to facilitate the passage of ingested food.

Pharmacological therapy with agents that reduce LES pressure, such as nitrates and calcium antagonists, has yielded unsatisfactory results and has been associated with significant side effects [3]. Endoscopic delivery of botulinum toxin into the LES muscle decreases sphincter tone by inhibiting acetylcholine release from smooth muscle excitatory neurons. Unlike nitrates or calcium antagonists, botulinum toxin injection has been widely used because of its adequate immediate response (success rates of over 90%) and overall safety profile. However, long-term results have been disappointing, with only half of all patients benefiting for more than 1 year [4]. Thus, in clinical practice, this therapy is mainly confined to treating older patients or those with unacceptable surgical risks [4, 5].

Given the relatively low efficacy of pharmacological therapies to date, definitive treatment has focused on the mechanical disruption of the LES. Endoscopic disruption of the LES involves pneumatic dilation of the sphincter with an air-filled balloon. The balloon is inflated, most often under fluoroscopic guidance, until the waist caused by the LES is obliterated. A recent meta-analysis of 29 studies by Katzka and Castell [6], evaluating pneumatic dilation for achalasia with Rigiflex balloons, revealed an 88% 1-year efficacy, gradually decreasing with time to 70 and 29% after 5 and 10 years, respectively. While the results suggested a decline in efficacy and symptom recurrence with time, periodic redilation was associated with sustained response rates of 81–93% after 6–10 years [6, 7]. Alternatively, from a surgical perspective, disruption of the LES can be achieved by myotomy of the smooth muscle sphincter. Several retrospective studies on laparoscopic Heller myotomy (LHM) have reported high rates of symptomatic resolution (80–84%) in patients at a mean follow-up of 5 to 6 years [8, 9]. Congruent with these results, in a meta-analysis including 3086 patients, Campos et al. described success rates with surgical myotomy as high as 89% (range 77–100%) after a mean follow-up of 35 months [10]. Because of these favorable outcomes, LHM is considered the operative gold standard of care by many authorities [11]. However, the disadvantages of LHM are that it is an invasive surgical procedure, necessitates complete mobilization of the gastroesophageal junction, and often requires an adjunctive antireflux operation.

With the exponential advance in natural orifice translumenal endoscopic surgery (NOTES), an interesting novel endoscopic method for the treatment of achalasia was first described by Pasricha and colleagues in a porcine model [12]. The authors demonstrated the feasibility of endoscopic myotomy by directly approaching the esophageal muscular layer through a submucosal tunnel. Subsequently, this technique of peroral endoscopic myotomy (POEM) was translated into clinical practice by Inoue et al. in 2010 [13]. Since then, there have been several prospective studies evaluating the feasibility, efficacy, and safety of this innovative endoscopic technique for the treatment of achalasia [14–25].

2. Technical Aspects

Multiple centers have performed POEM as initially described by Inoue et al. in 2010, with some technical variations. We summarize the POEM technique based on the current prospective studies and recent results from the international POEM survey [26].

2.1. Preoperative Patient Preparation. Patients selected to undergo POEM should have a diagnosis of achalasia firmly established by different methods (esophageal manometry, esophagogastroduodenoscopy (EGD) and esophagram). Patients are generally maintained on a clear liquid diet for 24–48 hours prior to the procedure. Prophylactic antibiotics are universally initiated on the day of the procedure, continued for the length of postprocedural hospitalization, and, in some cases, extended to 7 days.

2.2. POEM Operative Technique

2.2.1. Submucosal Tunnel Creation. All reported POEM cases have been performed with the patient under general anesthesia. In general, the patient is placed in the supine position and EGD is performed with a forward-viewing upper endoscope and minimal carbon dioxide (CO_2) insufflation. In most institutions, a dissecting cap is fitted onto the tip of the endoscope to facilitate its insertion into the submucosal space. With 12 o'clock representing the most anterior aspect of the esophagus on endoluminal view, most practitioners favor a mucosal incision site in the 1 to 2 o'clock position on the right anterolateral esophagus, in order to aim for a straight tunnel ending at the lesser curvature of the stomach. However, some centers favor a posterior approach in the 5 o'clock orientation, which is often regarded as the preferred site in patients with previous surgical myotomy, as POEM could be complicated by scar tissue in the anterior plane [20]. The site for mucosotomy in the midesophagus is often selected to be approximately 14 cm from the GEJ. Water is instilled into the esophagus and pooling of saline posteriorly is used to confirm anterior-posterior orientations. An anterior submucosal "lift" is achieved by injecting saline, glycerol-based solutions, or hydroxypropyl methylcellulose + MESNA. A triangle-tip (TT) endoscopic cautery knife (Triangle Tip Knife; Olympus) or a T-type hybrid (HK) knife (ERBE) is used to make a 1.5–3 cm longitudinal mucosal incision at the site of the submucosal bleb. The endoscope is subsequently inserted into the newly created submucosal space. Using a combination of blunt dissection with the cap and electrocautery, a submucosal tunnel is created. CO_2 insufflation and saline infusion are performed to facilitate submucosal tunneling, while repeated injections of dye help identify the correct plane and mark progression. The blue dye is used as a guide as it stains the muscle layer but not the loose areolar tissue of the submucosa. As the GEJ is approached, the tunnel becomes distinctively narrower. After passing this anatomical landmark, the space in the tunnel widens with a change in the muscle structure from clear circular fibers to irregular fibers, corresponding to the transition to the gastric cardia. Once the submucosal tunnel has been extended caudally, more dye is injected and the endoscope is withdrawn from the tunnel and advanced into the gastric lumen to endoscopically confirm that the distal end of the tunnel is at least 3 cm past the GEJ (i.e., blue dye is seen endoscopically extending at least 3 cm beyond the GEJ).

2.2.2. Submucosal Dissection. The endoscope is reinserted into the submucosal tunnel and dissection of the circular muscle layer is initiated approximately 3-4 cm distal to the mucosal entry site (approximately 10 cm above the GEJ), assuring that the breach of the mucosa and the muscle is not at the same level so as to minimize risk of esophageal leak after POEM. Dissection proceeds from proximal to distal, with an effort to maintain the underlying longitudinal fibers undisturbed. Full myotomy with splitting of the longitudinal fibers is often inevitable but theoretically inconsequential as long as there is no mucosal breach. Coagulation forceps are utilized for hemostasis of submucosal vessels when needed. Upon completion of the myotomy, the endoscope is withdrawn from the submucosal space.

2.2.3. Closure of Mucosal Entry Site. The mucosal entry site is usually closed by endoscopic clips. The initial clip is placed at the most distal part of the incision to facilitate approximation of the incisional borders and placement of subsequent clips is done in a proximal direction to completely close the mucosotomy site. In cases in which the sides of the incision are difficult to approximate, over-the-scope clips have been employed [27].

2.3. Intraoperative Monitoring and Care. Inspiratory pressures (plateau pressures) and abdominal distension is monitored continuously during POEM. Elevation of the plateau pressure from baseline and, or abdominal distension is promptly treated by withdrawing the endoscope from the tunnel and advancing it into the gastric lumen to decompress the stomach by suctioning excess CO_2. Capno/pneumoperitoneum is decompressed by placing a 14 G angiocatheter into the abdomen.

2.4. Postoperative Care. Patients are kept nil per os (NPO) the night after the procedure and started on an intravenous proton-pump inhibitor (PPI) immediately postoperatively, which can be subsequently transitioned to oral therapy upon resumption of diet. A gastrografin esophagram is obtained the next day to assess the effect of myotomy and to identify complications such as leaks. There is no consensus on whether a "second look" EGD within 24–72 hours following POEM is indicated, as it often does not affect the management of these patients [26]. Patients are generally discharged within 3 days of postoperative care if no complications are seen clinically and on esophagram. A full liquid diet is recommended for one week after POEM and then gradually advanced.

3. Published Data

A literature search in Medline/PubMed was conducted to identify all studies in the English language on POEM for the treatment of achalasia up to May 2013. Keywords searched included peroral endoscopic myotomy, POEM, achalasia, Heller myotomy, pneumatic balloon dilation, and dysphagia.

3.1. POEM for the Treatment of Achalasia. Table 1 summarizes the published clinical data on POEM from various institutions. In the first clinical study of 17 patients, Inoue and colleagues described performing mucosotomy at the level of the midesophagus, allowing submucosal insertion of the endoscope [13]. Complete division of the inner circular muscle layer was achieved by combining blunt dissection and electrocautery and this was continued for a few centimeters distal to the GEJ in the proximal stomach. Upon completion of the myotomy, the mucosal entry site was closed with endoclips. The investigators showed that endoscopic myotomy was technically feasible by completing the procedure in all of the patients.

Pneumoperitoneum occurred in one patient, who was treated successfully by puncturing the abdominal wall with an 18-gauge needle. None of the 17 patients had postoperative subcutaneous emphysema on clinical grounds nor reported complications or problems during the follow-up period. The authors reported a significant reduction in the dysphagia symptom score (10 to 1.3; $P = 0.0003$) and the resting LES pressure from 52.4 (14.2–80.5) to 19.8 (9.3–42.7) ($P = 0.0001$) after POEM during short-term follow-up (mean 5 months).

There have been several studies since then, which have confirmed the high success rate with this technique as initially reported in the landmark study by Inoue and colleagues. In 2011, Swanström et al. reported their experience with POEM in 5 patients [14]. Technical success, based on completion of the procedure, was achieved in all 5 patients. At the 2-week clinical follow-up, all patients reported immediate symptom relief. Similarly, other centers have independently reported excellent short-term symptom resolution rates with POEM [15–20]. Using the Eckardt score, a validated symptom score for achalasia, the majority of patients (97%; range 91–100%) achieved an Eckardt score ≤3 after POEM at 3-month follow-up. Symptomatic improvement after POEM was also accompanied by a decrease in mean LES pressure on follow-up manometry (Table 1). In addition to favorable Eckardt scores and manometric outcomes, Chiu et al. [17] also suggested that POEM improved esophagogastric function, based on esophageal emptying on timed barium esophagram and esophagogastric junction distensibility on EndoFLIP (Crospon, Galway, Ireland).

In light of all these studies supporting the feasibility and safety profile of POEM, Hungness and colleagues published the results from their clinical trial comparing POEM and LHM [21]. In this study, 18 patients underwent POEM and were compared to a control group of 55 LHM patients enrolled in a prospective outcomes database. The authors demonstrated slightly shorter operative times for POEM compared to LHM (113 versus 125 minutes, $P < 0.001$) and less estimated blood loss (≤10 mL in all cases versus 50 (10–250) mL, $P < 0.001$). Surprisingly, pain scores were similar upon postanesthesia care unit arrival and postoperative day 1 but were higher at 2 hours for POEM patients (3.5 versus 2, $P < 0.03$). The authors reported no differences in minor complications and there were no mortalities in either group. In terms of treatment efficacy, high-resolution manometry in 16 patients showed decrease in both resting expiratory GEJ pressures and 4 s integrated pressures at 6 weeks after POEM compared to baseline. Furthermore, among POEM patients, there was a decrease in Eckardt scores from 7 (5–12) preoperatively to 1 (0–9; $P < 0.01$) at median 6 (1–18) months of follow-up. In conclusion, the authors demonstrated similar perioperative outcomes between POEM and LHM with excellent short-term results with the endoscopic approach.

Von Renteln and colleagues recently published the first international multicenter POEM study on 70 patients with achalasia from 5 different centers [22]. In their report, the mean length of the myotomy was 13 cm (range 5–23) and full thickness dissection into the mediastinum was observed in the majority of patients (69%). Treatment success, defined as Eckardt score of ≤3 at 3 months, was achieved in 97% of cases (95% CI 89–99), which persisted in 82.4% at 12 months. The authors reported a reduction in the mean LES pressure of 27.6 (24.2–31.0) to 8.9 (7.3–10.5) mmHg ($P < 0.001$) after POEM. This study demonstrates long-term symptomatic relief after POEM and confirms the efficacy of this technique as previously reported in single-center case series.

3.2. POEM for the Treatment of Refractory Achalasia Patients in Setting of Prior Intervention. Sharata et al. evaluated the safety and feasibility of POEM in 12 patients (9 achalasia) in the setting of prior endoscopic interventions (Botox injections, balloon dilations) [23]. POEM was successfully completed in all patients. The authors do report a single case of intramural bleeding requiring repeat endoscopy for hemostasis and another case of dehiscence at mucosotomy managed with endoscopic clipping. Overall, symptomatic relief was achieved in all patients based on a decrease in the median Eckardt score from 5 to 1 after POEM. When compared to

Table 1: Clinical trials evaluating POEM for the management of achalasia.

Authors	Study design	Patients (n)	Myotomy length; mean (range), cm	Dysphagia score		Eckardt score		LES pressure; mean (range), mm Hg		GERD symptoms	Follow-up; mean (range)
				Baseline; mean	Post-POEM; mean (n, %)	Baseline; mean	Post-POEM; mean (n, %)	Baseline	Post-POEM		
Inoue et al. [13]	Single-center prospective	17	8.1 (3–15)	10	1.3 (17, 100%)	N/A	N/A	52.4 (14.2–80.5)	19.8 (9.3–42.7)	N/A	5 (1–16) months
Swanström et al. [14]	Single-center prospective	5	10 (10–13)	N/A	0 or 1 (5, 100%)	N/A	N/A	36.5 (9.9– 39.8)	N/A	N/A	2 weeks
von Renteln et al. [15]	Single-center prospective	16	12 (8–17)	N/A	N/A	N/A	≤3 (15, 94%)	27.2	11.8	None	3 months
Costamagna et al. [16]	Single-center prospective	11	10.2 ± 2.8	N/A	N/A	7.1	1.1 (11, 100%)	45.1	16.9	None	3 months
Chiu et al. [17]	Single-center prospective	16	10.8	2 (range 0–2)	0 (range 0-1)	5.5 (range 0–8)	0 (range 0–3) (16, 100%)	43.6 ± 24.4	29.8 ± 22	1/16 (6.25%)	176.5 (98–230) days
Hungness et al. [21]	Single-center retrospective	18	9 (6–14)	N/A	N/A	7 (range 5–12)	1 (range 0–9) (18, 100%)	19 (7–51)	9 (0–23)	4/18 (22%) based on GerdQ score ≥7	6 (1–18) months
Zhou et al. [24]	Single-center prospective	12	10.1 (8–13)	N/A	N/A		≤3 (11, 91.7%)	29.4 (23.5–40.2)	13.5 (8.6–22.5)	1/12 (8.3%)	10.4 (5–14) months
Verlaan et al. [18]	Single-center prospective	10	N/A	N/A	N/A	8 (range 4–8)	1 (range 0-1) (10, 100%)	20.5 (15.8–24.3)	6.8 (4.0–12.0)	3/10 (30%)	3 months
Minami et al. [20]	Single-center retrospective	28	14.4 (10–18)	N/A	N/A	6.7 (range 2–12)	0.7 (range 0–3) (28; 100%)	71.2 (35.8–119.0)	21.0 (6.7–41.0)	6/28 (21.4%)	16 (3–28) months
Lee et al. [19]	Single-center prospective	13	8.5 (6–13)	N/A	N/A	6.4 (range 4–10)	0.4 (range 0–2) (13; 100%)	30.3 (14.4–57.1)	15.3 (9.6–22.3)	N/A	6.9 (1–14) months
Von Renteln et al. [22]	Multicenter prospective	70	13 (5–13)	N/A	N/A		≤3 (68, 97%) at 3 months	27.6 (24.2–31.0)	8.9 (7.3–10.5)	37%	10.1 (3–12) months

N/A: not available.

Table 2: Adverse events associated with POEM.

Authors	Patients (n)	Adverse events*, n	Additional treatment
Inoue et al. [13]	17	1 pneumoperitoneum	Veress needle
Swanström et al. [14]	5	2 small perforations in gastric cardia 3 capnoperitoneum	Endoscopic clips Veress needle
von Renteln et al. [15]	16	6 minor cutaneous emphysema 8 capnoperitoneum treated with Veress needle 1 small perforation at GEJ, treated with endoscopic clips	Veress needle Endoscopic clips
Costamagna et al. [16]	11	2 small perforations at junctional flap Asymptomatic pneumomediastinum in all patients 2 transient cervical emphysema	Endoscopic clips
Chiu et al. [17]	16	1 aspiration pneumonia 2 transient cervical emphysema	Hospital admission and monitoring
Hungness et al. [21]	18	7 capnoperitoneum 1 contained perforation at the EGJ	Veress needle
Ren et al. [25]	119	66 subcutaneous emphysema 30 pneumothorax 35 mediastinal emphysema 1 delayed hemorrhage 58 pleural effusions 59 inflammations/atelectases of the lungs 47 aeroperitonea	
Zhou et al. [24]	12	1 small perforation at GEJ, treated with endoscopic clips 3 capnoperitoneum, one treated with Veress needle 4 pneumothorax, one treated with thoracic tube 4 mediastinal emphysema 2 subcutaneous emphysema	Endoscopic clips Veress needle Thoracic tube
Verlaan et al. [18]	10	No complications reported	None
Minami et al. [20]	28	1 perforation at GEJ, treated with endoscopic clips 2 postoperative bleedings	Endoscopic clips
Lee et al. [19]	13	No complications reported	None
Von Renteln et al. [22]	70	3 clip dislocation at mucosal closure 1 perforation at mucosal entry site 3 mucosal injuries 1 bleeding requiring intervention 1 cap detached in submucosal tunnel 1 delayed bleeding (hematoma)	Endoscopic reclipping Endoscopic clips Endoscopic clips Endoscopic hemostasis Endoscopic removal Hospital admission and monitoring

*includes all reported outcomes, including nonclinically significant and asymptomatic adverse events.

28 patients with no previous endoscopic intervention who underwent POEM, there were no differences in perioperative outcomes. The authors concluded that previous endoscopic therapies with Botox injections or large caliber balloon dilations do not increase adverse intraoperative or postoperative outcomes with POEM.

Recurrence or persistence of symptoms occurs in approximately 10–20% of patients after Heller myotomy at 2 years of follow-up [11]. To date, there is no current consensus regarding optimal therapy for these patients. Sharata et al. [23] recently reported their experience on the efficacy and feasibility of POEM in patients after failed Heller myotomy. All 12 patients underwent successful POEM after a mean of 11.9 years (range 2–38 years) from the time of primary Heller myotomy. During a mean follow-up period of 10.4 months (range 5–14 months), treatment success was achieved in 11/12 patients (Eckardt score ≤3), with a reduction of pretreatment mean LES pressure of 29.4 mmHg to 13.5 mmHg following POEM ($P < 0.001$). There were no serious complications reported in the study, with only one case of small mucosal perforation at GEJ treated with endoclips, one case of pneumoperitoneum treated with needle decompression, and one patient requiring chest tube for symptomatic pneumothorax. In conclusion, the authors suggest that while endoscopic remyotomy is technically more challenging in this group of patients, POEM was still feasible and resulted in short-term symptom relief in >90% of the cases.

3.3. Adverse Events Associated with POEM. POEM is a safe endoscopic technique associated with low rates of perioperative and postoperative complications. Dissection of air or CO_2 into the mediastinum and/or peritoneum during submucosal tunneling and endoscopic myotomy has been commonly reported (Table 2). In most instances, pneumo-/capnoperitoneum can be followed clinically and when symptomatic, treated by decompression with Veress needle insertion [14, 15, 21]. There were 6 cases (out of a total of 94 patients) [14–21] of mucosal perforation at the gastroesophageal junction treated with endoscopic clipping without long-term adverse effects reported. Similarly, in their multicenter study of 70 patients, von Renteln et al. reported only one case of mucosal perforation at the mucosotomy site, which was managed successfully with endoscopic clipping. Perioperative bleeding is rare and endoscopic hemostasis is often successful. There have been some reports of delayed (several days following procedure) bleeding, which have been managed conservatively without requiring specific endoscopic or surgical intervention [20–22]. Cardiopulmonary complications are infrequent, although there was one case reported of aspiration pneumonia associated with prolonged postoperative recovery [17].

In contrast to these findings, in the largest published single-center POEM series to date, Zhou and colleagues [24] demonstrated a high incidence of POEM-specific complications. The authors analyzed the data of 119 patients with achalasia who underwent POEM from October 2010 to July 2011. Postoperative complications included pneumothorax (25.2%, 30/119), subcutaneous emphysema (55.5%, 66/119), mediastinal emphysema (29.4%, 35/119), pleural effusion (48.7%, 58/119), and pneumoperitoneum (39.5%, 47/119). The authors report that all post-POEM complications were managed effectively with traditional therapies without resorting to additional surgery. The discrepancy in the complication rate between this study and other series could potentially be attributed to differences on how the submucosal tunnel was created (posterior versus anterior esophageal wall) and the use of air versus CO_2 for insufflation during POEM.

Mucosotomy site closure can be technically challenging. Indeed, clip dislocation at the mucosal closure location requiring endoscopic reclipping was the most common complication reported by von Renteln in their multicenter study [22]. Recently, Saxena et al. [27] reported two cases in which closure of the mucosotomy could not be achieved with standard endoclips and proposed the use of over-the-scope clips (OTSC) for difficult cases. Similarly, it is our experience that OTSC may be an alternate method for closing the mucosal incision site when standard clipping has failed (Yang et al., Endoscopy 2013; ENDOS-2013-9120). Future studies evaluating the optimal approach and standardization of the technique in POEM are largely needed.

3.4. Incidence of Gastroesophageal Reflux following POEM. The reported short-term incidence of reflux symptoms following POEM is relatively low (range from 0% to 33%) [15–24]. This was primarily assessed based on patient self-reports of heartburn or reflux symptoms at follow-up, with one study using a validated questionnaire for GERD (Table 1). One study demonstrated high clinical reflux rates (37%) with 29% of patients still requiring maintenance therapy with proton-pump inhibitors [22]. In addition to clinical symptoms of reflux, Chiu et al. [17] demonstrated abnormal esophageal acid exposure on ambulatory pH monitoring in 20% (3/15 patients at 3-month follow-up).

4. POEM versus Other Treatment Modalities for Achalasia

Initial data from these POEM studies highlight some potential advantages of this technique compared to endoscopic pneumatic balloon dilation. First, the short-term symptomatic efficacy of POEM is excellent. By following the principle of LHM, POEM provides a high lasting success rate (82% at 1 year) [22] and decreased need of retreatment when compared to balloon dilation. Second, the risk of uncontrolled perforation that may occur during balloon dilation could be avoided with myotomy under direct visualization. Based on the available evidence on POEM, it is evident that the longitudinal fibers are very thin and inadvertent transmural dissection can occur during endoscopic myotomy. However, "true" perforation is rare when mucosal integrity is maintained and closure of the mucosotomy site. Furthermore, the vast majority of reported cases of contained perforation with POEM have not required any specific intervention or have been managed successfully with endoscopic clipping. Thus, while POEM is associated with higher rates of pneumoperitoneum and subcutaneous emphysema perioperatively, there have been no reported significant clinical implications. Therefore, this initial clinical data on POEM seem to indicate that this is a procedure with an adequate risk profile; however, studies comparing the outcomes between POEM (with partial or complete myotomy) and endoscopic balloon dilation are needed before more definite conclusions can be drawn regarding long-term safety.

The potential advantages of POEM over LHM are founded on the basis of a myotomy through a natural orifice. First, advocates of POEM suggest that this technique allows the option of performing a very long myotomy. High mediastinal dissection can be challenging laparoscopically; thus, a transoral submucosal approach could presumably represent an alternate method for the management of conditions that may require extended myotomy, such as, vigorous achalasia. Unfortunately, current studies have been underpowered to detect differences in treatment response among different subtypes of achalasia. Furthermore, the operative techniques employed in most studies have been based on that described initially by Inoue and colleagues, and therefore they have not focused on the feasibility of creating a more extensive myotomy compared to LHM. Thus, whether a longer myotomy can be successfully performed and whether this will actually result in symptomatic improvement in different variant forms of achalasia remain to be elucidated.

A second theoretical advantage of POEM over LMH is that the incisionless approach with the former technique should theoretically be associated with less operative risk and reduced postoperative pain. As previously described, Hungness et al. provided direct initial evidence that POEM has a safety profile comparable with LHM and is associated with shorter operative time and estimated blood loss. However, these improved parameters were minimal, and thus whether these differences translate into measureable clinical benefits is unclear. Interestingly, POEM was not associated with reduced postoperative pain compared to LHM. However, the caveats of this study include the nonrandomized and nonblinded nature of the study, which could have introduced bias or differences in baseline among the groups, accounting for some of the reported findings.

Thirdly, some initial studies have suggested a potential role of POEM in the management of patients with refractory symptoms after surgical myotomy. Zhou and colleagues reported successful POEM in 12 patients with prior Heller myotomy and demonstrated excellent short-term symptom resolution and improvement in manometric outcomes. While this represents a very small sample size, it supports the potential application of POEM for patients who have failed previous open or laparoscopic myotomy. The role of POEM as an alternative treatment for persistent symptoms after Heller myotomy appears promising, especially in patients in which revisional operation may be complicated by periesophageal fibrotic scar tissue. Additional studies are needed to corroborate these positive initial findings.

Lastly, a transoral approach for myotomy potentially obviates the need to manipulate several structures around the GEJ in order to dissect the muscle layers. Studies have demonstrated a high incidence of GERD (up to 60% of patients) following LHM, and thus an adjuvant antireflux procedure is generally recommended [28]. This requirement adds a layer of complexity and intuitively increases the risk of complications. Endoscopic myotomy through the luminal side with POEM theoretically maintains the integrity of the natural antireflux mechanisms, which may account for an acceptable incidence (0 to 37%) of symptomatic GERD after POEM during short-term follow-up as described in most studies [15–24]. Future studies, using standardized validated clinical scores for GERD and objective assessment of esophageal acid exposure, are needed to investigate the long-term effects of POEM on acid reflux.

5. Future Directions

Based on the initial clinical trials, POEM appears to be an effective therapy for achalasia with an acceptable safety profile. However, this procedure is both technically demanding and time consuming, even in the hands of experienced endoscopists [29]. Thus, further adaptations of this technique that may help accelerate the learning curve and reduce operative time are pivotal for promoting its applicability.

Khashab and colleagues recently published their initial experience on a novel technique of "auto-tunneling" during POEM in a swine model [30]. In their swine model study, the authors used a submucosal lifting gel (Cook Medical, Winston-Salem, NC) as a dissecting gel, which was injected into the submucosal bleb created at the site of mucosotomy. Their results demonstrated that a complete submucosal tunnel to the level of the GEJ was noted to be already formed upon insertion of the endoscope into the submucosal space in all 5 pigs. Theoretically, this could obviate the need to mechanically dissect the submucosal loose areolar tissue in the esophagus during tunneling and thus significantly reduce the time and risk associated with "manual" tunneling. While future clinical studies are needed to validate these preliminary experimental findings, this study highlights the evolving nature of this field and introduces innovative modifications that may potentially circumvent current technical hurdles.

The tunneling approach in the submucosal space during POEM may be extended to other sites in the GI tract as well, extending the application of this technique to other areas such as endoscopic mucosal resection (EMR) and endoscopic submucosal dissection (ESD) for epithelial and subepithelial gastrointestinal lesions. Similarly, it can be envisioned that this technique may be used at other sphincter sites such as the pylorus and anorectum.

6. Conclusion

In summary, POEM appears to be a feasible endoscopic procedure for achalasia with excellent short-term symptom resolution and improvement in manometric outcomes. Initial studies have demonstrated that POEM can be conducted efficiently with a safety profile comparable to LHM, with the most commonly reported complication being uncomplicated pneumomediastinum and/or pneumoperitoneum. POEM is a promising, yet very sophisticated and technically demanding procedure that should be performed in centers with expertise and thoracic surgery support. Further prospective randomized trials are required to compare the effectiveness of POEM with current treatment modalities and to establish its long-term effects for the management of achalasia.

References

[1] D. L. Francis and D. A. Katzka, "achalasia: update on the disease and its treatment," *Gastroenterology*, vol. 139, no. 2, pp. 369.e2–374.e2, 2010.

[2] P. M. Fisichella, D. Raz, F. Palazzo, I. Niponmick, and M. G. Patti, "Clinical, radiological, and manometric profile in 145 patients with untreated achalasia," *World Journal of Surgery*, vol. 32, no. 9, pp. 1974–1979, 2008.

[3] J. E. Pandolfino, S. K. Ghosh, J. Rice, J. O. Clarke, M. A. Kwiatek, and P. J. Kahrilas, "Classifying esophageal motility by pressure topography characteristics: a study of 400 patients and 75 controls," *The American Journal of Gastroenterology*, vol. 103, no. 1, pp. 27–37, 2008.

[4] P. J. Pasricha, W. J. Ravich, T. R. Hendrix, S. Sostre, B. Jones, and A. N. Kalloo, "Intrasphincteric botulinum toxin for the treatment of achalasia," *The New England Journal of Medicine*, vol. 332, no. 12, pp. 774–778, 1995.

[5] V. D'Onofrio, P. Miletto, G. Leandro, and G. Iaquinto, "Long-term follow-up of achalasia patients treated with botulinum toxin," *Digestive and Liver Disease*, vol. 34, no. 2, pp. 105–110, 2002.

[6] D. A. Katzka and D. O. Castell, "Review article: an analysis of the efficacy, perforation rates and methods used in pneumatic dilation for achalasia," *Alimentary Pharmacology and Therapeutics*, vol. 34, no. 8, pp. 832–839, 2011.

[7] M. Hulselmans, T. Vanuytsel, T. Degreef et al., "Long-term outcome of pneumatic dilation in the treatment of achalasia,"

Clinical Gastroenterology and Hepatology, vol. 8, no. 1, pp. 30–35, 2010.

[8] H. Bonatti, R. A. Hinder, J. Klocker et al., "Long-term results of laparoscopic Heller myotomy with partial fundoplication for the treatment of achalasia," *The American Journal of Surgery*, vol. 190, no. 6, pp. 874–878, 2005.

[9] A. Kilic, M. J. Schuchert, A. Pennathur, S. Gilbert, R. J. Landreneau, and J. D. Luketich, "Long-term outcomes of laparoscopic Heller myotomy for achalasia," *Surgery*, vol. 146, no. 4, pp. 826–833, 2009.

[10] G. M. Campos, E. Vittinghoff, C. Rabl et al., "Endoscopic and surgical treatments for achalasia: a systematic review and meta-analysis," *Annals of Surgery*, vol. 249, no. 1, pp. 45–57, 2009.

[11] G. E. Boeckxstaens, V. Annese, S. B. des Varannes et al., "Pneumatic dilation versus laparoscopic heller's myotomy for idiopathic achalasia," *The New England Journal of Medicine*, vol. 364, no. 19, pp. 1807–1816, 2011.

[12] P. J. Pasricha, R. Hawarl, I. Ahmed et al., "Submucosal endoscopic esophageal myotomy: a novel experimental approach for the treatment of achalasia," *Endoscopy*, vol. 39, no. 9, pp. 761–764, 2007.

[13] H. Inoue, H. Minami, Y. Kobayashi et al., "Peroral Endoscopic Myotomy (POEM) for esophageal achalasia," *Endoscopy*, vol. 42, no. 4, pp. 265–271, 2010.

[14] L. L. Swanström, E. Rieder, and C. M. Dunst, "A stepwise approach and early clinical experience in peroral endoscopic myotomy for the treatment of achalasia and esophageal motility disorders," *Journal of the American College of Surgeons*, vol. 213, no. 6, pp. 751–756, 2011.

[15] D. von Renteln, H. Inoue, H. Minami et al., "Peroral endoscopic myotomy for the treatment of achalasia: a prospective single center study," *The American Journal of Gastroenterology*, vol. 107, no. 3, pp. 411–417, 2012.

[16] G. Costamagna, M. Marchese, P. Familiari, A. Tringali, H. Inoue, and V. Perri, "Peroroal Endoscopic Myotomy (POEM) for oesophageal achalasia: preliminary results in humans," *Digestive and Liver Disease*, vol. 44, no. 10, pp. 827–832, 2012.

[17] P. W. Chiu, J. C. Wu, A. Y. Teoh et al., "Peroral endoscopic myotomy for treatment of achalasia: from bench to bedside (with video)," *Gastrointestinal Endoscopy*, vol. 5107, no. 12, pp. 02638–02637, 2012.

[18] T. Verlaan, W. O. Rohof, A. J. Bredenoord, S. Eberl, T. Rösch, and P. Fockens, "Effect of peroral endoscopic myotomy on esophagogastric junction physiology in patients with achalasia," *Gastrointestinal Endoscopy*, vol. 78, no. 1, pp. 39–44, 2013.

[19] B. H. Lee, K. Y. Shim, S. J. Hong et al., "Peroral endoscopic myotomy for treatment of achalasia: initial results of a Korean study," *Clinical Endoscopy*, vol. 46, pp. 161–167, 2013.

[20] H. Minami, H. Isomoto, N. Yamaguchi et al., "Peroral endoscopic myotomy for esophageal achalasia: clinical impact of 28 cases," *Digestive Endoscopy*, 2013.

[21] E. S. Hungness, E. N. Teitelbaum, B. F. Santos et al., "Comparison of perioperative outcomes between Peroral Esophageal Myotomy (POEM) and laparoscopic Heller myotomy," *Journal of Gastrointestinal Surgery*, vol. 17, no. 2, pp. 228–235, 2013.

[22] D. von Renteln, K. H. Fuchs, and P. Fockens, "Peroral endoscopic myotomy for the treatment of achalasia: an international prospective multicenter study," *Gastroenterology*, vol. 145, no. 2, pp. 309.e1–3011.e1, 2013.

[23] A. Sharata, A. A. Kurian, C. M. Dunst et al., "Peroral Endoscopic Myotomy (POEM) is safe and effective in the setting of prior endoscopic intervention," *Journal of Gastrointestinal Surgery*, vol. 17, no. 7, pp. 1188–1192, 2013.

[24] P. H. Zhou, Q. L. Li, L. Q. Yao et al., "Peroral endoscopic remyotomy for failed Heller myotomy: a prospective single-center study," *Clinical Endoscopy*, vol. 46, no. 1, pp. 54–58, 2013.

[25] Z. Ren, Y. Zhong, P. Zhou et al., "Perioperative management and treatment for complications during and after peroral endoscopic myotomy (POEM) for esophageal achalasia (EA) (data from 119 cases)," *Surgical Endoscopy*, vol. 26, no. 11, pp. 3267–3272, 2012.

[26] S. N. Stavropoulos, R. J. Modayil, D. Friedel, and T. Savides, "The International Per Oral Endoscopic Myotomy Survey (IPOEMS): a snapshot of the global POEM experience," *Surgical Endoscopy*, vol. 27, no. 9, pp. 3322–3338, 2013.

[27] P. Saxena, Y. H. Chavez, K. A. Valeshabad et al., "An alternative method for mucosal flap closure during peroral endoscopic myotomy using an over-the-scope clipping device," *Endoscopy*, vol. 45, no. 7, pp. 579–581, 2013.

[28] D. Stefanidis, W. Richardson, T. M. Farrell, G. P. Kohn, V. Augenstein, and R. D. Fanelli, "SAGES guidelines for the surgical treatment of esophageal achalasia," *Surgical Endoscopy and Other Interventional Techniques*, vol. 26, no. 2, pp. 296–311, 2012.

[29] A. A. Kurian, C. M. Dunst, A. Sharata et al., "Peroral endoscopic esophageal myotomy: defining the learning curve," *Gastrointestinal Endoscopy*, vol. 77, no. 5, pp. 719–725, 2013.

[30] M. A. Khashab, R. Z. Sharaiha, P. Saxena et al., "Novel technique of auto-tunneling during peroral endoscopic myotomy (with video)," *Gastrointestinal Endoscopy*, vol. 77, no. 1, pp. 119–122, 2013.

10

The Use of Endobronchial Ultrasound in the Diagnosis of Subacute Pulmonary Histoplasmosis

Katarine von Lang Egressy, Mohammed Mohammed, and J. Scott Ferguson

Division of Allergy, Pulmonary, and Critical Care Medicine, Department of Medicine, University of Wisconsin School of Medicine and Public Health, Madison, WI 53706, USA

Correspondence should be addressed to J. Scott Ferguson; jsferguson@medicine.wisc.edu

Academic Editor: P. J. O'Dwyer

Objective. Endobronchial ultrasound (EBUS) utility in diagnosis in malignant and granulomatous mediastinal disease has been well demonstrated. We propose to examine the role of EBUS transbronchial needle aspiration (EBUS-TBNA) in the diagnosis of subacute pulmonary histoplasmosis (SPH) with mediastinal lymphadenopathy in an area where histoplasmosis is endemic. *Methods.* A retrospective review was performed in a single academic institution between 2009 and 2012 of patients referred for EBUS-TBNA who had radiographic imaging and clinical symptomatology suspicious for SPH. Seven patients were reviewed. TBNA results showing granulomatous disease with areas of necrosis in the appropriate clinical setting were considered to be adequate for the diagnosis of SPH when alternative diagnosis was excluded. Patients underwent further clinical follow-up of 12 months to determine the final diagnosis. *Results.* All seven patients were felt to have SPH diagnosis reached by a combination of clinical presentation, EBUS-TBNA results, fungal serologies, and antigen testing. None of the patients needed further invasive procedures. *Conclusions.* EBUS-TBNA is a minimally invasive tool that can be used to support a diagnosis of SPH in patients with a high degree of clinical suspicion. EBUS-TBNA should be considered as an adjunctive diagnostic procedure for patients with SPH in an appropriate clinical setting.

1. Introduction

Histoplasmosis is the most common endemic fungal infection seen in humans. The Central River valleys in the Midwestern and South Central United States have endemicity for histoplasmosis. Approximately 250,000 individuals are infected annually but clinical manifestations of histoplasmosis occur in less than 5% [1]. Infections are sporadic, although large outbreaks of histoplasmosis may occur and histoplasmosis remains the most common cause for hospitalization amongst the endemic mycoses [2]. The morbidity and mortality of histoplasmosis are related to the duration and extent of systemic infection as well as underlying comorbidities. Around 1–5% may advance to subacute pulmonary histoplasmosis (SPH) [3].

Subacute pulmonary histoplasmosis (SPH) is defined by infection with *Histoplasma capsulatum* and the presence of symptoms for >1 month with a localized pulmonary opacity and/or hilar and mediastinal adenopathy. Clinical presentation may include protean symptoms of fevers, chills, malaise, weight loss, cough, and wheezing, symptoms that occur with multiple diseases. In addition, laboratory examination of serum, blood, and urine may result in wide spectrum of findings including anemia, leukocytosis, ESR and CRP elevation, and LFT abnormalities.

The diagnosis of histoplasmosis can be challenging. Cultures and identification of the organisms in tissue are often not helpful in SPH because of a low organism burden. Antigen detection is often variable in individuals with intact immune systems but can be useful if positive. Serology for histoplasmosis can be useful since the patient has often been infected for greater than one month allowing for a humoral immune response. High initial titers or rising titers over time are strongly suggestive of current or very recent infection, while a single low titer (<1 : 8) may suggest infections any time in the past [2].

Pulmonary physicians and thoracic surgeons are often asked to evaluate patients with hilar and mediastinal adenopathy. If SPH is suspected based on symptoms, the diagnosis may remain challenging because SPH unlike disseminated histoplasmosis tends to occur in immunocompetent individuals and presents with a variety of nonspecific symptoms that may be attributable to other causes [3].

EBUS-TBNA has emerged as an accurate, minimally invasive, safe technique for assessing undiagnosed mediastinal and hilar adenopathy, particularly in patients with lung cancer [4]. The use of EBUS-TBNA has not been reported for endemic fungal disease, although granulomatous inflammation has been reported especially in the evaluation of suspected sarcoidosis [5]. We hypothesized that EBUS-TBNA would provide additional confirmatory information for diagnosis in individuals with high suspicion of SPH in a geographical location with known endemic histoplasmosis and would complement the clinical exam in the elimination of other important causes of mediastinal and/or hilar adenopathy.

2. Methods

This study is a retrospective case review of seven patients referred to outpatient pulmonary clinic in a single academic institution for a workup of mediastinal/hilar lymphadenopathy. Inclusion criteria for our study consisted of hilar or mediastinal adenopathy with or without calcification, a clinical history suggestive of SPH and positive or indeterminate serology to *Histoplasma capsulatum*. In all seven patients a diagnosis of SPH was strongly considered prior to any invasive procedures based on epidemiologic, clinical, radiographic, and serological findings. Exclusion criteria consisted of the presence of an alternative diagnosis, immunocompromised state, or history of malignancy. On review of medical records between 2009 and 2012 in a single academic institution of patients referred to outpatient pulmonary clinic for workup of mediastinal/hilar adenopathy, seven patients were identified as meeting all the inclusion criteria and none of the exclusion criteria. Data was not collected on patients who did not meet inclusion criteria. All seven patients underwent a thorough clinical evaluation including urine and blood testing for fungal diseases and QuantiFERON TB Gold In-Tube test (Qiagen) and tuberculin skin testing for tuberculosis. Additional testing was performed as indicated by the clinical scenario. EBUS-TBNA was performed in all seven patients. Data were obtained from the procedure record, radiologic studies, pathology reports, clinical laboratory results, and clinic records. Institutional review board approval was obtained (UW–Madison IRB protocol number 2012-1164).

EBUS-TBNA was performed using a bronchoscope equipped with a distal 7.5 MHz linear ultrasound transducer probe (CP-EBUS, model XBF-UC260F; Olympus, Tokyo, Japan) and dedicated ultrasound image processor (model EU-ME1; Olympus). A dedicated aspiration needle (ViziShot, Olympus) was used to obtain specimens. The needle gauge, aspiration site, and the number of passes obtained [1, 2, 4] were performed at the discretion of the bronchoscopist. An on-site adequacy assessment was not available. A pair of slides was made for each aspirate: one was air-dried for Diff-Quick staining and one was fixed in 95% ethanol for Papanicolaou staining. Additional material was placed into saline for a cell block. All slides and the cell block material were examined by a cytopathologist. In cases where a suspicion for lymphoproliferative disease was present based on clinical or cytologic examination, additional specimens were sent for flow cytometry. In some cases, nodal aspirates were also sent for bacterial and fungal cultures. Subsequently, patients were followed clinically. Radiologic studies to confirm regression in lymphadenopathy were repeated at appropriate intervals for a period of up to 12 months.

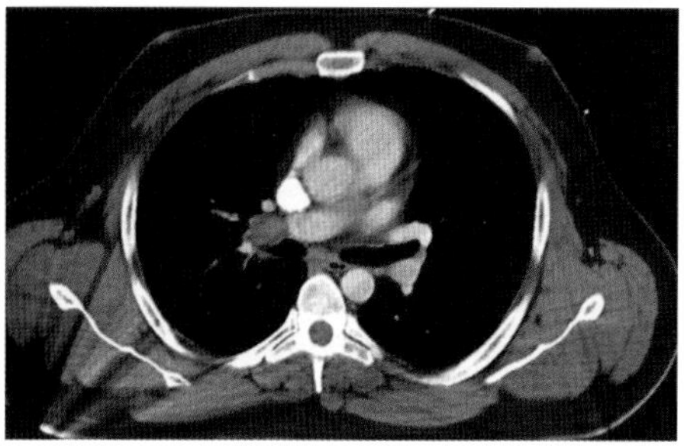

FIGURE 1: High resolution CT scan of hilar lymphadenopathy with pulmonary vein compression.

The final diagnosis of SPH was based on combination of clinical and radiographic follow-up, serologic and antigen testing, cytologic findings, and the absence of an identifiable malignancy or other infections (e.g., tuberculosis).

3. Results

Basic demographic data and clinical characteristics of the seven subjects are presented in Table 1. The average age of our patient series was 39 with a range of 26–58 years of age. All had clinical symptoms persistent for more than one month consisting primarily of cough, fevers, malaise, and weight loss. One patient presented with hemoptysis. None of the patients had a previous history of underlying malignancy or current infectious disease. Only one patient had an identifiable exposure to histoplasmosis while remodeling an old house that was contaminated with heavy bird droppings. Radiographic images showed mediastinal and/or hilar lymphadenopathy in seven out of seven patients, small pulmonary subcentimeter nodules in two out of seven patients, and pulmonary vein compression in one patient presumed due to postinflammatory fibrosis (Figure 1).

All patients had EBUS detectable mediastinal or hilar lymphadenopathy. Lymph node size measured from 15 mm to 35 mm in the short axis dimension (average 22 mm). Loosely organized granulomatous inflammation with areas of necrosis was present in five out of seven patients (Figure 2). Two patients had inadequate sampling. No fungal elements were identified in any of the patients' specimens.

All patients underwent urine and serum histoplasma and blastomycosis antigen testing, complement fixing antibody for histoplasma mycele and yeast forms, and blastomycosis antibody (Table 2). All patients had positive (>1 : 8 by complement fixation) serology for histoplasmosis. One patient had antigenemia and antigenuria and one patient

Table 1: Patient demographics and clinical features.

Case number	Age	Sex	Smoking Hx	Probable exposure to *Histoplasma capsulatum*	Clinical symptoms	Symptom duration	Radiographic findings
1	26	Male	None	Significant	Low grade fevers, cough, weight loss	4 months	Bilateral hilar and mediastinal adenopathy
2	30	Male	10 ppy	Minimal	fatigue	3 months	Right hilar adenopathy
3	50	Male	None	Minimal	Fevers, night sweats, cough, weight loss	1 year	Mediastinal and hilar adenopathy, small bilateral pulmonary nodules
4	34	Female	None	Minimal	Fevers, malaise, night sweats	9 months	Mediastinal and hilar adenopathy, small bilateral pulmonary nodules
5	57	Female	5 ppy	Minimal	Cough, fevers	8 months	Mediastinal adenopathy, small bilateral pulmonary nodules
6	36	Male	20 ppy	Minimal	Recurrent hemoptysis	3 months	Mediastinal and hilar adenopathy
7	29	Male	None	Minimal	Cough, fevers, fatigue	5 months	Left hilar adenopathy

Table 2: Diagnostic results.

Case number	Lymph node size	Stations sampled	Cultures	Infectious serologies	Histoplasmosis antigen	Cytology findings
1	35 mm	7	Negative	Acute 1 : 16 Convalescent 1 : 64	Negative	Loosely organized granuloma with necrotic debris
2	15 mm	11 R	Negative	Acute 1 : 32	Negative	Loosely organized granuloma with necrotic debris
3	15 mm	11 L	Negative	Acute 1 : 128	Positive urine Positive serum	Loosely organized granuloma with necrotic debris
4	25 mm	10 L	Negative	Acute 1 : 32	Positive urine	Nondiagnostic
5	20 mm	7	Negative	Acute 1 : 8 Convalescent 1 : 64	Negative	Nondiagnostic
6	30 mm	7	Negative	Acute 1 : 16	Negative	Loosely organized granuloma with necrotic debris
7	23 mm	11 L	Negative	Acute 1 : 16 Convalescent 1 : 512	Negative	Loosely organized granuloma with necrotic debris

had antigenuria alone. One patient had both positive histoplasma and blastomyces urinary antigens however due to high cross reactivity reactions of these fungi (as high as 90%) [6] as well as clinical picture; the patient was felt to have infectious process consistent with SPH. In one patient (case number 1), nodal material was sent for flow cytometry, which was negative for a monoclonal population of lymphocytes.

Four of the patients (cases 1, 3, 4, and 5) were treated with itraconazole for persistent or worsening symptoms. Infectious Disease Society of America guidelines were followed [7]. Clinical and radiographic follow-up was performed in all patients for up to 12 months. All patients in the series had improvement in symptoms (resolution of cough, fevers, and sweats) and radiographic findings (decreased nodal size and decreased nodules if present) over a 3-to-12-month period.

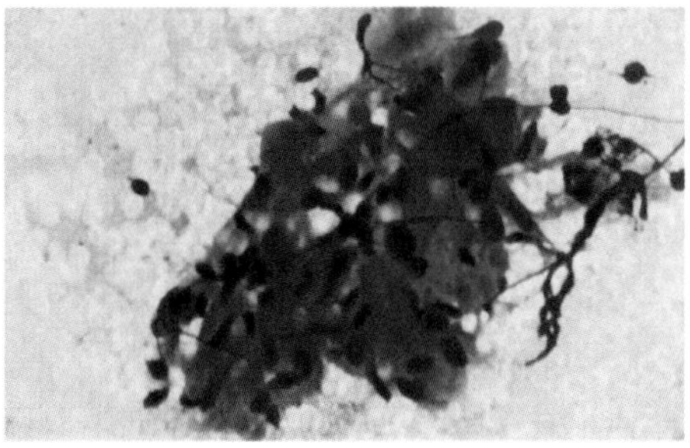

FIGURE 2: Diff-Quik stain of lymph node tissue with loosely organized granuloma.

None of the treated patients required retreatment, and none of the seven patients went on to further invasive procedures such as mediastinoscopy or video-assisted thoracoscopic surgery.

4. Discussion

Indeterminate mediastinal and hilar adenopathy in patients with nonspecific symptoms is often a clinical challenge for the treating pulmonologist or thoracic surgeon. In selected patients with a high index of clinical suspicion, indeterminate or weakly positive serology for histoplasmosis and cytologic confirmation of granulomatous inflammation may reduce the need for further invasive testing. This study demonstrates that EBUS-TBNA can be used in the evaluation of mediastinal and hilar adenopathy when histoplasmosis is suspected. Although our study is limited by number and nature of a retrospective review, our data show that mediastinal and hilar lymph nodes in the setting of suspected histoplasmosis are evaluable by EBUS and that cytologic findings are consistent with this diagnosis in most cases. Further, culture of nodal material obtained by EBUS-TBNA was negative for histoplasmosis in all cases. None of the patients were diagnosed with an alternative disease, even after careful radiographic and clinical follow-up.

The diagnosis of SPH in this study was made using a combination of clinical suspicion along with focused laboratory testing, the absence of alternative diseases, and follow-up. We feel that this is a valid model in an area where histoplasmosis is endemic. In other parts of the USA and world, practitioners would have to consider the epidemiology of the endemic mycoses for their region. The most frequently cited study that describes areas of endemicity for histoplasmosis in the United States was published in 1969 by Edwards et al. The study identified histoplasmosis endemicity on the basis of histoplasma skin testing, a diagnostic method of unknown sensitivity and probably poor specificity [8].

In the United States, an estimated 60% to 90% of people who live in areas surrounding the Ohio and Mississippi River Valleys (where *Histoplasma* is common in the environment) have been exposed to the fungus at some point during their lifetime [9]. One study calculated the incidence of histoplasmosis in adults aged 65 years and older in the USA to be 3.4 cases per 100,000 population. Rates were highest in the Midwest, with estimated 6.1 cases per 100,000 population [10].

Although findings of EBUS-TBNA were consistent with SPH, they were not confirmatory (no fungal elements observed in any specimen and negative fungal cultures). Pathologic findings in SPH may overlap or closely resemble such disease states as sarcoidosis or tuberculosis as well as malignancy in some cases, and interpretation of pathology may be very challenging as observation of fungal organisms in aspirate smears is unusual [11, 12]. Accordingly, serological workup and clinical/radiographic data and follow-up played an important role in reaching the final diagnosis in all seven patients.

In this selected patient population where the risk of SPH was considered to be much higher than the risk of malignancy, cytopathology obtained by EBUS-TBNA combined with additional testing was considered adequate and no further invasive testing was performed. However, in a patient population where the pretest probability for malignancy is higher, additional invasive testing would likely be warranted depending on the clinical circumstances. Additionally, other causes of granulomatous inflammation (e.g., metastatic cancers, lymphoma, and sarcoidosis) should always be carefully considered based on the clinical situation. A retrospective review of patients referred for mediastinal lymph node sampling in a large academic center demonstrated that despite presence of mediastinal calcification (56%) and lymph nodal enlargement in an area with known endemic histoplasmosis, EBUS-TBNA nodal sampling was not affected, and positive and negative predictive values of this test were comparable to other previously published studies [13].

Current recommendations for the diagnosis of *Histoplasma capsulatum* infection include a combination of several different modalities to achieve the highest yield depending on the presenting symptoms and timing of the exposure [5]. In SPH, the diagnosis can be challenging as most often these patients have nonspecific symptoms and findings that have a broad differential diagnosis. Although >90% of histoplasmosis infections are asymptomatic, mediastinal/hilar lymphadenopathy and associated nonspecific symptoms may be present in 5–10% of immunocompetent patients [2]. Currently, testing for antibodies by immunodiffusion or complement fixation technique is considered more sensitive for SPH than tests for an antigen, as fungal burden is low and pulmonary infection is often very localized in immunocompetent patients [3].

There are significant limitations of this study. First, this is a retrospective review of selected patient group who were strongly suspected of having SPH. As such, there is an intentional selection bias, and there are variables that we do not have control over, such as the skill of the bronchoscopist, the skill of the cytologist, and the exact methods used to perform diagnostic testing. Therefore, we are not able to conclude that EBUS-TBNA has a high utility in discriminating one cause of adenopathy from another. However we can conclude that, in this patient population, EBUS-TBNA should result in granulomatous inflammation in most cases.

Prospective studies with greater number of patients as well as more controlled data acquisition and uniform follow-up that include this population and others may be able to define the discriminant function of EBUS-TBNA in SPH. However, the precise incidence of SPH is not known [9]. These seven cases were accumulated over the course of 3 years in a busy academic pulmonary clinic. The likelihood that a prospective trial of EBUS for SPH could be accomplished is low without collaborations from multiple institutions.

Furthermore, 2 of 7 patients had inadequate sampling. Unfortunately this study is too small for us to determine if a value of 2 of 7 is significant. No currently available studies directly address inadequate sampling of EBUS-TBNA in patients with suspected infections. Inadequate sampling or nondiagnostic aspirates occur with variable frequency [14] and are potentially related to needle size, cytology procedures, operator technique, the specific target disease, and the prevalence of the disease in question [15]. Further study will be necessary to answer these questions. In the two patients who had inadequate samples by EBUS-TBNA, one had high urinary antigen positivity and the other had rising titers of antibody to histoplasmosis. Therefore, we feel that both of these individuals had SPH.

The body of literature accumulates on the use of EBUS-TBNA in diagnosis of mediastinal lymphoma [16], tuberculosis, sarcoidosis [5], and malignancy [17]. Although diagnosis of lymphoma by EBUS-TBNA technique remains a subject of controversy due to the small available retrospective studies as well as a minimal tissue yield that is available for pathologic analysis by EBUS-TBNA, future advances such as the use of miniforceps may improve the diagnostic yield and establish EBUS-TBNA as an initial procedure of choice [18].

Our study provides evidence that EBUS may be helpful in the evaluation of infectious diseases as well. We believe that in situations where there is a high suspicion of SPH (clinical symptoms, serology), EBUS-TBNA is useful in the elimination of alternative diseases and can provide compatible pathologic findings. If a presumptive diagnosis of SPH is made by a combination of clinical signs, serology, and EBUS, patients should be followed for response to treatment or resolution of the clinical findings. Further prospective studies are anticipated that will define the utility and efficacy of EBUS-TBNA in the evaluation of patients with mediastinal/hilar adenopathy and a high likelihood of infection.

5. Conclusion

The use of EBUS-TBNA is becoming widespread in diagnosis and staging of lung malignancies. No current literature exists on the role of EBUS-TBNA in infectious causes of mediastinal/hilar lymphadenopathy. This study demonstrates that EBUS-TBNA is a minimally invasive adjunctive procedure that can be used in patients in whom clinical, radiographic, and serological data raise a high index of suspicion for SPH. Furthermore, EBUS-TBNA with clinical and radiographic follow-up appears to have avoided additional invasive diagnostic testing. Further studies are needed to examine the efficacy and utility of EBUS-TBNA in patients with suspected infections and presence of mediastinal/hilar adenopathy.

References

[1] J. H. Chu, C. Feudtner, K. Heydon, T. J. Walsh, and T. E. Zaoutis, "Hospitalizations for endemic mycoses: a population-based national study," *Clinical Infectious Diseases*, vol. 42, no. 6, pp. 822–825, 2006.

[2] L. J. Wheat, D. Conces, S. D. Allen, D. Blue-Hnidy, and J. Loyd, "Pulmonary histoplasmosis syndromes: recognition, diagnosis, and management," *Seminars in Respiratory and Critical Care Medicine*, vol. 25, no. 2, pp. 129–144, 2004.

[3] S. Swartzentruber, L. Rhodes, K. Kurkjian et al., "Diagnosis of acute pulmonary histoplasmosis by antigen detection," *Clinical Infectious Diseases*, vol. 49, no. 12, pp. 1878–1882, 2009.

[4] B. L. McComb, M. B. Wallace, J. M. Pascual, and M. O. Othman, "Mediastinal staging of nonsmall cell lung carcinoma by endoscopic and endobronchial ultrasound-guided fine needle aspiration," *Journal of Thoracic Imaging*, vol. 26, no. 2, pp. 147–161, 2011.

[5] S. Garwood, M. A. Judson, G. Silvestri, R. Hoda, M. Fraig, and P. Doelken, "Endobronchial ultrasound for the diagnosis of pulmonary sarcoidosis," *Chest*, vol. 132, no. 4, pp. 1298–1304, 2007.

[6] C. A. Hage, J. A. Ribes, N. L. Wengenack et al., "A multicenter evaluation of tests for diagnosis of histoplasmosis," *Clinical Infectious Diseases*, vol. 53, article 448, 2011.

[7] L. J. Wheat, A. G. Freifeld, M. B. Kleiman et al., "Clinical practice guidelines for the management of patients with histoplasmosis: 2007 Update by the Infectious Diseases Society of America," *Clinical Infectious Diseases*, vol. 45, no. 7, pp. 807–825, 2007.

[8] L. B. Edwards, F. A. Acquaviva, V. T. Livesay, F. W. Cross, and C. E. Palmer, "An atlas of sensitivity to tuberculin, PPD-B, and histoplasmin in the United States," *The American Review of Respiratory Disease*, vol. 99, no. 4, supplement, pp. 1–132, 1969.

[9] N. E. Manos, S. H. Ferebee, and W. F. Kerschbaum, "Geographic variation in the prevalence of histoplasmin sensitivity," *Diseases of the Chest*, vol. 29, no. 6, pp. 649–668, 1956.

[10] J. W. Baddley, K. L. Winthrop, N. M. Patkar et al., "Geographic distribution of endemic fungal infections among older persons, United States," *Emerging Infectious Diseases*, vol. 17, no. 9, pp. 1664–1669, 2011.

[11] N. Navani, D. R. Lawrence, S. Kolvekar et al., "Endobronchial ultrasound-guided transbronchial needle aspiration prevents mediastinoscopies in the diagnosis of isolated mediastinal lymphadenopathy: a prospective trial," *American Journal of Respiratory and Critical Care Medicine*, vol. 186, no. 3, pp. 255–260, 2012.

[12] Z. S. DePew, W. I. Gonsalves, A. C. Roden, A. O. Bungum, J. J. Mullon, and F. Maldonado, "Granulomatous inflammation detected by endobronchial ultrasound-guided transbronchial needle aspiration in patients with a concurrent diagnosis of cancer: a clinical conundrum," *Journal of Bronchology & Interventional Pulmonology*, vol. 19, no. 3, pp. 176–181, 2012.

[13] Y. R. Shweihat, R. S. Samant, M. Joshi, H. Shah, P. C. Moore, and M. P. Kennedy, "Endobronchial ultrasound-guided transbronchial needle aspiration in a geographical region with endemic histoplasmosis infection," *Journal of Bronchology and Interventional Pulmonology*, vol. 17, no. 4, pp. 295–300, 2010.

[14] G. P. Currie, M. E. Mckean, K. M. Kerr, A. R. Denison, and M. Chetty, "Endobronchial ultrasound-transbronchial needle aspiration and its practical application," *QJM: An International Journal of Medicine*, vol. 104, no. 8, pp. 653–662, 2011.

[15] Z. S. DePew, E. S. Edell, D. E. Midthun et al., "Endobronchial ultrasound-guided transbronchial needle aspiration: determinants of sampling adequacy," *Journal of Bronchology and Interventional Pulmonology*, vol. 19, no. 4, pp. 271–276, 2012.

[16] M. P. Kennedy, C. A. Jimenez, J. F. Bruzzi et al., "Endobronchial ultrasound-guided transbronchial needle aspiration in the diagnosis of lymphoma," *Thorax*, vol. 63, no. 4, pp. 360–365, 2008.

[17] I. Kokkonouzis, A. S. Strimpakos, I. Lampaditis, S. Tsimpoukis, and K. N. Syrigos, "The role of endobronchial ultrasound in lung cancer diagnosis and staging: a comprehensive review," *Clinical Lung Cancer*, vol. 13, no. 6, pp. 408–415, 2012.

[18] A. Chrissian, D. Misselhorn, and A. Chen, "Endobronchial-ultrasound guided miniforceps biopsy of mediastinal and hilar lesions," *Annals of Thoracic Surgery*, vol. 92, no. 1, pp. 284–288, 2011.

11

Is It Possible to Predict the Presence of Intestinal Angioectasias?

Tiago Cúrdia Gonçalves,[1] Joana Magalhães,[1] Pedro Boal Carvalho,[1] Maria João Moreira,[1] Bruno Rosa,[1] and José Cotter[1,2,3]

[1] *Gastroenterology Department, Centro Hospitalar do Alto Ave, 4831-044 Guimarães, Portugal*
[2] *Life and Health Sciences Research Institute, University of Minho, 4710-057 Braga/Guimarães, Portugal*
[3] *ICVS/3B's, PT Government Associate Laboratory, 4710-057 Braga/Guimarães, Portugal*

Correspondence should be addressed to Tiago Cúrdia Gonçalves; tiagogoncalves@chaa.min-saude.pt

Academic Editor: Spiros D. Ladas

Background and Aim. Angioectasias are the most common vascular anomalies found in the gastrointestinal tract. In small bowel (SB), they can cause obscure gastrointestinal bleeding (OGIB) and in this setting, small bowel capsule endoscopy (SBCE) is an important diagnostic tool. This study aimed to identify predictive factors for the presence of SB angioectasias, detected by SBCE. *Methods.* We retrospectively analyzed the results of 284 consecutive SBCE procedures between April 2006 and December 2012, whose indication was OGIB, of which 47 cases with SB angioectasias and 53 controls without vascular lesions were selected to enter the study. Demographic and clinical data were collected. *Results.* The mean age of subjects with angioectasias (70.9 ± 14.7) was significantly higher than in controls (53.1 ± 18.6; $P < 0.001$). The presence of SB angioectasias was significantly higher when the indication for the exam was overt OGIB versus occult OGIB (13/19 versus 34/81, $P = 0.044$). Hypertension and hypercholesterolemia were significantly associated with the presence of SB angioectasias (38/62 versus 9/38, $P < 0.001$ and 28/47 versus 19/53, $P = 0.027$, resp.). Other studied factors were not associated with small bowel angioectasias. *Conclusions.* In patients with OGIB, overt bleeding, older age, hypercholesterolemia, and hypertension are predictive of the presence of SB angioectasias detected by SBCE, which may be used to increase the diagnostic yield of the SBCE procedure and to reduce the proportion of nondiagnostic examinations.

1. Introduction

Obscure gastrointestinal bleeding (OGIB) remains one of the most challenging issues for gastroenterologists. It is defined as bleeding from gastrointestinal (GI) tract that persists or recurs without obvious etiology after esophagogastroduodenoscopy (EGD), colonoscopy, and radiologic evaluation of the small bowel (SB). OGIB accounts for about 5% of the cases of gastrointestinal bleeding [1]. The source of bleeding is located in the SB in about 75% of cases, where lesions can be scarcely accessed by standard endoscopy [1, 2]. These patients frequently require several blood transfusions and repeated hospital admissions, being at risk for complications not only related to anemia, but also caused by numerous exploratory procedures [3]. As a consequence, OGIB negatively affects patients' quality of life and represents a significant burden of healthcare resources [3].

Small bowel capsule endoscopy (SBCE) has become a particularly useful tool in the management of OGIB, which remains the most common indication for the procedure [4]. Several studies have confirmed the higher diagnostic yield of SBCE in diagnosing the cause of OGIB when compared to other investigative procedures [2, 5–10].

The causes of GI bleeding originating in the SB include tumours, chemical/radiation injuries, vascular diseases, inflammatory diseases, systemic diseases, or infectious diseases [3]. The prevalence of those types of lesions varies with patient's age; for instance, SB tumours (such as gastrointestinal stromal cell tumours, carcinoid tumours, adenocarcinomas, and lymphomas), Dieulafoy's lesion, inflammatory bowel disease, and Meckel's diverticulum are the most common causes at younger ages [1, 11, 12], while older patients are more likely to bleed from vascular lesions or nonsteroidal anti-inflammatory drug (NSAID) induced SB disease [1, 12]. Overall, angioectasias are the most common origin of OGIB, being responsible for approximately 30–40% of the cases [3, 13, 14]. Angioectasias consist of dilated, ectatic, tortuous, thin-walled vessels of the mucosa or submucosa, without inflammation or fibrosis [13, 15].

The clinical significance of angioectasias has not been fully elucidated, and the optimal approach to these lesions is still controversial, although it is reasonable to assume that it is important to detect angioectasias in order to plan medical or endoscopic treatment when indicated. However, despite being the most common lesions found during OGIB investigation, there are still a considerable number of cases in which neither angioectasias nor other potentially bleeding lesions can be found after a SBCE examination. Those cases of non-diagnostic SBCE represent increased costs and an undesirable expenditure of healthcare resources, which could theoretically be reduced if predictive factors of lesions such as angioectasias could be identified and used to properly select patients to undergo SBCE.

The aim of this study was to collect demographic and clinical data of patients who were investigated for OGIB with SBCE and analyze whether any of those factors could be used to predict the presence of SB angioectasias.

2. Methods

This study was designed as a single-center, retrospective cohort investigation. All patients referred to our center for investigation of OGIB with SBCE between April 2006 and December 2012 were reviewed. OGIB was defined according to the published medical position statement of the American Gastroenterological Association (AGA) [1]. This condition was further divided on occult OGIB (positive fecal occult blood test or iron deficient anemia) and overt OGIB (passage of visible blood) [1]. Demographic characteristics (namely, age, gender, and race) and relevant medical history (such as indication for SBCE, hypertension, diabetes mellitus, hypercholesterolemia, tobacco use, chronic kidney disease (CKD), chronic liver disease, aortic stenosis, previous abdominal surgery, antiplatelet, or anticoagulant drugs use) were obtained by consultation of patients' medical records.

2.1. SBCE Procedure. All the procedures were performed using PillCam SB or PillCam SB2 capsules from GIVEN Imaging (Yoqneam, Israel). Before the procedure, each patient received general instructions and informed consent was obtained. Patients had a clear liquid diet the day before capsule ingestion and an overnight 12-hour fast. Patients were allowed to drink fluids after 2 hours and to have a light meal after 4 hours. Consensual contraindications for SBCE procedure were respected and have been described elsewhere [16–18].

2.2. Analysis of SBCE Findings. The complete video obtained in each SBCE was reviewed by two gastroenterologists with vast experience in capsule endoscopy. Angioectasias were identified as flat to slightly elevated, clearly demarcated, bright red vascular lesions, with variable size.

2.3. Inclusion Criteria. Patients with OGIB submitted to SBCE during the evaluation of OGIB with at least one SB angioectasia were included. Those patients investigated with SBCE for the same reason and without any finding during the examination were also included and used as the control group.

2.4. Exclusion Criteria. To minimize bias, patients with vascular lesions of the SB other than angioectasias, such as phlebectasias, portal enteropathy, or SB varices, were not included in the study. Patients in which the capsule detected other potentially bleeding lesions such as ulcers, erosion, or tumours were also excluded. Other patients had an incomplete SBCE and were not considered eligible for this study.

2.5. Data Analysis. Statistical analysis was performed using the Statistical Packages for Social Sciences software (SPSS) version 17.0. Differences between groups were evaluated using Student's t-test for quantitative variables and χ^2 test for nominal variables. A P Value <0.05 was considered statistically significant.

3. Results

3.1. Population Description. From April 2006 to December 2012, a total of 284 patients underwent SBCE examination in our center for etiologic investigation of OGIB. Of those, 100 patients met the inclusion criteria and were selected to enter the study. All patients swallowed the capsule without difficulty and none had any complication related to the procedure. SBCE detected at least one SB angioectasia in 47 patients. On the other hand, 53 patients were found to have no abnormalities and were included in the control group.

3.2. Demographic Data. We found that the mean age in the control group was 53.1 ± 18.6 years (range, 28–87), while, in the angioectasia group, it was 70.9 ± 14.7 years (range, 19–91). This difference was found to be statistically significant ($P < 0.001$). As for gender, the control group was composed of 18 men (34%) and 35 women (66%), whereas the angioectasia group had 23 men (49%) and 24 women (51%). In contrast to what was found with age, there were no significant differences between genders ($P = 0.156$). Lastly, all patients included in our study were Caucasian, so comparison between different races and the presence of angioectasias was not possible.

3.3. Relevant Medical History Data. The indication for the SBCE was one of the studied points, so division of patients between those with occult OGIB and those with overt OGIB was done. Globally, 81 patients were submitted to SBCE for the study of occult OGIB and the other 19 performed the capsule examination because they had overt OGIB. When subdivided, we found out that, in the control group, 47 patients (89%) had occult OGIB and only 6 (11%) had overt OGIB. By contrast, in the angioectasia group, 34 patients (72%) presented with occult OGIB and 13 patients (28%) had overt OGIB. There was a statistic difference between the two groups ($P = 0.044$).

From the conditions considered relevant in patients' past medical history, special attention should be put towards hypertension and hypercholesterolemia. Regarding hypertension, 29 patients (55%) in the control group had normal blood pressure values and 24 patients (45%) had diagnosis of hypertension, while, in the angioectasia group, however, 38 patients (81%) had hypertension but only 9 patients (19%) were normotensive. This result reached statistical significance ($P < 0.001$). As far as hypercholesterolemia is concerned, 34 patients (64%) in the control group had a normal lipid panel and 19 (36%) had altered lipid values. On the opposite side, in the angioectasia group, 19 patients (40%) had no lipid changes while 28 patients (60%) had diagnosed hypercholesterolemia. This finding was also statistically significant ($P = 0.027$).

As mentioned previously, other conditions were searched in the studied patients. In this investigation, the diagnoses of diabetes mellitus, chronic kidney or liver diseases, aortic stenosis, as well as previous abdominal surgery, or tobacco use were not significantly different between the two groups. In addition, regarding medication use, namely, antiplatelet or anticoagulant drugs, no differences were found among the control or the angioectasia groups.

The results are summarized in Table 1.

Table 1: Demographic and clinical characteristics of patients.

Characteristic	Control group	Angioectasia group	*P* value
Mean Age (±SD)	53.1 (±18.6)	70.9 (±14.7)	**<0.001***
Gender			
Men (%)	18 (34%)	23 (49%)	0.156
Women (%)	35 (66%)	24 (51%)	
SBCE indication			
Occult OGIB (%)	47 (89%)	34 (72%)	**0.044***
Overt OGIB (%)	6 (11%)	13 (28%)	
Hypertension			
Yes (%)	24 (45%)	38 (81%)	**<0.001***
No (%)	29 (55%)	9 (19%)	
Diabetes mellitus			
Yes (%)	13 (25%)	17 (36%)	0.275
No (%)	40 (75%)	30 (64%)	
Hypercholesterolemia			
Yes (%)	19 (36%)	28 (60%)	**0.027***
No (%)	34 (64%)	19 (40%)	
Tobacco use			
Yes (%)	7 (13%)	13 (28%)	0.084
No (%)	46 (87%)	34 (72%)	
Chronic kidney disease			
Yes (%)	8 (15%)	13 (28%)	0.145
No (%)	45 (85%)	34 (72%)	
Chronic liver disease			
Yes (%)	4 (8%)	1 (2%)	0.367
No (%)	49 (92%)	46 (98%)	
Previous abdominal surgery			
Yes (%)	17 (32%)	20 (43%)	0.306
No (%)	36 (68%)	27 (57%)	
Aortic stenosis			
Yes (%)	2 (4%)	5 (11%)	0.249
No (%)	51 (96%)	42 (89%)	
Antiplatelet use			
Yes (%)	15 (28%)	19 (40%)	0.213
No (%)	38 (72%)	28 (60%)	
Anticoagulant use			
Yes (%)	8 (15%)	6 (13%)	0.781
No (%)	45 (85%)	41 (87%)	

SD: standard deviation. *statistically significant.

4. Discussion

Angioectasias can be found throughout the entire GI tract. They may be clustered in one single region or they may coexist in several different GI locations. The pathogenesis of GI angioectasias is not fully understood, but different theories had already been proposed. Some authors advocate that angioectasias should be regarded as degenerative lesions of aging, caused by chronic intermittent low-grade obstruction of veins, capillaries, and arterioles that supply the mucosa [19]. Other authors defend the theory of a neurohormonal abnormality in which sympathetic nerves may stimulate intestinal vascular smooth muscle relaxation in response to hypoperfusion. Chronically, local vascular overload, dilation, and ectasia may pathologically develop leading to permanent angioectasia [13, 19]. Overexpression of angiogenic factors and deficient production of type IV collagen have also been suggested as pathogenic factors [20, 21].

In our study, we observed that age was significantly associated with higher prevalence of SB angioectasias, which is in line with the results of other previous studies, endorsing the possibility of a degenerative process behind the pathogenesis of GI angioectasias [13, 15, 22]. No significant differences were observed between the two groups regarding gender. It is frequently reported that the diagnostic yield of SBCE is the highest for patients with ongoing overt OGIB, although it has not been consistent in all studies [23, 24]. Indeed, the diagnostic yield of SBCE seems to be closely related to the timing of the procedure and it has been recommended that it should be performed early in the work-up of patients with OGIB [25, 26]. In our study, we found a significant association between overt OGIB and the presence of SB angioectasias. However, the exact time interval between the bleeding episode and the SBCE examination was not analyzed in our study.

We analyzed some major vascular disease risk factors, particularly, hypertension, diabetes mellitus, hypercholesterolemia, and smoking. Hypertension is a very common clinical finding in patients with GI angioectasias [15, 27, 28]. In our study, about 80% of patients with angioectasias had a known diagnosis of hypertension, being reasonable to admit that, similarly to what happens in other vascular territories (like in brain, eye, kidney, or heart microcirculations), hypertension might have a role in the aging of GI blood vessel, leading to the development of identifiable vascular lesion such as angioectasias. Diabetes mellitus can recognizably damage both endothelial and smooth muscle cells, which chronically cause degenerative alterations in blood vessels and impair tissue healing [29]. In our study, we found that the prevalence of diabetes mellitus in both control and angioectasia groups was similar. We also analyzed hypercholesterolemia as a possible risk factor for angioectasias, not only because of its prevalence in western populations but also because of that it plays as well an important role in the pathogenesis of vascular dysfunction [30]. Although some studies report no association [28], we found that more than an half of patients with SB angioectasias had hypercholesterolemia versus about one third of patients in the control group, which was statistically significant. Regarding smoking, it has been proven to have deleterious effects on the regulation of gastric microcirculation, consequently leading to some recognized causes of GI bleeding such peptic ulcer disease [31, 32]. While some studies report higher rates of tobacco use among patients with angioectasias, others could not support such an association [33, 34]. In our study, smoking was twice as common in the angioectasia group, although it did not reach statistical significance.

We also investigated some other conditions possibly associated with the presence of GI angioectasias, such as chronic kidney disease (CKD). Angioectasias have been reported to be a common cause of upper GI bleeding in patients with CKD [35] and some studies identified angioectasias as the leading cause of recurrent lower GI bleeding in those patients [36]. The reason for this association is still unknown, although a possible explanation is that angioectasias may not be more common but could bleed more easily due to uremia-induced platelet dysfunction. In our study, few patients with CKD were included and the differences between groups were not significant. It has also been suggested as an association between GI bleeding from angioectasias and aortic stenosis, also known as Heyde's syndrome [37]. In our study, very few patients had aortic stenosis and there were no significant differences between groups. Chronic liver disease, especially with associated portal hypertension, has also been linked to the presence of GI angioectasias and, as reported by some authors, they could be reversed after transjugular intrahepatic portosystemic shunt [34, 38, 39]. We found no significant differences between the two groups concerning the presence of chronic liver disease, which can be partly explained by the small number of patients included. Previous abdominal surgery has also been linked to vascular lesions in the GI tract, such as jejunal varices [40, 41]. However, in our study, we have not found any significant association. We also investigated whether factors known to interfere with hemostasis, such as antithrombotic therapy (antiplatelet or anticoagulant drugs), would be associated with the detection of GI angioectasias. The use of antithrombotic therapy has been associated with a higher diagnostic yield of SBCE, but the possible causal effects with the presence of angioectasias, as well as the risk of recurrent bleeding, are controversial [42, 43]. In our study, the use of antithrombotic therapy was similar between patients in the control group and those with angioectasias.

In conclusion, this study reinforces the importance of evaluating patients' baseline demographic and clinical features before they are selected to undergo SBCE. We confirmed, as reported in previous studies, age and overt OGIB as predictive factors of SB angioectasias. Moreover, we also observed additional associations with some vascular disease risk factors, such as hypertension and hypercholesterolemia. The abovementioned factors should be considered in the process of patients' selection to undergo SBCE. When present, patients should be submitted to SBCE and these factors should be taken into account in the valorization of angioectasias as origin of bleeding. Furthermore, these patients' SBCE recordings may benefit from the use of some new software tools such as flexible spectral imaging color enhancement (FICE), particularly, if the initial study with conventional white light is negative, because it has been shown to increase the detection rate of some SB lesions such angioectasias, as reported in several studies [44–46]. On the other hand, in patients in which all these predictive factors are absent, a more expectant attitude may be followed. It may be acceptable to defer the use of SBCE and insist in the identification of other potential causes of iron deficient anemia (e.g., coeliac disease, *H. pylori* colonization, inflammatory bowel disease, NSAID enteropathy), leaving SBCE as a subsequent possibility. Applying the proposed strategy, the identified predictive factors may be used to increase the diagnostic yield of the SBCE procedure and to reduce the proportion of nondiagnostic examinations.

References

[1] G. S. Raju, L. Gerson, A. Das, and B. Lewis, "American Gastroenterological Association (AGA) Institute Technical Review on Obscure Gastrointestinal Bleeding," *Gastroenterology*, vol. 133, no. 5, pp. 1697–1717, 2007.

[2] A. de Leusse, K. Vahedi, J. Edery et al., "Capsule endoscopy or push enteroscopy for first-line exploration of obscure gastrointestinal bleeding?" *Gastroenterology*, vol. 132, no. 3, pp. 855–862, 2007.

[3] F. Li, J. A. Leighton, and V. K. Sharma, "Capsule endoscopy in the evaluation of obscure gastrointestinal bleeding: a comprehensive review," *Gastroenterology and Hepatology*, vol. 3, no. 10, pp. 777–785, 2007.

[4] Z. Liao, R. Gao, C. Xu, and Z.-S. Li, "Indications and detection, completion, and retention rates of small-bowel capsule endoscopy: a systematic review," *Gastrointestinal Endoscopy*, vol. 71, no. 2, pp. 280–286, 2010.

[5] S. L. Triester, J. A. Leighton, G. I. Leontiadis et al., "A meta-analysis of the yield of capsule endoscopy compared to other diagnostic modalities in patients with obscure gastrointestinal bleeding," *The American Journal of Gastroenterology*, vol. 100, no. 11, pp. 2407–2418, 2005.

[6] W. A. Voderholzer, M. Ortner, P. Rogalla, J. Beinhölzl, and H. Lochs, "Diagnostic yield of wireless capsule enteroscopy in comparison with computed tomography enteroclysis," *Endoscopy*, vol. 35, no. 12, pp. 1009–1014, 2003.

[7] E. Saperas, J. Dot, S. Videla et al., "Capsule endoscopy versus computed tomographic or standard angiography for the diagnosis of obscure gastrointestinal bleeding," *The American Journal of Gastroenterology*, vol. 102, no. 4, pp. 731–737, 2007.

[8] D. Hartmann, H. Schmidt, G. Bolz et al., "A prospective two-center study comparing wireless capsule endoscopy with intra-operative enteroscopy in patients with obscure GI bleeding," *Gastrointestinal Endoscopy*, vol. 61, no. 7, pp. 826–832, 2005.

[9] S. K. Gölder, A. G. Schreyer, E. Endlicher et al., "Comparison of capsule endoscopy and magnetic resonance (MR) enteroclysis in suspected small bowel disease," *International Journal of Colorectal Disease*, vol. 21, no. 2, pp. 97–104, 2006.

[10] M. Nakamura, Y. Niwa, R. Miyahara et al., "Preliminary comparison of capsule endoscopy and double-balloon enteroscopy in patients with suspected small-bowel bleeding," *Endoscopy*, vol. 38, no. 1, pp. 59–66, 2006.

[11] K. Liu and A. J. Kaffes, "Review article: the diagnosis and investigation of obscure gastrointestinal bleeding," *Alimentary Pharmacology and Therapeutics*, vol. 34, no. 4, pp. 416–423, 2011.

[12] G. Bresci, "Occult and obscure gastrointestinal bleeding: Causes and diagnostic approach in 2009," *World Journal of Gastrointestinal Endoscopy*, vol. 1, pp. 3–6, 2009.

[13] J. Regula, E. Wronska, and J. Pachlewski, "Vascular lesions of the gastrointestinal tract," *Best Practice and Research*, vol. 22, no. 2, pp. 313–328, 2008.

[14] M. Kovacs, P. Pak, G. Pak, J. Feher, and K. Huttl, "Multiple angiodysplasias diagnosed by capsule endoscopy," *Orvosi Hetilap*, vol. 148, pp. 2435–2440, 2007.

[15] A. T. DeBenedet, S. D. Saini, M. Takami, and L. R. Fisher, "Do clinical characteristics predict the presence of small bowel angioectasias on capsule endoscopy?" *Digestive Diseases and Sciences*, vol. 56, no. 6, pp. 1776–1781, 2011.

[16] S. D. Ladas, K. Triantafyllou, C. Spada et al., "European Society of Gastrointestinal Endoscopy (ESGE): Recommendations (2009) on clinical use of video capsule endoscopy to investigate small-bowel, esophageal and colonic diseases," *Endoscopy*, vol. 42, no. 3, pp. 220–227, 2010.

[17] D. S. Mishkin, R. Chuttani, J. Croffie et al., "ASGE Technology Status Evaluation Report: Wireless capsule endoscopy," *Gastrointestinal Endoscopy*, vol. 63, no. 4, pp. 539–545, 2006.

[18] A. K. Hara, J. A. Leighton, V. K. Sharma, R. I. Heigh, and D. E. Fleischer, "Imaging of small bowel disease: comparison of capsule endoscopy, standard endoscopy, barium examination, and CT," *Radiographics*, vol. 25, no. 3, pp. 697–711, 2005.

[19] T. Yamada and D. H. Alpers, *Textbook of Gastroenterology*, Lippincott Williams and Wilkins, Philadelphia, Pa, USA, 4th edition, 2003.

[20] F. Junquera, E. Saperas, I. De Torres, M. T. Vidai, and J.-R. Malagelada, "Increased expression of angiogenic factors in human colonic angiodysplasia," *The American Journal of Gastroenterology*, vol. 94, no. 4, pp. 1070–1076, 1999.

[21] D. E. Roskell, S. C. Biddolph, and B. F. Warren, "Apparent deficiency of mucosal vascular collagen type IV associated with angiodysplasia of the colon," *Journal of Clinical Pathology*, vol. 51, no. 1, pp. 18–20, 1998.

[22] P. Tsibouris, C. Kalantzis, P. Apostolopoulos, G. Alexandrakis, P. Mavrogianni, and N. Kalantzis, "Capsule endoscopy findings in patients with occult or overt bleeding older than 80 years," *Digestive Endoscopy*, vol. 24, no. 3, pp. 154–158, 2012.

[23] M. Pennazio, R. Santucci, E. Rondonotti et al., "Outcome of patients with obscure gastrointestinal bleeding after capsule endoscopy: report of 100 consecutive cases," *Gastroenterology*, vol. 126, no. 3, pp. 643–653, 2004.

[24] W. Selby, "Can clinical features predict the likelihood of finding abnormalities when using capsule endoscopy in patients with GI bleeding of obscure origin?" *Gastrointestinal Endoscopy*, vol. 59, no. 7, pp. 782–787, 2004.

[25] M. Pennazio, G. Eisen, and N. Goldfarb, "ICCE consensus for obscure gastrointestinal bleeding," *Endoscopy*, vol. 37, no. 10, pp. 1046–1050, 2005.

[26] M. Esaki, T. Matsumoto, S. Yada et al., "Factors associated with the clinical impact of capsule endoscopy in patients with overt obscure gastrointestinal bleeding," *Digestive Diseases and Sciences*, vol. 55, no. 8, pp. 2294–2301, 2010.

[27] S. Ueno, H. Nakase, K. Kasahara et al., "Clinical features of Japanese patients with colonic angiodysplasia," *Journal of Gastroenterology and Hepatology*, vol. 23, no. 8, pp. e363–e366, 2008.

[28] J. MacDonald, V. Porter, N. W. Scott, and D. McNamara, "Small bowel lymphangiectasia and angiodysplasia: a positive association; Novel clinical marker or shared pathophysiology?" *Journal of Clinical Gastroenterology*, vol. 44, no. 9, pp. 610–614, 2010.

[29] M. A. Creager, T. F. Lüscher, F. Cosentino, and J. A. Beckman, "Diabetes and vascular disease: pathophysiology, clinical consequences, and medical therapy. Part I," *Circulation*, vol. 108, no. 12, pp. 1527–1532, 2003.

[30] H. K. Saini, A. S. Arneja, and N. S. Dhalla, "Role of cholesterol in cardiovascular dysfunction," *Canadian Journal of Cardiology*, vol. 20, no. 3, pp. 333–346, 2004.

[31] M. Battistel, M. Plebani, F. Di Mario, M. Jocic, I. T. Lippe, and P. Holzer, "Chronic nicotine intake causes vascular dysregulation in the rat gastric mucosa," *Gut*, vol. 34, no. 12, pp. 1688–1692, 1993.

[32] M. Moshkowitz, S. Brill, F. M. Konikoff, M. Averbuch, N. Arber, and Z. Halpern, "Additive deleterious effect of smoking on gastroduodenal pathology and clinical course in Helicobacter pylori-positive dyspeptic patients," *Israel Medical Association Journal*, vol. 2, no. 12, pp. 892–895, 2000.

[33] M. S. Cappell and A. Gupta, "Changing epidemiology of gastrointestinal angiodysplasia with increasing recognition of clinically milder cases: angiodysplasia tend to produce mild chronic gastrointestinal bleeding in a study of 47 consecutive patients admitted from 1980–1989," *The American Journal of Gastroenterology*, vol. 87, no. 2, pp. 201–206, 1992.

[34] Y. Sekino, H. Endo, E. Yamada et al., "Clinical associations and risk factors for bleeding from colonic angiectasia: a case-controlled study," *Colorectal Disease*, vol. 14, pp. 740–746, 2012.

[35] N. Chalasani, G. Cotsonis, and C. M. Wilcox, "Upper gastrointestinal bleeding in patients with chronic renal failure: role of vascular ectasia," *The American Journal of Gastroenterology*, vol. 91, no. 11, pp. 2329–2332, 1996.

[36] G. Galanopoulos, "Angiodysplastic lesions as a cause of colonic bleeding in patients with chronic renal disease: is there an association?" *Saudi Journal of Kidney Diseases and Transplantation*, vol. 23, pp. 925–928, 2012.

[37] A. Vaz, A. Correia, B. Martins et al., "Heyde syndrome: the link between aortic stenosis and gastrointestinal bleeding," *Revista Portuguesa de Cardiologia*, vol. 29, no. 2, pp. 309–314, 2010.

[38] S. Naveau, P. Bedossa, T. Poynard, B. Mory, and J.-C. Chaput, "Portal hypertensive colopathy: a new entity," *Digestive Diseases and Sciences*, vol. 36, no. 12, pp. 1774–1781, 1991.

[39] C. Balzer, E. Lotterer, G. Kleber, and W. E. Fleig, "Transjugular intrahepatic portosystemic shunt for bleeding angiodysplasia-like lesions in portal-hypertensive colopathy," *Gastroenterology*, vol. 115, no. 1, pp. 167–172, 1998.

[40] N. Yuki, M. Kubo, Y. Noro et al., "Jejunal varices as a cause of massive gastrointestinal bleeding," *The American Journal of Gastroenterology*, vol. 87, no. 4, pp. 514–517, 1992.

[41] Y.-E. Joo, H.-S. Kim, S.-K. Choi, J.-S. Rew, H.-R. Kim, and S.-J. Kim, "Massive gastrointestinal bleeding from jejunal varices," *Journal of Gastroenterology*, vol. 35, no. 10, pp. 775–778, 2000.

[42] S. J. B. Van Weyenberg, S. T. Van Turenhout, M. A. Jacobs, G. Bouma, and C. J. J. Mulder, "Video capsule endoscopy for previous overt obscure gastrointestinal bleeding in patients using anti-thrombotic drugs," *Digestive Endoscopy*, vol. 24, pp. 247–254, 2012.

[43] T. Matsumura, M. Arai, S. Sazuka et al., "Negative capsule endoscopy for obscure gastrointestinal bleeding is closely associated with the use of low-dose aspirin," *Scandinavian Journal of Gastroenterology*, vol. 46, no. 5, pp. 621–626, 2011.

[44] H. Imagawa, S. Oka, S. Tanaka et al., "Improved detectability of small-bowel lesions via capsule endoscopy with computed virtual chromoendoscopy: a pilot study," *Scandinavian Journal of Gastroenterology*, vol. 46, no. 9, pp. 1133–1137, 2011.

[45] Y. Kobayashi, H. Watabe, A. Yamada et al., "Efficacy of flexible spectral imaging color enhancement on the detection of small intestinal diseases," *Journal of Diagnostic Diseases*, vol. 13, pp. 614–620, 2012.

[46] G. Duque, N. Almeida, P. Figueiredo et al., "Virtual chromoendoscopy can be a useful software tool in capsule endoscopy," *Revista Espanola de enfermedades Digestivas*, vol. 104, no. 5, pp. 231–236, 2012.

12

Treatment of Internal Hemorrhoids by Endoscopic Sclerotherapy with Aluminum Potassium Sulfate and Tannic Acid

Yuichi Tomiki, Seigo Ono, Jun Aoki, Rina Takahashi, Shun Ishiyama, Kiichi Sugimoto, Yukihiro Yaginuma, Yutaka Kojima, Michitoshi Goto, Atsushi Okuzawa, and Kazuhiro Sakamoto

Department of Coloproctological Surgery, Faculty of Medicine, Juntendo University, 2-1-1 Hongo, Bunkyo-ku, Tokyo 113-8421, Japan

Correspondence should be addressed to Yuichi Tomiki; tomiki@juntendo.ac.jp

Academic Editor: P. J. O'Dwyer

Objective. A new sclerosing agent for hemorrhoids, aluminum potassium sulfate and tannic acid (ALTA), is attracting attention as a curative treatment for internal hemorrhoids without resection. The outcome and safety of ALTA sclerotherapy using an endoscope were investigated in the present study. *Materials and Methods.* Subjects comprised 83 internal hemorrhoid patients (61 males and 22 females). An endoscope was inserted and retroflexed in the rectum, and a 1st-step injection was applied to the upper parts of the hemorrhoids. The retroflexed scope was returned to the normal position, and 2nd–4th-step injections were applied to the middle and lower parts of the hemorrhoids under direct vision. The effects of endoscopic ALTA sclerotherapy were determined by evaluating the condition of the hemorrhoids using an anoscope and interviewing the patient 28 days after the treatment. *Results.* A cure, improvement, and failure were observed in 54 (65.1%), 27 (32.5%), and 2 (2.4%) patients, respectively, treated with ALTA. Complications developed in 4 patients (mild fever in 3 and hematuria in 1). Recurrence occurred in 9.6%. *Conclusions.* The results of the present study suggest that endoscopic ALTA has the potential to become a useful and minimally invasive approach for ALTA sclerotherapy.

1. Introduction

Hemorrhoids are a very common anal disease and, when formed on the upper and lower sides of the dentate line, are classified as internal and external hemorrhoids, respectively. Internal hemorrhoids are the most common anal disease, the symptoms of which include hemorrhage and prolapse.

Internal hemorrhoids are resolved in part by conservative treatments with suppositories and ointments, in addition to lifestyle improvements and the avoidance of straining on defecation; however, subsequent treatments may be necessary when symptoms become aggravated and interfere with daily living activities. The treatment of this disease without resection is desirable because internal hemorrhoids are mostly benign.

Several treatment options are available for patients who do not respond to conservative medical management [1–4]. Rubber band ligation and injection sclerotherapy have been the mainstay of nonsurgical treatments for more than a century and are considered to sufficiently treat hemorrhoids. A meta-analysis of 18 randomized trials that compared various treatment methods for hemorrhoids concluded that rubber band ligation was more effective than sclerotherapy and also that patients who underwent ligation were less likely to need subsequent therapy [5]. However, injection sclerotherapy represents a simple and safe palliative treatment for hemorrhoids. The most common sclerosing agent used is 5% phenol almond oil, which is mainly effective for hemorrhage; however, its effects on prolapse are considered to be insufficient [5].

A new sclerosing agent for hemorrhoids, aluminum potassium sulfate and tannic acid (ALTA: Zione; Mitsubishi Pharma Corporation, Osaka, Japan), is effective for not only hemorrhaging from, but also the prolapse of internal hemorrhoids and is expected to replace surgical treatments [6–8].

Injection sclerotherapy with ALTA for hemorrhoids is now performed in Japan, and its efficacy has been reported [6]. ALTA resolves prolapse and hemorrhage after defecation and has several advantages over surgery in that it is associated with fewer complications, such as pain and hemorrhage after treatment, and shortens the treatment period. Therefore, ALTA has been attracting attention as a new hemorrhoid treatment method without resection.

On the other hand, ALTA damages tissue, and complications, such as rectal ulcer and rectal stenosis, have been reported due to the misplacement of injections [9]. Thus, it has been recommended at workshops that ALTA injections be performed after acquiring sufficient knowledge of anal diseases and fully understanding the surgical procedure. Injection sclerotherapy with ALTA is performed through a procedure termed "4-step injections," which differs from that of conventional injection sclerotherapy in that the agent is injected into 4 regions of the hemorrhoids (upper, deep middle, shallow middle, and lower parts) using an injection needle exclusive for ALTA. Since ALTA is mainly injected into the submucosa, we considered that endoscopic injections using a colonoscope are applicable to ensure submucosal injections [10]. Furthermore, since the injection needle for ALTA is too long to be used for injections into the submucosal layer, an endoscopic injection needle may assist in preventing misplacement of the injection [11].

In the present study, we investigated the outcomes of endoscopic ALTA sclerotherapy and its safety with a literature review.

2. Materials and Methods

2.1. Patients. Subjects comprised 83 patients with internal hemorrhoids (61 males and 22 females) who required treatment for hemorrhage or prolapse between January 2009 and December 2011 and were unsatisfied with conservative steroid suppository treatments.

ALTA was only indicated for internal hemorrhoids, and acute, thrombosed, strangulated, and external hemorrhoids were excluded from the indication. Concomitant resection of anal polyps and skin tags was not performed.

Since the endoscopic administration of ALTA was not included among the procedures recommended at workshops, this study was performed following approval by the Ethics Committee of our hospital (approval number 488) and obtaining informed consent.

2.2. Technique of Endoscopic ALTA Sclerotherapy. Endoscopic ALTA sclerotherapy was performed on all patients at the outpatient clinic (day procedure), and a pretreatment was applied following that for colonoscopy. A thin endoscope was used, and its tip was covered with a transparent hood. A blunt needle (25G, 3 mm in length, Top Corporation, Tokyo, Japan) was used as the endoscopic injection needle (Figure 1).

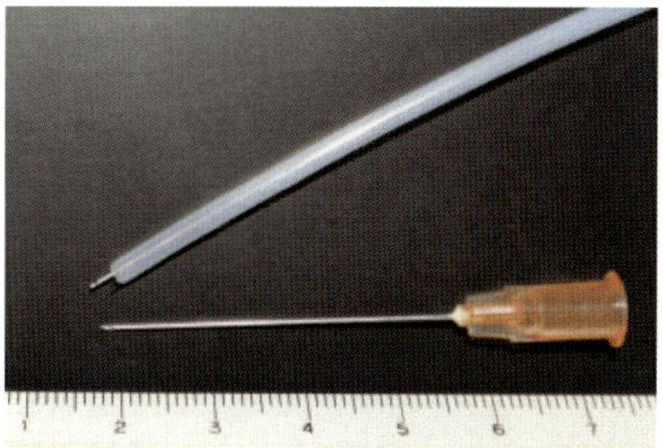

FIGURE 1: Injection needle. Upper: endoscopic injection needle (25G blunt needle with a length of 3 mm, Top Corporation). Lower: injection needle exclusive for ALTA (25G blunt needle with a length of 38 mm, Nipro Corporation).

The treatment was conducted in the left lateral decubitus position after attaching an electrocardiograph and oxygen monitor, and no anesthesia was applied around the anus.

An endoscope was inserted and retroflexed in the rectum. After observations, the 1st-step injection was applied to the upper pole of the hemorrhoids (Figure 2(a)).

The 1st-step injection was applied to 2-3 sites (3 mL/injection) while keeping the endoscope retroflexed. The retroflexed scope was then returned to the normal position, and the 2nd–4th-step injections (2-3 mL/injection) were applied under direct vision (Figure 2(b)). When the endoscope could not be retroflexed in the rectum, the 1st-step injection was applied under direct vision. Injections were applied while confirming that ALTA had been injected into the submucosa on the monitor. Injections were immediately discontinued when the patient complained of pain [10]. The mean dose of the agent per patient was 14.4 ± 4.0 mL.

The scope was removed after the injections. The local region was then massaged with the index finger to diffuse ALTA throughout the region in order to avoid retention at the injection site, and the procedure was completed [6].

2.3. Investigation Items. Patient backgrounds (age, gender, Goligher's classification, ALTA injection dose, and adverse events) and outcomes (treatment effects and recurrence) were investigated.

The effects of ALTA sclerotherapy were determined by evaluating the condition of the hemorrhoids using an anoscope and interviewing the patient 28 days or more after the treatment based on the following evaluation criteria: When the internal hemorrhoid size had decreased on anoscopy and prolapse and hemorrhage after defecation had resolved, the treatment was judged to be markedly effective (cure). When the internal hemorrhoid size had decreased on anoscopy and prolapse and hemorrhage after defecation had remitted but not completely, the treatment was judged to be effective (improvement). When symptoms remained the same after ALTA sclerotherapy regardless of the extent of internal hemorrhoid size reductions, the treatment was determined to be ineffective (failure). During the follow-up, 52 patients who went to the hospital as outpatients were interviewed and examined, while 31 patients who did not go

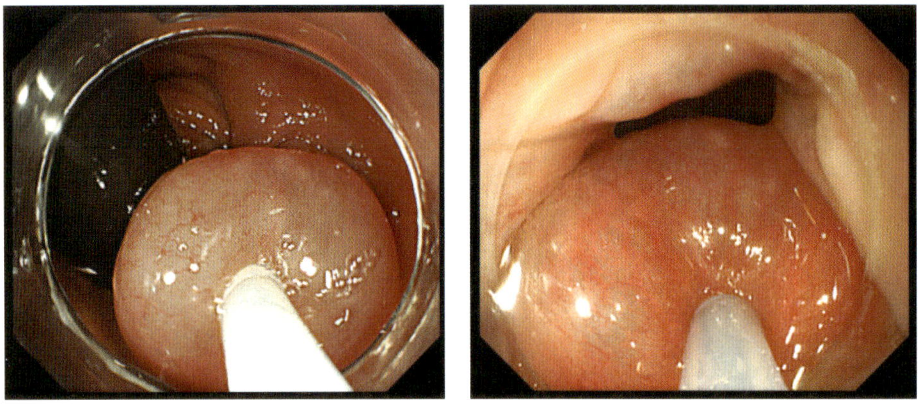

Figure 2: (a) ALTA injection with retroflection of the endoscope as the first step. (b) ALTA injection with a forward-viewing direction as the second to fourth steps.

to hospital were interviewed by the surgeon over the phone one year after ALTA sclerotherapy. The follow-up period ranged from 10 to 62 months with a median of 27 months.

2.4. Safety of Endoscopic ALTA Sclerotherapy. In ALTA sclerotherapy, the agent is mainly injected into the submucosa; however, misplacement of the injection into the muscular layer may occur. In order to verify the safety of endoscopic ALTA sclerotherapy, normal anal regions without tumor infiltration were collected from specimens resected from 12 rectal cancer patients who underwent abdominoperineal resection at our department and were subjected to Elastica van Gieson staining. The distance between the mucosa and muscular layer was measured at 1-2 cm on the oral side from the dentate line, the location at which the rectal venous plexus causing internal hemorrhoids is present, in order to investigate the safety of the endoscopic injections (Figure 3).

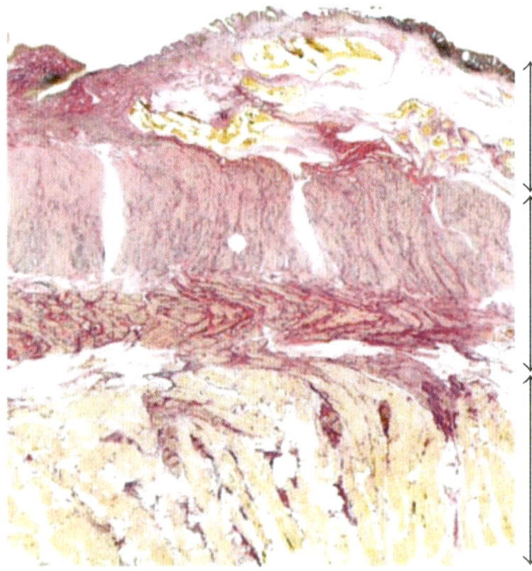

Figure 3: Distance between the mucosa and muscular layer in the lower rectum.

2.5. Comparison with Conventional Injection Sclerotherapy. Conventional injection sclerotherapy with 5% phenol almond oil (sclerosing agent) was compared with ALTA using previous findings [12–15]. Furthermore, conventional ALTA sclerotherapy with an anoscope was similarly examined based on a literature review [6, 7, 16–19].

3. Results

3.1. Background of Endoscopic ALTA Sclerotherapy. ALTA was endoscopically injected into 61 male and 22 female patients (mean age: 60.4 years). The most common Goligher's classification grade of the internal hemorrhoids was III, accounting for 81.9% (68 patients), followed by grade II in 12 patients (14.5%). Three grade IV cases (3.6%) were not complicated by thrombosed external hemorrhoids. ALTA sclerotherapy was conducted to ameliorate prolapse.

No symptoms, such as bradycardia, blood pressure reductions, or discomfort, developed during the procedure. Complications developed in 4 patients (4.8%): fever between 37 and 38°C was observed in 3 patients, and hematuria developed 17 days after the procedure in other patients but was remitted by conservative treatment (Table 1).

3.2. Therapeutic Effects of Endoscopic ALTA. Among the patients treated with endoscopic ALTA, a cure, improvement, and failure were observed in 54 (65.1%), 27 (32.5%), and 2 (2.4%) patients, respectively, treated with ALTA. Goligher's classification of the 2 failure cases' grade was IV. ALTA was not injected into external hemorrhoids. The two failed cases showed soiling of the underwear after the ALTA injection and no improvements were observed in discomfort or itching. Efficacy was noted in 97.6% when cured and improved cases were combined, suggesting that the short-term outcome of ALTA sclerotherapy was favorable (Table 2). ALTA was fast-acting, with its effects being observed immediately after the injections had been performed in some patients.

Table 1: Patient characteristics.

	Endoscopic ALTA (n = 83)
Sex (male : female)	61 : 22
Age	60.4 ± 14.0
Grade of hemorrhoids	
Goligher's classification	
I	0 (0.0%)
II	12 (14.5%)
III	68 (81.9%)
IV	3 (3.6%)
Injection dose (mL)	14.4 ± 4.0
Complications	4 (4.8%)

Table 2: Short-term outcomes of ALTA sclerotherapy.

	Effectiveness of ALTA			
	Cure	Improvement	Failure	Recurrence
Endoscopic ALTA (n = 83)	54 (65.1%)	27 (32.5%)	2 (2.4%)	8 (9.6%)

Recurrence occurred in 8 patients (9.6%), and hemorrhoids recurred within one year in 4. In the fastest case, prolapse was noted after 91 days.

Endoscopic ALTA sclerotherapy was repeated in 6 out of the 8 recurrence cases. In the other 2 cases, one patient requested surgery and the other continued suppository treatment.

Recurrence was not detected in 5 out of the 6 patients retreated with endoscopic ALTA; however, one patient was not satisfied with the effects and underwent surgery at another institution 3 months after second ALTA sclerotherapy.

3.3. Distance between the Mucosa and Muscular Layer in the Lower Rectum. In the 12 rectal cancer patients (8 males and 4 females, mean age: 64.3 years) who underwent abdominoperineal resection, the distance between the mucosa and muscular layer at 1-2 cm on the oral side from the dentate line was 3.3 ± 0.4 mm.

3.4. Comparison with Conventional Injection Sclerotherapy. The short-term outcomes of ALTA appeared to be superior to those of 5% phenol in many studies. However, previous findings suggested that ALTA was more effective than 5% phenol. Anal pain was previously reported to be the main complication of these agents [6, 13, 14]. Previous studies also indicated that recurrence was more common and additional therapy was required more frequently with ALTA than with 5% phenol. However, a 4-year follow-up study by Yano et al. showed no significant difference in effectiveness or the need for additional therapy between ALTA and 5% phenol.

The results of the present study, which were obtained with a flexible endoscope, suggested that no significant differences existed between 5% phenol and ALTA sclerotherapy with an anoscope (Table 3).

4. Discussion

Hemorrhoids are the most common anal disease. Hemorrhoidectomy is often performed as a surgical treatment for internal hemorrhoids but is associated with postoperative pain, longer recovery times, and complications such as bleeding and anal stricture. Therefore, less invasive treatments are desired for the treatment of this disease without resection. Pile suture by the Farag method has traditionally been employed as a nonexcisional method for hemorrhoids [20]. Various treatment methods, such as procedure for prolapse and hemorrhoids (PPH) and transanal hemorrhoidal dearterialization (THD), have recently been developed and employed [21, 22]. Rubber band ligation and injection sclerotherapy have traditionally been employed as effective treatments and have been the mainstay of nonsurgical treatments for more than a century. Previous studies reported that injection sclerotherapy was less effective than rubber band ligation at controlling symptoms and achieving long-term outcomes [4, 5, 15]. Furthermore, the recurrence rate was lower with rubber band ligation than with injection sclerotherapy. Since the advent of aluminum potassium sulfate and tannic acid (ALTA), ALTA sclerotherapy has been employed as a major nonexcisional method in Japan.

ALTA was prepared by partially changing the additives of Xiaozhiling, a sclerosing agent that was approved for injection sclerotherapy for internal hemorrhoids in 2005 in China. The active ingredient of ALTA, aluminum potassium sulfate, induces aseptic acute inflammation after being injected into hemorrhoids. Fibrosis of the hemorrhoid occurs in the repair process and the hemorrhoid scleroses and recesses. Vascular constriction occurs immediately after the injection, which reduces blood flow to the hemorrhoid and stops hemorrhage. On the other hand, tannic acid inhibits excess acute inflammation induced by aluminum potassium sulfate, thereby reducing secondary tissue damage [23]. ALTA is only indicated for internal hemorrhoids; thus, acute, strangulated, and external hemorrhoids are excluded from the indication.

ALTA is injected using a procedure termed "4-step injections." Anesthesia may be applied around the anus (preinjection anesthesia). After insertion of the anoscope, ALTA is injected into the submucosa of internal hemorrhoids. At workshops, practitioners have been instructed to shake the needle tip to confirm that it has not been inserted into the muscular layer when its contact with the muscular layer is felt and then inject ALTA. The injection of ALTA into the narrow submucosa by operating an anoscope with one hand and adjusting a light with the other hand requires skill; therefore, we considered application of the endoscopic mucosal resection technique using an endoscopic injection needle to be safer for submucosal injections. Since this is not instructed at workshops, we carefully performed this procedure by applying a pretreatment following that for colonoscopy to prevent accidents, covering the endoscope tip with a transparent hood to add an anoscopic function and ensuring that ALTA was injected into the submucosa by observing a bulge in the injected regions on a monitor.

The distance between the mucosa and muscular layer was previously reported to be 3.3 ± 0.4 mm in resected

TABLE 3: Comparison with conventional injection sclerotherapy.

References	Patients (n)	Follow-up (months)	Sclerosing agents	Effectiveness (%)	Complications (%)	Recurrence (%)	Additional therapy (%)
Greca et al. 1981 [27]	43	12	5% phenol	70.0	0	30.2	14.0
Gartell et al. 1985 [12]	109	33	5% phenol	70.0	0	—	25.7
Walker et al. 1990 [13]	28	48	5% phenol	35.7	70.2	64.2	14.3
Santos et al. 1993 [14]	189	48	5% phenol	60.3	0.5	8.5	22.2
Kanellos et al. 2003 [15]	80	48	5% phenol	17.5	36.3	63.0	30.0
Shi 1997 [16]	21,361	36	Xiaozhiling	99.0	4.6	1.0	—
Takano et al. 2006 [6]	95	12	ALTA	94.0	49.0	16.0	—
Tokunaga et al. 2010 [17]	784	4–30	ALTA	96.0	1.8	—	—
Hachiro et al. 2011 [7]	448	29	ALTA	—	3.1	—	3.1
Miyamoto et al. 2012 [18]	28	8–21	ALTA	100	21.4	10.7	—
Yano et al. 2014 [19]	57	48	ALTA	53	—	—	22.8
Present study 2015	83	27	ALTA	97.6	4.8	9.6	8.4

—: results absent or not clearly reported in the text.

rectal cancer preparations [24]. Therefore, the possibility of misplacing injections into the muscular layer using an endoscopic injection needle with a length of 3 mm is low unless the needle is strongly pressed into hemorrhoids. Inversely, an injection into a shallow submucosal region with the endoscopic injection needle is also a matter of concern, and it may be important to carefully massage the treated region after injections in order to sufficiently diffuse the drug solution.

The effectiveness of endoscopic injections of sclerosing agents into internal hemorrhoids has already been reported [25, 26], and the principle of endoscopic ALTA sclerotherapy is the same as that of conventional ALTA sclerotherapy, excluding the use of a flexible endoscope.

Endoscopic ALTA sclerotherapy does not require anesthesia, the visual field is favorable, the operative field may be shared through a monitor, and deep insertion of the needle is prevented. Furthermore, the screening step of colorectoanal neoplasia is not necessary. However, this procedure requires a pretreatment with laxatives and the cost of endoscopy cannot be calculated.

In order to determine the therapeutic effects of endoscopic ALTA, its clinical outcomes were compared with those of conventional anoscopic ALTA sclerotherapy. A combination of cured and improved cases showed that endoscopic ALTA remitted symptoms in 97.6%. The incidence of complications was 4.8%; this value was slightly higher when mild symptoms, such as discomfort of the anus, were included and appeared to be slightly lower than that caused by conventional ALTA sclerotherapy, suggesting that this is a less invasive and more effective method than conventional ALTA sclerotherapy. Hematuria developed 17 days after ALTA injections in one patient. Urological complications have been suggested to result from an anteriorly misplaced injection into the prostate, urethra, or periprostatic venous plexus [11]. Even though the endoscopic injection needle was used, injections may have been deep; therefore, injections need to be closely observed in order to ensure submucosal injections on the monitor, and the immediate discontinuation of injections is necessary when the patient complains of pain. In addition, it is important to sufficiently massage the treated region to prevent the local retention of injected ALTA, thereby reducing the risk of complications.

Recurrence occurred in 9.6% of patients. The standard dose of ALTA was 9–13 mL per hemorrhoid and 27–39 mL for 3 hemorrhoids. The endoscopic dose of ALTA applied was low (14 mL per patient), which may have been the cause of recurrence [6]. We set the dose at a lower level as a cautionary measure because endoscopic ALTA is different to the recommended procedure; however, elevations in the dose while paying attention to complications may be necessary. In the present study, sufficient therapeutic effects were achieved for grade II and III internal hemorrhoids at the low dose. A higher ALTA dosage and subsequent treatments, including surgery, may be needed for grade IV internal hemorrhoids. Since ALTA sclerotherapy is not a radical treatment for hemorrhoids and it is positioned between conservative suppository treatments and surgery, a recurrence rate of approximately 10% may be acceptable.

Regarding the long-term outcomes of ALTA, a symptom-free rate of 53% after 4 years has been reported [19]; however, since ALTA is also known to be effective for recurrence, endoscopic ALTA sclerotherapy, which is applicable as a day procedure, may be used as the first-line treatment for recurrent cases.

The present study had the following limitations: a conventional ALTA method with an anoscope and a randomized prospective trial were not conducted. Therefore, further investigations are warranted.

5. Conclusions

Subsequent treatments, including surgery, have been recommended for many cases of internal hemorrhoids for which conservative suppository treatments were ineffective. The results of the present study suggest that the therapeutic effects of ALTA were similar to those of surgery and also that it has the potential to become a breakthrough treatment method for curing internal hemorrhoids without resection. Therefore, endoscopic ALTA has the potential to become a minimally invasive and useful approach for ALTA sclerotherapy.

References

[1] C. G. Solomon and D. Jacobs, "Hemorrhoids," *The New England Journal of Medicine*, vol. 371, no. 10, pp. 944–951, 2014.

[2] D. E. Rivadeneira, S. R. Steele, C. Ternent, S. Chalasani, W. D. Buie, and J. L. Rafferty, "Practice parameters for the management of hemorrhoids (revised 2010)," *Diseases of the Colon & Rectum*, vol. 54, no. 9, pp. 1059–1064, 2011.

[3] D. F. Altomare, A. Roveran, G. Pecorella, F. Gaj, and E. Stortini, "The treatment of hemorrhoids: guidelines of the Italian Society of Colo-Rectal Surgery," *Techniques in Coloproctology*, vol. 10, no. 3, pp. 181–186, 2006.

[4] S. Buntzen, P. Christensen, A. Khalid et al., "Diagnosis and treatment of haemorrhoids," *Danish Medical Journal*, vol. 60, no. 12, Article ID B4754, 2013.

[5] H. M. MacRae and R. S. McLeod, "Comparison of hemorrhoidal treatment modalities. A meta-analysis," *Diseases of the Colon & Rectum*, vol. 38, no. 7, pp. 687–694, 1995.

[6] M. Takano, J. Iwadare, H. Ohba et al., "Sclerosing therapy of internal hemorrhoids with a novel sclerosing agent: comparison with ligation and excision," *International Journal of Colorectal Disease*, vol. 21, no. 1, pp. 44–51, 2006.

[7] Y. Hachiro, M. Kunimoto, T. Abe, M. Kitada, and Y. Ebisawa, "Aluminum potassium sulfate and tannic acid (ALTA) injection as the mainstay of treatment for internal hemorrhoids," *Surgery Today*, vol. 41, no. 6, pp. 806–809, 2011.

[8] S. W. Lim, "Aluminum potassium sulfate and tannic acid injection for hemorrhoids," *Journal of the Korean Society of Coloproctology*, vol. 28, no. 2, pp. 73–77, 2012.

[9] Y. Hachiro, M. Kunimoto, T. Abe, S. Muraki, and M. Kusano, "Strangulation of internal hemorrhoids complicating sclerosing therapy with injection of OC-108 (Zione)," *International Journal of Colorectal Disease*, vol. 22, no. 7, pp. 851–852, 2007.

[10] Y. Tomiki, S. Ono, J. Aoki, R. Takahashi, and K. Sakamoto, "Endoscopic sclerotherapy with aluminum potassium sulfate and tannic acid for internal hemorrhoids," *Endoscopy*, vol. 46, article E114, 2014.

[11] R. Al-Ghnaniem, A. J. M. Leather, and J. A. Rennie, "Survey of methods of treatment of haemorrhoids and complications of injection sclerotherapy," *Annals of the Royal College of Surgeons of England*, vol. 83, no. 5, pp. 325–328, 2001.

[12] P. C. Gartell, R. J. Sheridan, and F. P. McGinn, "Out-patient treatment of haemorrhoids: a randomized clinical trial to compare rubber band ligation with phenol injection," *British Journal of Surgery*, vol. 72, no. 6, pp. 478–479, 1985.

[13] A. J. Walker, R. J. Leicester, R. J. Nicholls, and C. V. Mann, "A prospective study of infrared coagulation, injection and rubber band ligation in the treatment of haemorrhoids," *International Journal of Colorectal Disease*, vol. 5, no. 2, pp. 113–116, 1990.

[14] G. Santos, J. R. Novell, G. Khoury, M. C. Winslet, and A. A. M. Lewis, "Long-term results of large-dose, single-session phenol injection sclerotherapy for hemorrhoids," *Diseases of the Colon & Rectum*, vol. 36, no. 10, pp. 958–961, 1993.

[15] I. Kanellos, I. Goulimaris, E. Christoforidis, T. Kelpis, and D. Betsis, "A comparison of the simultaneous application of sclerotherapy and rubber band ligation, with sclerotherapy and rubber band ligation applied separately, for the treatment of haemorrhoids: a prospective randomized trial," *Colorectal Disease*, vol. 5, no. 2, pp. 133–138, 2003.

[16] Z. Shi, "Xiazhiling four-step injection in treating hemorrhoids of stages III and IV-A sclerotherapeutic approach of thrombosing branches of artery rectalis superior," *Journal of Traditional Chinese Medicine*, vol. 3, pp. 246–249, 1997.

[17] Y. Tokunaga, H. Sasaki, and T. Saito, "Evaluation of sclerotherapy with a new sclerosing agent and stapled hemorrhoidopexy for prolapsing internal hemorrhoids: retrospective comparison with hemorrhoidectomy," *Digestive Surgery*, vol. 27, no. 6, pp. 469–472, 2010.

[18] H. Miyamoto, M. Asanoma, H. Miyamoto, and M. Shimada, "ALTA injection sclerosing therapy: non-excisional treatment of internal hemorrhoids," *Hepato-Gastroenterology*, vol. 59, no. 113, pp. 77–80, 2012.

[19] T. Yano, M. Asano, S. Tanaka, N. Oda, and Y. Matsuda, "A prospective study comparing the new sclerotherapy and hemorrhoidectomy in terms of therapeutic outcomes at 4 years after the treatment," *Surgery Today*, vol. 44, no. 3, pp. 449–453, 2014.

[20] A. El-Meguid Farag, "Pile suture: a new technique for the treatment of haemorrhoids," *British Journal of Surgery*, vol. 65, no. 4, pp. 293–295, 1978.

[21] S. Festen, M. J. van Hoogstraten, A. A. W. van Geloven, and M. F. Gerhards, "Treatment of grade III and IV haemorrhoidal disease with PPH or THD. A randomized trial on postoperative complications and short-term results," *International Journal of Colorectal Disease*, vol. 24, no. 12, pp. 1401–1405, 2009.

[22] P. Giordano, J. Overton, F. Madeddu, S. Zaman, and G. Gravante, "Transanal hemorrhoidal dearterialization: a systematic review," *Diseases of the Colon and Rectum*, vol. 52, no. 9, pp. 1665–1671, 2009.

[23] T. Ono, K. Goto, S. Takagi, S. Iwasaki, and H. Komatsu, "Sclerosing effect of OC-108, a novel agent for hemorrhoids,

is associated with granulomatous inflammation induced by aluminum," *Journal of Pharmacological Sciences*, vol. 99, no. 4, pp. 353–363, 2005.

[24] S. A. Pilkington, A. C. Bateman, S. Wombwell, and R. Miller, "Anatomical basis for impotence following haemorrhoid sclerotherapy," *Annals of the Royal College of Surgeons of England*, vol. 82, no. 5, pp. 303–306, 2000.

[25] ASGE Technology Committee, U. D. Siddiqui, B. A. Barth et al., "Devices for the endoscopic treatment of hemorrhoids," *Gastrointestinal Endoscopy*, vol. 79, no. 1, pp. 8–14, 2014.

[26] J. L. Ponsky, J. D. Mellinger, and I. B. Simon, "Endoscopic retrograde hemorrhoidal sclerotherapy using 23.4% saline: a preliminary report," *Gastrointestinal Endoscopy*, vol. 37, no. 2, pp. 155–158, 1991.

[27] F. Greca, M. M. Hares, E. Nevah, J. Alexander-Williams, and M. R. Keighley, "A randomized trial to compare rubber band ligation with phenol injection for treatment of haemorrhoids," *British Journal of Surgery*, vol. 68, no. 4, pp. 250–252, 1981.

13

Capsule Endoscopy for Obscure Gastrointestinal Bleeding in Patients with Comorbid Rheumatic Diseases

Neal Shahidi,[1] George Ou,[1] Jessica Tong,[1] Ricky Kwok,[1] Cherry Galorport,[1] Joanna K. Law,[1,2] and Robert Enns[1,3]

[1] *Department of Medicine, Division of Gastroenterology, University of British Columbia, Vancouver, BC, Canada V5Z 1M9*
[2] *Department of Medicine, Division of Gastroenterology, Johns Hopkins University, Baltimore, MD 21205, USA*
[3] *St. Paul's Hospital, University of British Columbia, Pacific Gastroenterology Associates, 770-1190 Hornby Street, Vancouver, BC, Canada V6Z 2K5*

Correspondence should be addressed to Robert Enns; rob.enns@ubc.ca

Academic Editor: Tony C. K. Tham

Background and Aim. We evaluated the association between patients with rheumatic diseases (RD) suffering from obscure gastrointestinal bleeding (OGIB) and positive capsule endoscopy (CE) findings. *Methods.* All CE procedures performed on patients with RD and OGIB were assessed from a large database at St. Paul's Hospital (Vancouver, BC, Canada) between December 2001 and April 2011. A positive finding on CE was defined as any pathology, including ulcers/erosions, vascular lesions, and mass lesions, perceived to be the source of bleeding. *Results.* Of the 1133 CEs performed, 41 (4%) complete CEs were for OGIB in patients with RD. Of these, 54% presented with overt bleeding. Mean age was 66 years. Positive findings were seen in 61% of patients. Ulcerations/erosions (36%) and vascular lesions (36%) were the most common findings. Significant differences between the RD versus non-RD populations included: inpatient status, nonsteroidal anti-inflammatory drug (NSAIDs) use, oral steroid use, and mean Charlson index score (all $P \leq 0.008$). Similar nonsignificant trends were seen between positive and negative CEs among the RD population. *Conclusions.* The correlation between RD and positive CE findings is likely influenced by ongoing anti-inflammatory drug use, poorer health status, and a predisposition for angiodysplastic lesions.

1. Introduction

Capsule endoscopy (CE) is a novel diagnostic technique which allows assessment of the entire small bowel that is not feasible with conventional endoscopy. Its noninvasive nature together with its documented high sensitivity and specificity [1–3] has encouraged its use most notably in obscure gastrointestinal bleeding (OGIB). With OGIB comprising approximately 5% of all gastrointestinal bleeds, it represents a significant economic burden with multiple studies attempting to optimize investigational algorithms through cost-effectiveness analyses [4–7]. While identifying the source of OGIB early is characteristically uncommon, CE has led to an increased feasibility for identifying pathology allowing for superior patient outcomes, alongside a potential reduction in resource utilization [1, 2, 8] from repeated, expensive investigations.

With the emergence of CE as a pivotal tool in current investigational algorithms for OGIB, consequent studies [1, 8–11] have attempted to identify predictors of positive findings on CE with the goal of refining patient selection to optimize diagnostic yield. In a recent study assessing this correlation, we identified comorbid rheumatic diseases (RD) as a significant correlate to positive findings on CE [11]. While studies exist describing the association between gastrointestinal bleeding and RD, there is an overall deficit in the literature focusing on patients with RD suffering specifically from OGIB [12–14]. Therefore, we sought to further evaluate this correlation between patients with RD being evaluated for OGIB and positive pathology on CE.

2. Methods

2.1. Population Description. All CE cases performed between December 2001 and April 2011 at St. Paul's Hospital (Vancouver, British Columbia, Canada) for the evaluation of OGIB in patients with comorbid RD were considered for inclusion. These cases were a specific subpopulation of a previous retrospective evaluation of all CE procedures performed for the evaluation of OGIB [11]. Written approval was obtained from our institutional ethics committee. Obscure gastrointestinal bleeding was defined as gastrointestinal bleeding with no apparent source subsequent to evaluation of the upper and lower gastrointestinal tracts by conventional endoscopic methods. Bleeding was stratified into overt bleeding (hematemesis, hematochezia, or melena) and occult bleeding (positive fecal occult blood test, iron deficiency anemia, or an acute drop in hemoglobin). Cases were excluded if patients had significant findings on conventional endoscopy and CE was undertaken to confirm that there were no other potential sources within the small bowel. The Charlson index [15, 16] was used as a framework for the definition of RD.

2.2. Capsule Endoscopy Procedure and Interpretation. Included CE procedures were performed using PillCam (Given Imaging, Yoqneam, Isreal), EndoCapsule (Olympus, Tokyo, Japan), or MiroCam (IntroMedic, Seoul, Korea). Informed consent was obtained prior to all CE procedures. All participants were instructed to stop oral iron supplementation 5 days prior to CE and to undergo bowel preparation which included adherence to a clear fluid diet and ingestion of 2 L of polyethylene glycol-electrolyte solution. Patients were allowed to drink and eat at 2 and 4 hours after ingestion of the capsule camera, respectively.

Subsequent to administration, the capsule assistant, the gastrointestinal therapeutics fellow, and a single experienced gastroenterologist reviewed each CE procedure independently with any discrepancy in findings being resolved by consensus. Positive findings on CE were defined as any definitive pathology (e.g., ulcers/erosions, vascular lesions, and mass lesions) perceived to be the source of bleeding. Fresh blood was also considered a positive finding as it suggests proximity of the lesion. In cases where multiple findings were identified, the most prominent lesion was recorded alongside its location. CE which (1) did not enter the small bowel, (2) traversed the small bowel for less than 1 hour in an unremarkable study, or (3) had excessive debris obscuring the examination warranting repeat procedure was considered incomplete.

2.3. Data Collection and Statistical Analysis. Data was extracted by two independent authors (NS, GO) retrospectively, with discrepancy being resolved by consensus with a third author (RE). Comorbid status was assessed utilizing definitions outlined by the Charlson Index [15, 16]. Identical definitions for covariables were utilized as in our previous study [11]. Further covariables were extracted including the use of selective serotonin reuptake inhibitors (SSRIs), immunomodulators (azathioprine, hydroxychloroquine, cyclosporine, penicillamine, gold therapy, leflunomide, methotrexate, minocycline, and sulfasalazine), and biologic therapies. Follow-up data were obtained in a retrospective manner up to 1 year after CE or after confirmatory testing.

Differences in demographic characteristics and comorbid disease states between both CE positive (CE+) and CE negative (CE−) cases among the RD population and between the RD and non-RD populations [11] were evaluated using Fisher's exact test, chi-square test, or t-test as appropriate. A P value of <0.05 was deemed to be statistically significant.

3. Results

A total of 1133 CE procedures were performed between December 2001 and April 2011, with 42 CE cases for the indication of OGIB in patients with comorbid RD. One case was incomplete which was subsequently excluded from analysis leaving 41 complete CE cases. The most common diagnoses were rheumatoid arthritis ($n = 18$), polymyalgia rheumatica ($n = 6$), scleroderma ($n = 5$), systemic lupus erythematosus ($n = 5$), and dermatomyositis ($n = 2$). Mean age was 66 years with 27% being male (Table 1). Most cases were completed on an outpatient basis (80%). Twenty-two patients presented with a history of overt bleeding, with melena being the most common overt symptomatic presentation. Among those who presented with occult bleeding, 11 tested positive for fecal occult blood, 7 were confirmed to simply have iron deficiency anemia, and 1 had an acute decline in hemoglobin with suspected gastrointestinal etiology. The majority of cases (78%) had symptoms for greater than 24 weeks. Concerning precapsule endoscopic assessment, the mean number of esophagogastroduodenoscopies (EGDs), enteroscopies, and colonoscopies was 1.8, 0.5, and 1.6, respectively. The most common comorbidities in this cohort included chronic pulmonary disease (15%), diabetes with or without end-organ complications (12% each), and moderate to severe renal disease (15%) (Table 2). As for medications, proton pump inhibitors (66%), immunomodulators (39%), oral steroids (29%), antiplatelet/coagulants (22%), nonsteroidal anti-inflammatory drugs (NSAIDs) (22%), and SSRIs (12%) were common. Biologic therapy was seen in 1 case. Only 27% of cases had no history of transfusion requirements.

Of the 41 complete CE procedures, 61% identified a definitive source of gastrointestinal bleeding (Table 3). The most common findings were erosions/ulcerations (36%) and angiodysplastic/vascular lesions (36%). Sources of pathology were frequently located in the small bowel (84%) as expected given negative precapsule evaluations. However, gastric pathologies were identified in 3 cases and cecal pathology in 1 case. No capsule related adverse events were seen but 6 CEs did not reach the cecum by the end of the camera battery life and 1 was retained in the stomach due to a stricture/lesion.

Following identification of positive findings, further intervention was recommended in 15/25 of cases. Follow-up data were available for 13/15 of cases with pathology

TABLE 1: Demographic and clinical characteristics of included cases.

Characteristics	Negative CE (N = 16)		Positive CE (N = 25)		P value	RHEUM CE (N = 41)		Non-RHEUM CE (N = 627)		P value
	N (%)	SD	N (%)	SD		N (%)	SD	N (%)	SD	
Mean age (years)	64.50	17.05	67.68	9.59	0.449	66.44	12.91	63.19	15.26	0.183
Gender (male)	3 (18.8)		8 (32.0)		0.478	11 (26.8)		321 (51.2)		0.003
Status (inpatient)	2 (12.5)		6 (24.0)		0.448	8 (19.5)		42 (6.7)		0.008
Indication for CE					0.121					0.483
Occult	5 (31.3)		14 (56.0)			19 (46.3)		326 (52.0)		
Overt	11 (68.8)		11 (44.0)			22 (53.7)		301 (48.0)		
Occult breakdown										
Anemia	1 (20.0)		0 (0)			1 (5.3)		18 (2.9)		
IDA	3 (60.0)		4 (28.6)			7 (36.8)		130 (20.7)		
FOBT+	1 (20.0)		10 (71.4)			11 (57.9)		178 (28.4)		
Overt breakdown										
Hematemesis	1 (6.3)		0 (0)			1 (2.4)		9 (1.4)		
Hematochezia	4 (25.0)		4 (16.0)			8 (19.5)		124 (19.8)		
Melena	6 (37.5)		8 (32.0)			14 (34.2)		193 (30.8)		
Duration of problem					0.865					0.309
0–8 weeks	2 (12.5)		3 (12.0)			5 (12.2)		44 (7.0)		
9–24 weeks	2 (12.5)		2 (8.0)			4 (9.8)		51 (8.1)		
>24 weeks	12 (75.0)		20 (80.0)			32 (78.1)		532 (84.9)		
Mean EGDs	1.63	0.96	1.96	1.81	0.507	1.83	1.53	1.84	1.09	0.956
Mean enteroscopies	0.38	0.50	0.52	0.51	0.393	0.46	0.50	0.56	1.07	0.553
Mean colonoscopies	1.56	0.81	1.56	0.71	1.000	1.56	0.74	1.90	1.17	0.067
Excessive alcohol	0 (0)		1 (4.0)		1.000	1 (2.4)		43 (6.9)		0.510
Smoking	0 (0)		1 (4.0)		1.000	1 (2.4)		65 (10.4)		0.169
NSAIDs	2 (12.5)		7 (28.0)		0.441	9 (22.0)		23 (3.7)		<0.001
Antiplatelet/coagulation	4 (25.0)		5 (20.0)		0.717	9 (22.0)		97 (15.5)		0.271
Oral steroids	4 (25.0)		8 (32.0)		0.734	12 (29.3)		16 (2.6)		<0.001
Proton pump inhibitors	12 (75.0)		15 (60.0)		0.323	27 (65.9)		252 (40.2)		0.001
Number of transfusions					0.623					0.842
0 units	6 (37.5)		5 (20.0)			11 (26.8)		177 (28.2)		
1-2 units	1 (6.3)		3 (12.0)			4 (9.8)		68 (10.9)		
3–9 units	4 (25.0)		6 (24.0)			10 (24.4)		181 (28.9)		
≥10 units	5 (31.3)		11 (44.0)			16 (39.0)		201 (32.0)		

CE: capsule endoscopy; EGDs: esophagogastroduodenoscopies; FOBT+: fecal occult blood test positive; IDA: iron deficiency anemia; NSAIDs: nonsteroidal anti-inflammatory drugs; SD: standard deviation.

Table 2: Comorbid diseases of included cases.

Characteristics	Negative CE (N = 16)		Positive CE (N = 25)		P value	RHEUM CE (N = 41)		Non-RHEUM CE (N = 627)		P value
	N (%)	SD	N (%)	SD		N (%)	SD	N (%)	SD	
Myocardial infarction history	1 (6.3)		1 (4.0)		1.000	2 (4.9)		45 (7.2)		0.760
Congestive heart failure	0 (0)		1 (4.0)		1.000	1 (2.4)		59 (9.4)		0.164
Peripheral vascular disease	2 (12.5)		1 (4.0)		0.550	3 (7.3)		26 (4.2)		0.413
Cerebrovascular disease	1 (6.3)		1 (4.0)		1.000	2 (4.9)		47 (7.5)		0.760
Dementia	0 (0)		0 (0)		1.000	0 (0)		3 (0.5)		1.000
Chronic pulmonary disease	3 (18.8)		3 (12.0)		0.662	6 (14.6)		66 (10.5)		0.432
History of ulcer disease	2 (12.5)		2 (8.0)		0.637	4 (9.8)		53 (8.5)		0.771
Mild liver disease	0 (0)		4 (16.0)		0.143	4 (9.8)		21 (3.4)		0.060
Diabetes w/o end-organ damage	2 (12.5)		3 (12.0)		1.000	5 (12.2)		100 (16.0)		0.522
Hemiplegia or paraplegia	0 (0)		0 (0)		1.000	0 (0)		3 (0.5)		1.000
Diabetes w/end-organ damage	1 (6.3)		4 (16.0)		0.632	5 (12.2)		48 (7.7)		0.362
Moderate-severe renal disease	1 (6.3)		5 (20.0)		0.376	6 (14.6)		60 (9.6)		0.280
Any tumor	3 (18.8)		4 (16.0)		1.000	7 (17.1)		96 (15.3)		0.762
Leukemia	0 (0)		0 (0)		1.000	0 (0)		5 (0.8)		1.000
Lymphoma	0 (0)		1 (4.0)		1.000	1 (2.4)		10 (1.6)		0.505
Moderate-severe liver disease	0 (0)		1 (4.0)		1.000	1 (2.4)		11 (1.8)		0.535
Metastatic solid tumor	0 (0)		0 (0)		1.000	0 (0)		7 (1.1)		1.000
AIDS	0 (0)		0 (0)		1.000	0 (0)		0 (0)		1.000
Mean Charlson index	2.31	1.54	2.88	1.56	0.258	2.66	1.56	1.50	1.93	<0.001

AIDS: acquired immunodeficiency syndrome.

TABLE 3: Capsule endoscopy results.

Characteristics	N (%)
CE system	
PillCam	29 (70.7)
EndoCapsule	10 (24.4)
MiroCam	2 (4.9)
CE results	
Negative	16 (39.0)
Positive	25 (61.0)
Type of positive findings	
Mass lesion	3 (12.0)
Blood on CE	4 (16.0)
Erosions/ulcerations	9 (36.0)
Angiodysplastic/vascular lesions	9 (36.0)
Location of findings	
Esophagus	0 (0.0)
Stomach	3 (12.0)
Small bowel	21 (84.0)
Large bowel	1 (4.0)

CE: capsule endoscopy.

confirmed in 8/13 of cases. This included 2 mass lesions and 1 ulcerated lesion at an anastomotic site which were surgically excised. Alternatively, 4 angiodysplastic lesions and 1 case of gastric antral vascular ectasia were identified on subsequent upper endoscopy and were treated with argon plasma coagulation. Follow-up data were available in all 8 cases subsequent to intervention for a mean of 10 months, with rebleeding occurring in 63% of cases.

Among the 10 CE+ cases where conservative management was recommended, follow-up was available in 3/10 of cases, over a mean of 6 months with 67% suffering from rebleeding. Concerning the CE− cases, all 16 cases underwent conservative management. Follow-up data were available among 10/16 of cases over a mean of 5 months with 60% suffering from rebleeding.

In comparing the RD versus non-RD populations, statistically significant differences were noted concerning male gender, inpatient status, mean Charlson index, NSAID use, oral steroid use, and proton pump inhibitor use (all $P \leq 0.008$). Similar trends, albeit not statistically significant, were seen comparing the CE+ versus CE− RD cases concerning inpatient status, mean Charlson index, NSAID use, and oral steroid use.

4. Discussion

The evaluation of OGIB continues to become increasingly complex, with a myriad of costly diagnostic procedures. Consequently, not only does inappropriate diagnostic selection impair early diagnosis but also incurs increased costs placing onus on the refinement of current investigational algorithms. Recently, studies have surfaced evaluating the association of clinical and demographic factors with positive outcomes in CE [1, 8–11, 17]. With the recent emergence of RD as a novel significant predictor of positive findings, we sought to further elucidate this association. Our study shows that the correlation between RD and positive CE findings is influenced in a multifactorial manner; specifically, ongoing anti-inflammatory drug use, overall poorer health status, and a predisposition to vascular lesions may be pivotal factors driving this association.

Anti-inflammatory medications, specifically NSAIDs, are a cornerstone in the management of RD [18], with their gastrointestinal adverse effects well recognized in the literature [19, 20]. Specific to the small bowel, previously documented NSAID-induced lesions include erosions, ulcerations, mucosal diaphragms, strictures, and NSAID-associated enteropathy [21, 22]. As highlighted in our study, a potentially significant contributing factor for the correlation between RD and positive CE findings is the ongoing utilization of NSAIDs. Patients with comorbid RD were significantly more likely to consume NSAIDs compared to patients without RD suffering from OGIB described in our previous study (22% versus 4%, resp.) [11]. Furthermore, analyses within the RD subpopulation showed that regular NSAID use was more prevalent among CE+ cases (28%) compared to CE− cases (13%). Interestingly, NSAID use has not been shown in the literature to be a significant correlate with positive CE findings and this is surprising since it is well known that NSAIDs commonly result in small bowel mucosal breaks for which current methods of cytoprotection are not beneficial. However, perhaps the lack of reporting that NSAIDs increase the yield of positive findings on CE may be due to a lack of patient-reported NSAID use [23, 24].

In a recent study by Sidhu et al. [25] evaluating the surreptitious use of NSAIDs including aspirin in patients undergoing CE, 10/76 (14%) of patients were found to have urinalysis suggestive of NSAID use. Only 10% of these cases declared their utilization. Of the 10 cases with suspected NSAID use, 8 had positive findings on CE including erosions ($n = 5$), ulcerations ($n = 2$), and ulceration with early stricturing ($n = 1$). The findings by Sidhu et al. are supported by 3 CE+ cases within our study where suspected NSAID-induced pathology was identified despite patients' denial of regular NSAID use. This highlights the importance of rigorous questioning regarding the use of NSAIDs on history, specifically over-the-counter forms of these medications.

An interesting finding of our study is that multiple comorbid disease states (diabetes with end-organ damage, mild liver disease, and moderate to severe renal disease) were more prevalent not only within the RD population, but also on subanalyses among CE+ cases compared to CE− cases. A statistically significant difference was noted concerning the Charlson index as well as inpatient status. In isolation, inpatient status [10] and liver disease [17] have been shown to significantly correlate with positive CE findings on multivariate analyses. Comparable trends have been found for diabetes with end-organ damage [11], renal disease, [17] and Charlson index scores [11], albeit solely on univariate analyses. By all things in consideration, we feel that these isolated comorbid states may have played a potentially additive or synergistic role in conjunction with overall poorer health status within the RD population predisposing them to more readily apparent gastrointestinal lesions on CE.

Another potential factor driving the correlation between RD and positive CE findings was a predisposition to vascular/angiodysplastic lesions. Vascular lesions are common findings on CE, with a recent systematic review identifying angiodysplasia as the most prevalent finding on CE in patients with OGIB [3]. In our study, vascular lesions were the most common finding at 36%, which was equal to erosions/ulcerations. Notably, this was greater than the overall general population of OGIB cases (26%) extracted over the same time period [11]. Among those suffering from scleroderma, all positive findings were vascular/angiodysplastic in nature. This correlation between scleroderma and gastrointestinal vascular lesions has been documented in the literature [12], with case reports focusing on this relationship in patients with OGIB [13, 14].

Unfortunately, our study was not devoid of limitations. Specifically, it is retrospective in design and data were obtained from a single tertiary health centre. Furthermore, due to small sample size, statistical analysis that aimed at identifying significant correlations was limited, specifically when comparing CE+ versus CE− cases among the RD population. Lastly, our assessment of rebleeding after CE was limited, as our database was not initially designed to collect this data; therefore, it may overestimate the rebleeding risk given that patients without rebleeding were likely not commonly seen in follow-up.

In summary, optimization of current investigational algorithms through the identification of clinical correlates with positive CE findings is critical. In our study, we show that the previously identified correlation between RD and positive CE findings is likely driven by ongoing anti-inflammatory drug use, poor overall health status, and a predisposition to vascular lesions within the small bowel. This highlights the importance of minimizing the use of anti-inflammatory medications in this patient population as endoscopic and surgical management have limited benefit. Further analyses, specifically prospective studies that aim at further elucidating this correlation, are needed. Moreover, cost-effectiveness analyses are needed to assess the already identified correlates with positive CE findings to see whether further modification to diagnostic algorithms is warranted.

Acknowledgments

The authors would like to thank Terry Lee and Joel Singer for their assistance with statistical analysis.

References

[1] M. Pennazio, R. Santucci, E. Rondonotti et al., "Outcome of patients with obscure gastrointestinal bleeding after capsule endoscopy: report of 100 consecutive cases," *Gastroenterology*, vol. 126, no. 3, pp. 643–653, 2004.

[2] M. Delvaux, I. Fassler, and G. Gay, "Clinical usefulness of the endoscopic video capsule as the initial intestinal investigation in patients with obscure digestive bleeding: validation of a diagnostic strategy based on the patient outcome after 12 months," *Endoscopy*, vol. 36, no. 12, pp. 1067–1073, 2004.

[3] Z. Liao, R. Gao, C. Xu, and Z. S. Li, "Indications and detection, completion, and retention rates of small-bowel capsule endoscopy: a systematic review," *Gastrointestinal Endoscopy*, vol. 71, no. 2, pp. 280–286, 2010.

[4] C. Cellier, "Obscure gastrointestinal bleeding: role of videocapsule and double-balloon enteroscopy," *Best Practice and Research: Clinical Gastroenterology*, vol. 22, no. 2, pp. 329–340, 2008.

[5] L. Gerson and A. Kamal, "Cost-effectiveness analysis of management strategies for obscure GI bleeding," *Gastrointestinal Endoscopy*, vol. 68, no. 5, pp. 920–936, 2008.

[6] J. Vlachogiannakos, K. Papaxoinis, N. Viazis et al., "Bleeding lesions within reach of conventional endoscopy in capsule endoscopy examinations for obscure gastrointestinal bleeding: is repeating endoscopy economically feasible?" *Digestive Diseases and Sciences*, vol. 56, no. 6, pp. 1763–1768, 2011.

[7] M. Somsouk, I. M. Gralnek, and J. M. Inadomi, "Management of obscure occult gastrointestinal bleeding: a cost-minimization analysis," *Clinical Gastroenterology and Hepatology*, vol. 6, no. 6, pp. 661–670, 2008.

[8] E. J. Carey, J. A. Leighton, R. I. Heigh et al., "A single-center experience of 260 consecutive patients undergoing capsule endoscopy for obscure gastrointestinal bleeding," *American Journal of Gastroenterology*, vol. 102, no. 1, pp. 89–95, 2007.

[9] W. Selby, "Can clinical features predict the likelihood of finding abnormalities when using capsule endoscopy in patients with GI bleeding of obscure origin?" *Gastrointestinal Endoscopy*, vol. 59, no. 7, pp. 782–787, 2004.

[10] L. Lepileur, X. Dray, M. Antonietti et al., "Factors associated with diagnosis of obscure gastrointestinal bleeding by video capsule enteroscopy," *Clinical Gastroenterology and Hepatology*, vol. 10, no. 12, pp. 1376–1380, 2012.

[11] N. C. Shahidi, G. Ou, S. Svarta et al., "Factors associated with positive findings from capsule endoscopy in patients with obscure gastrointestinal bleeding," *Clinical Gastroenterology and Hepatology*, vol. 10, no. 12, pp. 1381–1385, 2012.

[12] A. Duchini and S. L. Sessoms, "Gastrointestinal hemorrhage in patients with systemic sclerosis and CREST syndrome," *American Journal of Gastroenterology*, vol. 93, no. 9, pp. 1453–1456, 1998.

[13] H. Khanlou, A. Malhotra, F. Friedenberg, and K. Rothstein, "Jejunal telangiectasias as a cause of massive bleeding in a patient with scleroderma," *Revue du Rhumatisme*, vol. 66, no. 2, pp. 119–121, 1999.

[14] G. Vautier, E. McDermott, J. E. Carty, and B. B. Scott, "Small bowel telangiectasia in scleroderma.," *Annals of the Rheumatic Diseases*, vol. 54, no. 1, article 78, 1995.

[15] M. E. Charlson, P. Pompei, K. A. Ales, and C. R. MacKenzie, "A new method of classifying prognostic comorbidity in longitudinal studies: development and validation," *Journal of Chronic Diseases*, vol. 40, no. 5, pp. 373–383, 1987.

[16] H. Quan, V. Sundararajan, P. Halfon et al., "Coding algorithms for defining comorbidities in ICD-9-CM and ICD-10 administrative data," *Medical Care*, vol. 43, no. 11, pp. 1130–1139, 2005.

[17] R. Sidhu, D. S. Sanders, K. Kapur, J. S. Leeds, and M. E. McAlindon, "Factors predicting the diagnostic yield and intervention

in obscure gastrointestinal bleeding investigated using capsule endoscopy," *Journal of Gastrointestinal and Liver Diseases*, vol. 18, no. 3, pp. 273–278, 2009.

[18] C. Baum, D. L. Kennedy, and M. B. Forbes, "Utilization of nonsteroidal antiinflammatory drugs," *Arthritis and Rheumatism*, vol. 28, no. 6, pp. 686–692, 1985.

[19] J. M. Scheiman, "NSAID-induced peptic ulcer disease: a critical review of pathogenesis and management," *Digestive Diseases*, vol. 12, no. 4, pp. 210–222, 1994.

[20] D. J. Bjorkman and M. B. Kimmey, "Nonsteroidal antiinflammatory drugs and gastrointestinal disease: pathophysiology, treatment and prevention," *Digestive Diseases*, vol. 13, no. 2, pp. 119–129, 1995.

[21] M. C. Allison, A. G. Howatson, C. J. Torrance, F. D. Lee, and R. I. Russell, "Gastrointestinal damage associated with the use of nonsteroidal antiinflammatory drugs," *New England Journal of Medicine*, vol. 327, no. 11, pp. 749–754, 1992.

[22] I. Bjarnason, J. Hayllar, A. J. MacPherson, and A. S. Russell, "Side effects of nonsteroidal anti-inflammatory drugs on the small and large intestine in humans," *Gastroenterology*, vol. 104, no. 6, pp. 1832–1847, 1993.

[23] T. Ong, C. J. Hawkey, and K. Y. Ho, "Nonsteroidal antiinflammatory drug use is a significant cause of peptic ulcer disease in a tertiary hospital in Singapore: a prospective study," *Journal of Clinical Gastroenterology*, vol. 40, no. 9, pp. 795–800, 2006.

[24] B. I. Hirschowitz and A. Lanas, "Intractable upper gastrointestinal ulceration due to aspirin in patients who have undergone surgery for peptic ulcer," *Gastroenterology*, vol. 114, no. 5, pp. 883–892, 1998.

[25] R. Sidhu, S. Morley, L. Brunt, D. S. Sanders, and M. E. McAlindon, "PTH-095 Surreptitious use of non-steroidal antiinflammatory drugs and aspirin may be responsible for small bowel injury seen by capsule endoscopy," *Gut*, vol. 59, article A162, 2010.

14

Narrow Band Imaging with Magnification Endoscopy for Celiac Disease: Results from a Prospective, Single-Center Study

L. De Luca,[1] L. Ricciardiello,[2] M. B. L. Rocchi,[3] M. T. Fabi,[1] M. L. Bianchi,[1] A. de Leone,[1] S. Fiori,[1] and D. Baroncini[1]

[1] *Gastroenterology and Digestive Endoscopy Unit, "San Salvatore" Hospital, Piazzale Cinelli, I-61121 Pesaro, Italy*
[2] *Department of Clinical Medicine, University of Bologna, Via Massarenti 9, 40138 Bologna, Italy*
[3] *Department of SUAN, University of Urbino, Via Ca le Suore 2/4, 61029 Urbino, Italy*

Correspondence should be addressed to L. De Luca; lucadeluca1210@gmail.com

Academic Editor: Lars Aabakken

In celiac disease (CD), the intestinal lesions can be patchy and partial villous atrophy may elude detection at standard endoscopy (SE). Narrow Band Imaging (NBI) system in combination with a magnifying endoscope (ME) is a simple tool able to obtain targeted biopsy specimens. The aim of the study was to assess the correlation between NBI-ME and histology in CD diagnosis and to compare diagnostic accuracy between NBI-ME and SE in detecting villous abnormalities in CD. Forty-four consecutive patients with suspected CD undergoing upper gastrointestinal endoscopy have been prospectively evaluated. Utilizing both SE and NBI-ME, observed surface patterns were compared with histological results obtained from biopsy specimens using the k-Cohen agreement coefficient. NBI-ME identified partial villous atrophy in 12 patients in whom SE was normal, with sensitivity, specificity, and accuracy of 100%, 92.6%, and 95%, respectively. The overall agreement between NBI-ME and histology was significantly higher when compared with SE and histology (kappa score: 0.90 versus 0.46; $P = 0.001$) in diagnosing CD. NBI-ME could help identify partial mucosal atrophy in the routine endoscopic practice, potentially reducing the need for blind biopsies. NBI-ME was superior to SE and can reliably predict *in vivo* the villous changes of CD.

1. Introduction

Standard endoscopy (SE) does not usually allow the visualization of duodenal villous patterns and may be inaccurate in patients with celiac disease (CD) [1–4]. In CD the intestinal damages can have a patchy, "stain-like" distribution, and the macroscopic features can be more or less dependent on the degree/severity of the histological lesions [2]. Indeed, at SE, partial villous atrophy may elude detection, and a normal endoscopic appearance of the mucosa does not necessarily imply normal histology.

Several endoscopic features observed during SE reflect the presence of villous atrophy; however their sensitivity varies from 50% to 94% [5, 6]. Sensitivity is particularly low in patients with subclinical CD, partial villous atrophy, or patchy disease [1, 2, 7]. Improved visual identification of suspected mucosal atrophy could assist in targeting biopsies and thereby increasing the sensitivity of endoscopy [8]. Different emerging techniques have been evaluated, alone or in combination, to enhance the ability of the endoscopist to detect mucosal abnormalities, including chromoendoscopy, water-immersion techniques, magnification endoscopy (ME), alone or combined with acetic-acid instillation, and optimal band imaging [8–12].

A previous observation reported the combination of high-resolution Narrow Band Imaging (NBI) with ME (NBI-ME) to obtain targeted biopsy specimens indicating a higher simplicity (with the switch of a button) than chromoendoscopy, thus reducing the procedure time [13]. In fact, NBI-ME is a simple tool that allows detection of the subepithelial microvascular architecture and mucosal microsurface structure in a variety of pathological conditions [14, 15]. To our knowledge there is not a prospective study that addresses the performance of NBI-ME in evaluating patients with suspected CD. The aim of this study was to assess the correlation between NBI-ME and histology and to compare the diagnostic accuracy between NBI-ME and SE using histology as gold standard in detecting villous abnormalities in CD.

2. Materials and Methods

2.1. Subjects and Endoscopic Procedures. Forty-four consecutive patients (17 males, 27 females, age range 14–73 years, mean age 36.5 years) with clinical history suggestive of malabsorption (weight loss, chronic diarrhea, iron-deficiency anemia, etc.) and serologic suspicion for CD as positive or borderline antiendomysial (normal values are absent for both IgA and IgG) and antitransglutaminase antibodies (normal values 0–10 U/mL) were prospectively enrolled in the study. The presence of severe gastrointestinal or systemic disease was considered as an exclusion criterion (e.g., chronic pancreatitis, liver cirrhosis, and blood coagulation disorders). The study was performed under the local ethics committee approval.

Prior to endoscopy, a written informed consent was obtained from all participants. In order to prolong the procedure for the evaluation of the duodenal mucosa with NBI-ME, a conscious sedation with intravenous midazolam (0.05–0.1 mg/Kg) was used before undergoing upper gastrointestinal (UGI) endoscopy together with induction of gastrointestinal hypotony (with hyoscine N-butylbromide 10–20 mg i.v.).

All procedures were performed with an Olympus GIFQ 160Z, Exera II (Olympus, America Corp., Melville, NY, USA), a high-resolution endoscope with adjustable image magnification to ×115 which included the NBI system. A disposable polyethylene cap was applied on the distal end of the endoscope to prevent slippage of the mucosa and to help secure a single area for focus, thus maintaining an optimum depth from the mucosa. A physician interviewed and selected the patients. All UGI endoscopies were performed by a single endoscopist who was blinded to the laboratory data of all patients. A regular inspection of the duodenum with SE was performed before switching to the NBI vision. A judgement on the villous appearance (abnormalities or not) for SE and for NBI-ME was then expressed. The various duodenal villous patterns at NBI-ME inspection were classified as follows: normal, abnormal (partial villous atrophy), or absent (marked villous atrophy) (Figure 1).

To avoid insufficient sampling, as recommended by previous investigators [16], 4 to 6 biopsy specimens were taken from the descending duodenum and from any other area of irregular appearing duodenal mucosa by using standard biopsy forceps. If no abnormality was macroscopically evident, random biopsy specimens were obtained. The histopathological evaluation was performed according to the Marsh classification, modified by Oberhuber [17]. Samples were evaluated by a pathologist who was blinded to the clinical data and the endoscopic findings.

2.2. Statistical Analysis. The relationship between NBI-ME and SE findings was compared with histology using the k-Cohen agreement coefficient. Sensitivity, specificity, and positive and negative predictive values (PPV-NPV) for both techniques were calculated using histology reports as the gold standard. The efficacy of NBI-ME for predicting villous abnormalities in CD was evaluated by the area under the Receiver Operating Characteristic (ROC) curve analysis. Statistical significance was established at $P < 0.05$ for all the analyses.

3. Results and Discussion

3.1. Results. A diagnosis of CD was histologically made in 17 (38.6%) of 44 enrolled patients, while the remaining 27 (61.4%) had a normal villous pattern. Among those diagnosed with CD, 7 (41%) showed endoscopic features of disease during SE.

After switching to NBI-ME, a diagnosis of mucosal abnormalities was made in 19 patients. Among these, 7, which were the same as those found at SE, had a complete absent duodenal villous pattern, while 12 displayed an abnormal duodenal villous pattern. Two cases showing abnormal villous patterns at NBI-ME were subsequently classified as negative for CD at histology (Table 1). NBI-ME identified patchy areas of partial villous atrophy in 12 patients with a sensitivity, specificity, PPV, and NPV of 100%, 93%, 89%, and 100%, respectively. The corresponding values for SE were 41%, 100%, 100%, and 73%, respectively (Table 2). The area under the ROC curve for NBI-ME was 0.978 ($P = 0.0005$), indicating an excellent agreement with the histological results. The area under the ROC was 0.706 for SE ($P = 0.023$) (Figure 2). The overall agreement between NBI-ME and histology was significantly higher when compared with SE and histology (kappa score: 0.90 versus 0.46; $P = 0.001$) in determining CD (Table 3). Among 27 subjects without CD, the diagnoses were functional dyspepsia, irritable bowel syndrome, or overlap syndromes.

The mean additional time for single NBI-ME procedure was 4 minutes and 30 seconds (±1 minute).

3.2. Discussion. The first report on the use of ME with chromoendoscopy to highlight duodenal villous pattern was published by Siegel et al. [18] demonstrating an increased detection rate of focal villous atrophy as well as partial villous atrophy compared with SE in patients with malabsorption. However, some limitations of this technique related to difficulty in achieving a complete and an even coating of the mucosal surface with the dye [12], increased cost and procedure time, and the lack of visualization of the vascular pattern have prevented the widespread use of vital dye staining chromoendoscopy techniques. Recently a new technology called "Fuji Intelligent Color Enhancement," a virtual chromoendoscopy, was introduced to enhance the contrast of the mucosal surface without the use of dyes,

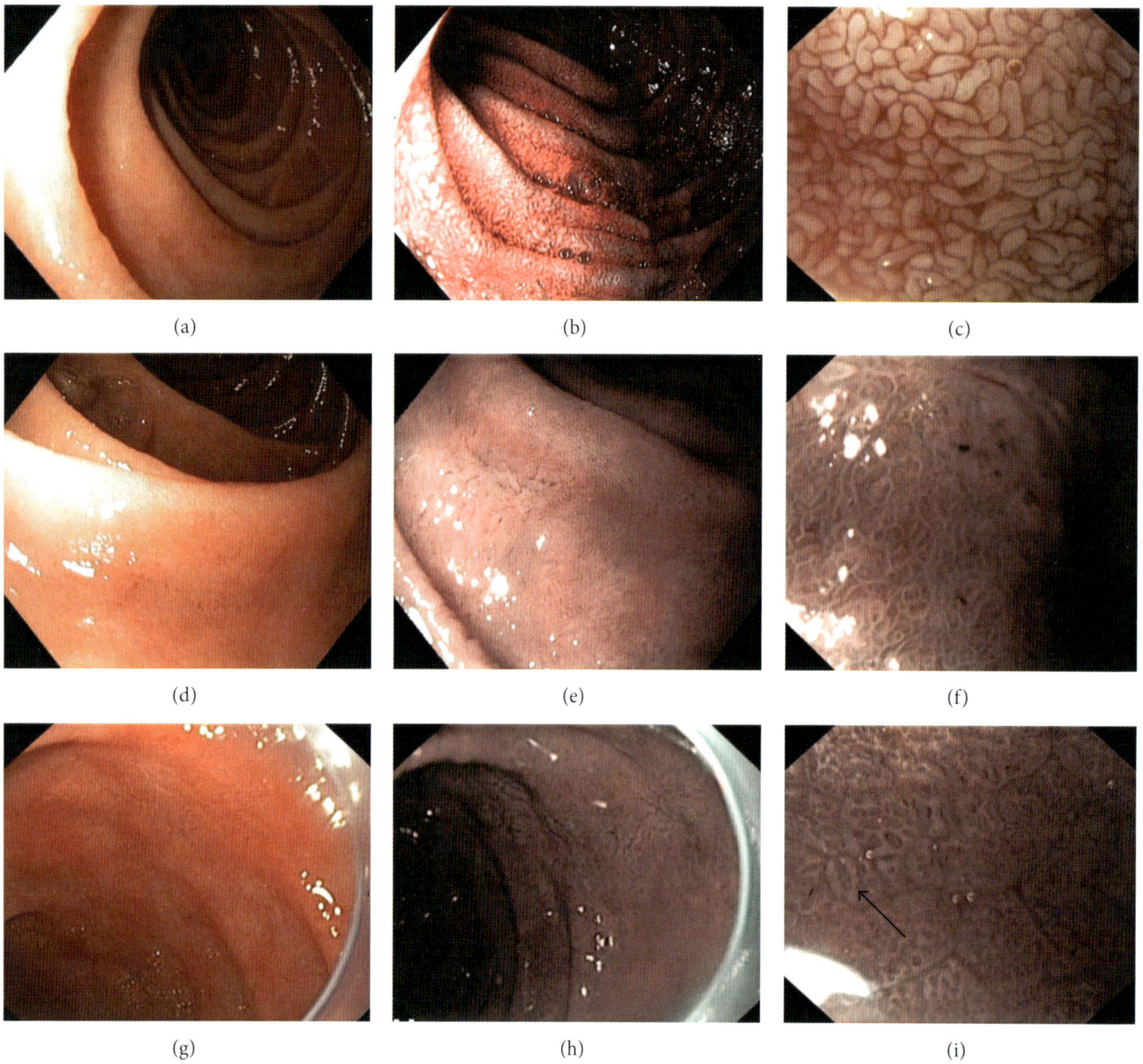

FIGURE 1: (a, b, and c) Normal villous patterns. Visualization of normal duodenal mucosa at white light SE (a). Regular villi appear well represented, thick, with a finger-like appearance at NBI system and ME (b and c). (d, e, and f) Abnormal villous patterns. Partial villous atrophy view at SE (d); NBI-ME showing a low-density of villi which appear irregular, disoriented, and with an initial pattern of surface destruction (e and f). (g, h, and i) Absent villous patterns. Marked villous atrophy with NBI system and ME (g); the surface is flat (h), "foveolar-like," with total villi absence and wide circles (i: black arrow).

through the ability to select better spectral images decomposed from ordinary endoscopic images [19]. Cammarota et al. [12] published an original open, prospective, single-centre trial on the potential of a similar system, the optimal band imaging (OBI), for predicting the duodenal villous morphologic characteristics in patients with suspected CD. The authors concluded that the OBI system, in association with ME, allows clear visualization of the duodenal pattern, with a potential role in optimizing the diagnostic accuracy of endoscopy in CD.

In the present study we show that the NBI system, associated with ME, has provided superior performance than conventional endoscopy in detecting mucosal abnormalities on otherwise normal appearing duodenal mucosa. We found high sensitivity and specificity values with an overall agreement between NBI-ME and histology significantly higher when compared with SE and histology in determining duodenal villous pattern features. Moreover, the ROC curve analysis demonstrated that the NBI-ME performance was greater than SE, showing an excellent agreement with the histological results.

The NBI system consists of a sequential electronic endoscope system that can select better spectral images using particular luminous bands, thus enabling to filter incidence light resulting in some kind of "coloration without coloring." Since the gastrointestinal tract is mainly composed of blood vessels and mucosa, narrow band illumination, which is strongly absorbed by hemoglobin and penetrates only the surface of tissues, is ideal for enhancing the contrast between the two.

However, our results have some limitations. First, we did not assess the inter- or intraobserver reliability of the

TABLE 1: Histological diagnosis and corresponding endoscopic findings.

		Endoscopic findings	
	n° patients	SE	NBI + ME
CD	17	7	19$
Normal	27	37	25

$7 absent villous patterns.
12 abnormal villous patterns.: 2 negative, histology for CD.

TABLE 2: Diagnostic accuracy of SE and NBI with ME.

	Sensitivity (%)	Specificity (%)	PPV (%)	NPV (%)
NBI + ME	100	93	89	100
SE	41	100	100	73

TABLE 3: Overall agreement (k-Cohen coefficient) between endoscopic findings and histology reports.

NBI + ME and histology	0.90*
SE and histology	0.46

*$P = 0.001$ (Student's t-test).

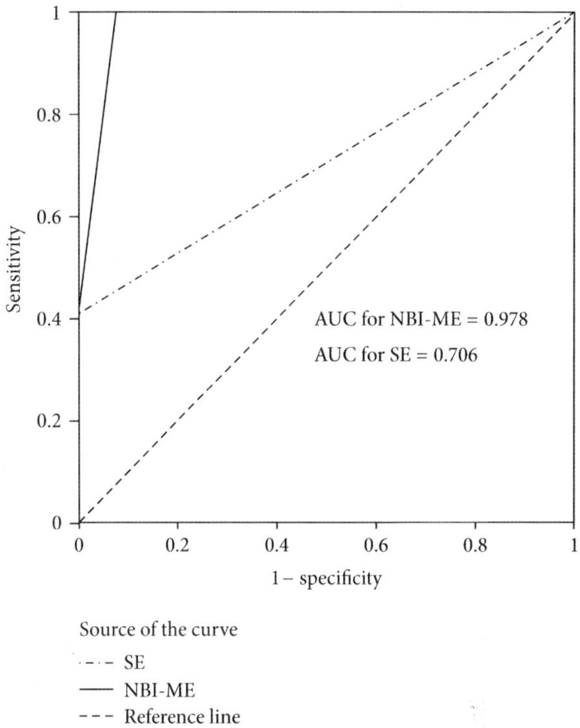

FIGURE 2: Receiver operating characteristic curves of NBI-ME and SE for diagnosing CD.

mucosal patterns. Consequently, although duodenal villous classified patterns were normal, abnormal, or absent, we have not evaluated the correlation between partial or marked villous atrophy with histological score. In fact, our main objective was to establish the presence or absence of CD. A previous report by Badreldin et al. [10] on the potential role of zoom endoscopy for the diagnosis of the various degrees of villous atrophy showed a sensitivity of 90.7% and specificity of 63%. In their study the main disagreement between zoom endoscopy and histopathology was the distinction between normal tall villi and morphologically normal but shortened villi, which depends on the assessment of villus height. More recently another study, using a simplified classification, demonstrated the feasibility of using NBI-ME for the detection of villous atrophy in patients presenting with suspected CD [20].

Second, among the criticisms that have been raised for the use of NBI-ME was the slightly increased procedure time, including conscious sedation, for routine application. We observed an additional mean procedure time of 4 minutes and 30 seconds.

Third, as reported by other authors [12], all patients who underwent UGI endoscopy had clinical history of malabsorption or serologic suspicion for CD, thus having a high pretest probability for duodenal abnormalities.

Fourth, we have found two false-positive cases at NBI-ME which reduced the specificity. It is possible that this approach could lead to an overestimation of the findings, and the results could be influenced by the high pretest probability for duodenal disease. It is widely known that the prevalence of CD in open access endoscopy is likely to be underestimated, with missed diagnose, ranging from less than 1% to 16% [21]. The ideal diagnostic technique approach for CD should increase accuracy and sensitivity and be easy to perform, cost saving, and repeatable, and not be time consuming [22].

Furthermore, other endoscopic options, such as confocal endomicroscopy [23] and optical coherence tomography [24], that were studied in patients with suspected CD achieved good results. However, these techniques are hampered by technical problems. In particular, difficulty of image acquisition/stability, with potential distortion and artifacts, and a long learning curve would restrict their wide use on the basis of the local availability of equipment and expertise. Moreover, according to Fedeli and colleagues [25], the combination of two or more simple new endoscopic approaches, such as OBI together with ME, during water-immersion would obtain outstanding images of the villous pattern.

Using these new endoscopic techniques, the same authors have proposed an algorithm to minimize the need for duodenal biopsy in patients with suspected CD in particular for those with total villous atrophy [22], or in such circumstances that could involve patients who are on anticoagulation therapy and that cannot be safely interrupted [26]. As suggested in a correspondence [27], we believe that it is not possible, at present, to avoid biopsies in CD, both for the initial diagnosis and for followup. In fact it is not possible to make a precise differential diagnosis of *Giardia lamblia* infection or Crohn's disease (where there could also be changes of serological markers) [28] and eosinophilic jejunitis or HIV enteropathy [29]; furthermore, the histological evaluation is fundamental because it allows verifying improvement of duodenal lesions after gluten-free diet or the absence of mucosal recovery that needs an analysis of molecular markers in the suspicion of a T-cell dysplasia lymphoma [30].

4. Conclusions

In conclusion, our findings show that the NBI with ME represents a simple technique that could help identify patchy areas of partial mucosal atrophy and then estimate the extension, even considering frequently mixed patterns. With these tools it is also possible to predict, in a reliable manner, "minimal changes" of duodenal villi in CD occurring *in vivo* and, importantly, improve biopsy sampling by potentially reducing the need for blind biopsies and false-negative cases.

References

[1] W. Dickey and D. Hughes, "Prevalence of celiac disease and its endoscopic markers among patients having routine upper gastrointestinal endoscopy," *American Journal of Gastroenterology*, vol. 94, no. 8, pp. 2182–2186, 1999.

[2] W. Dickey and D. Hughes, "Disappointing sensitivity of endoscopic markers for villous atrophy in a high-risk population: implications for celiac disease diagnosis during routine endoscopy," *American Journal of Gastroenterology*, vol. 96, no. 7, pp. 2126–2128, 2001.

[3] S. Lecleire, F. Di Fiore, M. Antoniette et al., "Endoscopic markers of villous atrophy are not useful for the detection of celiac disease in patients with dyspeptic symptoms," *Endoscopy*, vol. 38, no. 7, pp. 696–701, 2006.

[4] W. Dickey, "Endoscopic markers for celiac disease," *Nature Clinical Practice Gastroenterology & Hepatology*, vol. 3, no. 10, pp. 546–551, 2006.

[5] M. T. Bardella, G. Minoli, F. Radaelli, M. Quatrini, P. A. Blanchi, and D. Conte, "Reevaluation of duodenal endoscopic markers in the diagnosis of celiac disease," *Gastrointestinal Endoscopy*, vol. 51, no. 6, pp. 714–715, 2000.

[6] E. Maurino, H. Capizzano, S. Niveloni et al., "Value of endoscopic markers in celiac disease," *Digestive Diseases and Sciences*, vol. 38, no. 11, pp. 2028–2033, 1993.

[7] A. Tursi, G. Brandimarte, G. M. Giorgetti, and A. Gigliobianco, "Endoscopic features of celiac disease in adults and their correlation with age, histological damage, and clinical form of the disease," *Endoscopy*, vol. 34, no. 10, pp. 787–792, 2002.

[8] A. Lo, M. Guelrud, H. Essenfeld, and P. Bonis, "Classification of villous atrophy with enhanced magnification endoscopy in patients with celiac disease and tropical sprue," *Gastrointestinal Endoscopy*, vol. 66, no. 2, pp. 377–382, 2007.

[9] R. Kiesslich, K. Mergener, C. Naumann et al., "Value of chromoendoscopy and magnification endoscopy in the evaluation of duodenal abnormalities: a prospective, randomized comparison," *Endoscopy*, vol. 35, no. 7, pp. 559–563, 2003.

[10] R. Badreldin, P. Barrett, D. A. Wooff, J. Mansfield, and Y. Yiannakou, "How good is zoom endoscopy for assessment of villous atrophy in coeliac disease?" *Endoscopy*, vol. 37, no. 10, pp. 994–998, 2005.

[11] R. Banerjee, A. Shekharan, C. Ramji et al., "Role of magnification endoscopy in the diagnosis and evaluation of suspected celiac disease: correlation with histology," *Indian Journal of Gastroenterology*, vol. 26, no. 2, pp. 67–69, 2007.

[12] G. Cammarota, P. Cesaro, A. Cazzato et al., "Optimal band imaging system: a new tool for enhancing the duodenal villous pattern in celiac disease," *Gastrointestinal Endoscopy*, vol. 68, no. 2, pp. 352–357, 2008.

[13] R. Banerjee and D. N. Reddy, "High-resolution narrow-band imaging can identify patchy atrophy in celiac disease: targeted biopsy can increase diagnostic yield," *Gastrointestinal Endoscopy*, vol. 69, no. 4, pp. 984–985, 2009.

[14] L. M. Song, D. G. Adler, J. D. Conway et al., "Narrow band imaging and multiband imaging," *Gastrointestinal Endoscopy*, vol. 67, no. 4, pp. 581–589, 2008.

[15] K. Yao, Y. Takaki, T. Matsui et al., "Clinical application of magnification endoscopy and narrow-band imaging in the upper gastrointestinal tract: new imaging techniques for detecting and characterizing gastrointestinal neoplasia," *Gastrointestinal Endoscopy Clinics of North America*, vol. 18, no. 3, pp. 415–433, 2008.

[16] W. P. Pais, D. R. Duerksen, N. M. Pettigrew, and C. N. Bernstein, "How many duodenal biopsy specimens are required to make a diagnosis of celiac disease?" *Gastrointestinal Endoscopy*, vol. 67, no. 7, pp. 1082–1087, 2008.

[17] G. Oberhuber, G. Granditsch, and H. Vogelsang, "The histopathology of coeliac disease: time for a standardized report scheme for pathologists," *European Journal of Gastroenterology and Hepatology*, vol. 11, no. 10, pp. 1185–1194, 1999.

[18] L. M. Siegel, P. D. Stevens, C. J. Lightdale et al., "Combined magnification endoscopy with chromoendoscopy in the evaluation of patients with suspected malabsorption," *Gastrointestinal Endoscopy*, vol. 46, no. 3, pp. 226–230, 1997.

[19] J. Pohl, A. May, T. Rabenstein, O. Pech, and C. Ell, "Computed virtual chromoendoscopy: a new tool for enhancing tissue surface structures," *Endoscopy*, vol. 39, no. 1, pp. 80–83, 2007.

[20] R. Singh, G. Nind, G. Tucker et al., "Narrow-band imaging in the evaluation of villous morphology: a feasibility study assessing a simplified classification and observer agreement," *Endoscopy*, vol. 42, no. 11, pp. 889–894, 2010.

[21] E. Brocchi, G. R. Corazza, G. Caletti, E. A. Treggiari, L. Barbara, and G. Gasbarrini, "Endoscopic demonstration of loss of duodenal folds in the diagnosis of celiac diasease," *The New England Journal of Medicine*, vol. 319, no. 12, pp. 741–744, 1988.

[22] G. Cammarota, P. Fedeli, and A. Gasbarrini, "Emerging technologies in upper gastrointestinal endoscopy and celiac disease," *Nature Clinical Practice Gastroenterology and Hepatology*, vol. 6, no. 1, pp. 47–56, 2009.

[23] C. Trovato, A. Sonzogni, D. Ravizza et al., "Celiac disease: in vivo diagnosis by confocal endomicroscopy," *Gastrointestinal Endoscopy*, vol. 65, no. 7, pp. 1096–1099, 2007.

[24] E. Masci, B. Mangiavillano, L. Albarello, A. Mariani, C. Doglioni, and P. A. Testoni, "Pilot study on the correlation of optical coherence tomography with histology in celiac disease and normal subjects," *Journal of Gastroenterology and Hepatology*, vol. 22, no. 12, pp. 2256–2260, 2007.

[25] P. Fedeli, G. Gasbarrini, and G. Cammarota, "The combined application of advanced endoscopic imaging techniques may increase the duodenal villous morphology definition in suspected celiac disease," *Digestive and Liver Disease*, vol. 42, no. 8, pp. 595–596, 2010.

[26] A. Rubio-Tapia and J. A. Murray, "Novel endoscopic methods for the evaluation of the small-bowel mucosa," *Gastrointestinal Endoscopy*, vol. 66, no. 2, pp. 382–386, 2007.

[27] L. Elli, A. Bonura, and M. T. Bardella, "Avoiding duodenal endoscopic biopsies in celiac disease: are we going forward or looking to the past?" *Digestive and Liver Disease*, vol. 42, no. 2, p. 154, 2010.

[28] M. Di Tola, L. Sabbatella, M. C. Anania et al., "Anti-tissue transglutaminase antibodies in inflammatory bowel disease: new evidence," *Clinical Chemistry and Laboratory Medicine*, vol. 42, no. 10, pp. 1092–1097, 2004.

[29] V. H. Shah, H. Rotterdam, D. P. Kotler, A. Fasano, and P. H. R. Green, "All that scallops is not celiac disease," *Gastrointestinal Endoscopy*, vol. 51, no. 6, pp. 717–720, 2000.

[30] N. Krauss and D. Schuppan, "Monitoring nonresponsive patients who have celiac disease," *Gastrointestinal Endoscopy Clinics of North America*, vol. 16, no. 2, pp. 317–327, 2006.

15

Increased Incidence of Benign Pancreatic Pathology following Pancreaticoduodenectomy for Presumed Malignancy over 10 Years despite Increased Use of Endoscopic Ultrasound

Shadi S. Yarandi, Thomas Runge, Lei Wang, Zhijian Liu, Yueping Jiang, Saurabh Chawla, Kevin E. Woods, Steven Keilin, Field F. Willingham, Hong Xu, and Qiang Cai

Division of Digestive Diseases, Emory University School of Medicine, 1365 Clifton Road, B1262, Atlanta, GA 30322, USA

Correspondence should be addressed to Qiang Cai; qcai@emory.edu

Academic Editor: Lars Aabakken

Despite using imaging studies, tissue sampling, and serologic tests about 5–10% of surgeries done for presumed pancreatic malignancies will have benign findings on final pathology. Endoscopic ultrasound (EUS) is used with increasing frequency to study pancreatic masses. The aim of this study is to examine the effect of EUS on prevalence of benign diseases undergoing Whipple over the last decade. Patients who underwent Whipple procedure for presumed malignancy at Emory University Hospital from 1998 to 2011 were selected. Demographic data, history of smoking and drinking, history of diabetes and pancreatitis, imaging data, pathology reports, and tumor markers were extracted. 878 patients were found. 95 (10.82%) patients had benign disease. Prevalence of benign finding had increased over the recent years despite using more EUS. Logistic regression models showed that abdominal pain (OR: 5.829, 95% CI 2.681–12.674, $P \leq 0.001$) and alcohol abuse (OR: 3.221, CI 95%: 1.362–7.261, P: 0.002) were predictors of benign diseases. Jaundice (OR: 0.221, 95% CI: 0.084–0.58, P: 0.002), mass (OR: 0.145, 95% CI: 0.043–0.485, P: 0.008), and ductal dilation (OR: 0.297, 95% CI 0.134–0.657, P: 0.003) were associated with malignancy. Use of imaging studies, ERCP, and EUS has not decreased the percentage of benign findings after surgery for presumed pancreatic malignancy.

1. Introduction

Pancreatic cancer accounts for 2% of newly diagnosed malignancies, with pancreaticoduodenectomy (The Whipple procedure) being the only potentially curative treatment [1]. Differentiating between pancreatic carcinoma and benign diseases of the pancreas such as chronic pancreatitis is challenging. Pancreatic cancer can present with vague symptoms that overlap with the symptomatology of benign diseases and have an insidious course. The imaging findings also overlap between benign and malignant diseases and no single finding such as pancreatic duct dilation, focal mass, cyst, or abnormal enhancement pattern can reliably make the differentiation. In addition, secondary inflammatory changes are often seen in pancreatic cancer while chronic pancreatitis is associated with an increased risk of pancreatic carcinoma [2].

Although the outcome of the Whipple procedure has improved significantly over the past years and is associated with 1-2% mortality when performed in large volume centers, the morbidity of the procedure remains high [3]. Therefore, constant efforts are being made to improve available diagnostic tools in order to prevent performing Whipple for benign diseases. Despite the advances in imaging techniques, 5–10% of patients who undergo Whipple procedure for a presumed malignant disease will have benign pathology on the final pathologic review [4–12]. Usually a combination of computed tomography (CT), magnetic resonance imaging/magnetic resonance cholangiopancreatography (MRI/MRCP), endoscopic retrograde cholangiopancreatography (ERCP) with brushing, endoscopic ultrasound/fine needle aspiration (EUS/FNA), and serology testing is performed before the decision for surgery is made.

All of these methods have false negative results and relatively low negative predictive values, adding uncertainty to the decision making process. Given the high mortality of untreated pancreatic cancer, surgeons often decide to offer surgery to the patients in whom a malignant lesion is clinically suspected even if the results of tissue sampling are unconvincing for malignancy.

In the current study, we have reviewed Whipple procedures that have been performed for presumed malignant pancreatic disease over the past decade at Emory University Hospital. The aim of this study is to examine the effect of presurgical tissue sampling by EUS/FNA on the rate of finding benign pathology from Whipple procedure performed for presumed malignant disease. We also performed a multivariate binary logistic regression analysis to investigate if any of the collected data can help differentiating benign disease from malignant before surgery.

2. Patients and Methods

With approval of institutional review board at Emory University, the admitting and discharge diagnosis and procedure codes were queried from the electronic medical records at Emory University Hospital (EUH). The current procedural terminology (CPT) and International Classification of Diseases Ninth Revision (ICD-9) codes for "pancreaticoduodenectomy" were used to identify patients who underwent the surgery.

A retrospective review from January 1998 to December 2011 of the patients undergoing Whipple procedure for presumed malignant pancreatic disease at Emory University Hospital was conducted. Patients with a diagnosis of chronic pancreatitis undergoing resection for relief of the symptoms were excluded from the analysis. A total of 872 patients were identified. Electronic medical records were reviewed and the following data were collected: demographics, clinical presentation including weight loss (10% or more of body weight), jaundice, abdominal, pain, acute or chronic pancreatitis, diabetes mellitus, history of smoking, history of alcohol over use, radiographic findings including CT scan, MRI/MRCP, ERCP, EUS, diagnostic preoperative pathologic data including endoscopic and image-guided biopsies, and final pathologic report after surgery.

There was no universal preoperative imaging protocol over years and imaging studies were performed based on the evaluation of the case by the attending surgeons or the consulting gastroenterologists. CT scans were often performed before referral to our center and findings were documented in the surgeons note in all of the cases. MRI/MRCP, ERCP, and EUS/FNA were performed at EUH and the records of radiology and pathology reports in case of biopsy were reviewed. Preoperative specimens with conclusive evidence of malignancy or those suspicious for malignancy, showing dysplasia or evidence of neoplastic processes, were considered positive. Biopsies described as inflammatory, reactive, or atypical were considered nondiagnostic. All specimens were reviewed by experienced gastrointestinal pathologists at EUH. Patients with benign disease were characterized based on the histopathological findings. Chronic fibrosing

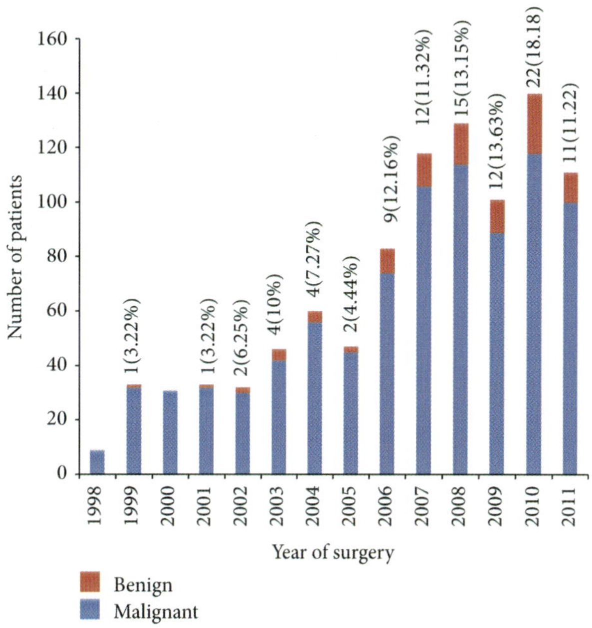

FIGURE 1: Distribution of number of surgeries and percentage of benign pathologic findings per year. Number of Whipple surgeries performed each year for presumed malignant disease at EUH from 1998 to 2011. Number and percentage of benign findings are listed above each bar. As illustrated in the figure, total number of surgeries and percentage of benign findings have been increased over the years.

pancreatitis was defined by pathologic findings including inflammatory changes, fat necrosis, fibrosis, and loss of acinar cells.

All continuous data were represented as mean +/− standard error of the mean. Frequency data was used otherwise. Binary logistic regression models were constructed to assess the potential predictor factors of benign disease in patients undergoing Whipple procedure.

3. Results

From 878 Whipple procedures performed between January 1998 and December 2011, 95 (10.8%) patients had benign pathology on the final pathology report. Number of benign findings as well as the percentage of benign finding to total number of operation performed each year has been increased over the years despite increased number of EUS/FNA performed in each year (Figure 1).

Out of 95 patients with benign findings, 43 (45.3%) were female and 52 (54.7%) were male. Age of the patients with benign findings ranges between 20 and 81 with mean of 53.66 (standard deviation: 11.54 years). 65 (68.4%) patients were Caucasian while 28 (29.5) were African American, 1 Hispanic, and 1 Asian. 57 (60%) patients had history of smoking and 42 (44.2%) had history of excessive alcohol use. Ten patients had history of DM (10.5%) and 40 (42.5%) had history of at least one episode of pancreatitis. Summary of this data is presented in Table 1.

TABLE 1: Demographic data of patients with benign disease.

Category	Number (percent)
Gender	
Male	52 (54.7)
Female	43 (45.3)
Race	
White	65 (68.4)
African American	28 (29.5)
Asian	1 (1.1)
Hispanic	1 (1.1)
Past medical history	
Diabetes	10 (10.5)
Pancreatitis	40 (42.1)
Social history	
Smoking	57 (60)
Alcohol	42 (44.2)
Presenting symptom	
Abdominal pain	91 (95.8)
Jaundice	25 (26.3)
Weight loss	69 (72.6)

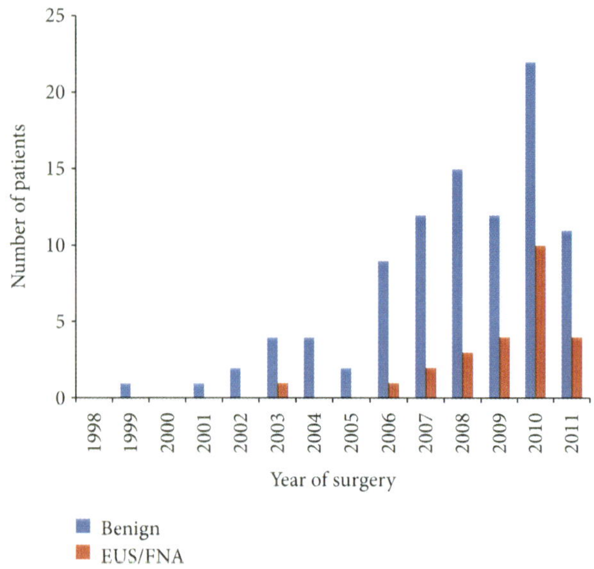

FIGURE 2: Number of EUS/FNA performed between 1998 and 2011 in patients with benign disease who underwent Whipple procedure for presumed malignancy. Number of EUS/FNA in patients with benign findings after Whipple procedure performed each year for presumed malignant disease at EUH from 1998 to 2011. As illustrated, number of EUS/FNA performed has increased over the years, but has not led to decreased number of Whipple procedures performed for benign diseases.

The most common complaint at the time of presentation among patients with benign finding was abdominal pain which was reported by 91 (95.8%) patients. 69 (72.6%) patients in benign group also reported some degree of weight loss. Jaundice that was reported to be more common in malignant pathology in some of the previous studies was reported by 25 (26.3%) patients with benign disease. As for imaging studies that were performed before surgery, 49 patients in benign group had CT scan at EUH and 46 had CT scan done before referral to EUH with reports available to review. MRI with or without MRCP was done in 85 (89.5%) of patients with benign pathology. EUS with FNA aspiration was done in 25 (26.3%) and ERCP with brushing was done in 32 (33.7%) of patients with benign pathology. Results of these tests were invariably nondiagnostic, leading the surgeon to pursue the surgery. Number of EUS/FNA and ERCPs done before surgery had increased over the years, as illustrated in Figure 2. Among 783 patients with malignant disease on final pathology, 274 (35%) had underwent ERCP and 92 (11.7%) had underwent EUS/FNA before the surgery. The same trend toward more EUS/FNAs over recent years was observed in patients with malignant disease as well. For example, 25 (27% of the total number of the EUS procedures) EUS/FNA was performed in 2011 and 22 was performed (23.9%) in 2010 alone.

Among these 95 patients, imaging studies including CT and MRI reported a solid mass within the head of pancreas in 56 (58.9%) of patients with the average size of 13.7 millimeter and standard deviation of 15.45 millimeter. 23 (24.2) patients were reported to have a cystic mass or cyst at the head of pancreas with the average size of 7.6 mm and standard deviation of 16.48 mm. An abnormal pattern of enhancement of the mass, or periductal enhancement without a mass, was reported in 62 (65.3%) patients. Abnormal enhancement was reported with multiple patterns including increased early enhancement, increased delayed enhancement, or decreased enhancement (Table 2). In the imaging studies of 32 (33.7%) patients there was evidence of inflammation; abnormally enlarged abdominal lymph nodes were reported in imaging of 6 (6.3%) patients; imaging studies of 62 (65.3%) patients showed some degree of pancreatic duct dilation and invasion or pressure to vascular structures including the portal vein or the superior mesenteric artery was seen in 10 (10.5%) patients.

The final histologic findings of these patients are listed in Table 3. The most common findings were chronic fibrosing pancreatitis with or without focal mass like fibrosis, paraduodenal pancreatitis, chronic pancreatitis, and focal pancreatitis. There were 6 cases of lymphoplasmacytic sclerosing autoimmune pancreatitis. Rare conditions such as arteriovenous malformation (AVM), thrombosed aneurism, xanthogranulomatosis chronic inflammation, and lipoma were reported in few cases.

Binary logical regression models were constructed using gender, race, smoking, alcohol abuse, chronic pancreatitis, presenting symptoms including abdominal pain, jaundice and weight loss, radiographic findings including presence of mass, ductal dilation, lymphadenopathy, and vascular invasion as independent predictors. This analysis showed that Odds ratio of benign disease in patients with abdominal pain (OR: 5.829, 95% CI 2.681–12.674, $P \leq 0.001$) as the main presenting symptom and alcohol abuse (OR: 3.221, CI 95%: 1.362–7.261, P: 0.002) was significantly higher compared to the patients with pancreatic cancer. On the other hand, OR of benign disease in patients presenting with jaundice

TABLE 2: Imaging modalities and findings of patients with benign disease.

Category	Number (percent)
Imaging type	
MRI	85 (89.5)
EUS	25 (26.3)
ERCP	32 (33.7)
Space occupying lesion	
Mass	56 (58.9)
Size	13.71 (15.43 SD)
Cyst	23 (24.2)
Size	7.6 (16.48)
Abnormal enhancement	
Periductal	7 (7.36)
Decreased enhancement	13 (13.68)
Increased early enhancement	24 (25.6)
Increased delayed enhancement	18 (18.94)
Other	
Inflammation	32 (33.7)
Duct dilation	62 (65.3)
Lymph node	6 (6.3)
Vascular involvement	10 (10.5)

TABLE 3: Frequency of Benign Findings.

Type	Number (percent)
PLSP autoimmune pancreatitis	6 (6.3)
Chronic fibrosing pancreatitis	20 (21)
Chronic pancreatitis	18 (18.94)
Focal active pancreatitis	11 (11.57)
Perideudonal pancreatitis	14 (14.73)
AVM	1 (1)
Chronic pancreatitis with infection	2 (2.1)
Granulomatose pancreatitis	1 (1)
Necrotizing pancreatitis	5 (5.26)
Pseudotumoral pancreatitis	6 (6.3)
Focal fat necrosis	2 (2.1)
Chronic pancreatitis with ductal stone	2 (2.1)
Lipoma	1 (1)
Lipomatose pseudohypertrophy	1 (1)
Intraductal adenoma	1 (1)
Xanthogranulomatous inflammation	1 (1)
Thrombosed pseudoaneurysm	1 (1)
Chronic pancreatitis with thrombosed vessels	1 (1)
Chronic pancreatitis due to deudonal diverticulum	1 (1)

(OR: 0.221, 95% CI: 0.084–0.58, *P* value: 0.002), with a mass present in imaging (OR: 0.145, 95% CI: 0.043–0.485, *P*: 0.008) and with ductal dilation (OR: 0.297, 95% CI 0.134–0.657, *P*: 0.003), was significantly lower compared to the malignant disease (Table 4).

TABLE 4: Logistic regression models for benign findings in patients undergoing Whipple procedure for presumed malignancy.

Variable	OR	95% CI	*P* value
Gender (female)	1.229	0.625–2.49	0.55
Race (African American)	0.804	0.390–1.66	0.55
Smoking	0.966	0.445–2.09	0.93
Chronic pancreatitis	1.072	0.184–1.168	0.102
Alcohol abuse	3.221	1.362–7.261	0.002
Abdominal pain	5.829	2.681–12.674	<0.001
Jaundice	0.221	0.084–0.58	0.002
Weight loss	1.566	0.94–1.89	0.078
Mass	0.145	0.043–0.485	0.008
Dilation of ducts	0.297	0.134–0.657	0.003
Lymphadenopathy	0.874	0.478–4.736	0.485
Vascular invasion	1.00	0.357–2.80	0.99

4. Discussion

In this study, out of 878 Whipple procedures performed on the patients with presumed pancreatic cancer over ten years, the percentage of benign finding was 10.8 with a trend toward increase over recent years despite increased number of EUS/FNA performed. The most common pathologic finding was chronic fibrosing pancreatitis, most likely in the setting of chronic pancreatitis secondary to alcohol abuse. Also, the results of this study showed that abdominal pain as main presenting symptom and a history of alcohol abuse is associated with benign pancreatic diseases while jaundice, presence of a mass in imaging studies, and bile duct/pancreatic duct dilation are associated with malignancies.

Previously, 11 academic institutions have published their experience with Whipple procedure and prevalence of unexpected benign findings. Thompson et al. initially reported 67 patients who underwent surgery between 1978 and 1993 at the University of Nebraska and reported 11 patients with benign findings [10]. They later published a follow-up report of 132 patients who underwent Whipple procedure between 1995 and 2008, with the prevalence of benign findings reported as 12.9%, most commonly chronic fibrosing pancreatitis. In this follow-up report, similar to our finding, incidence of benign pathology was increased over years [7]. They attributed this finding to decreased use of EUS in their center, however in our center EUS or ERCP was performed more frequently during the recent years.

Tessler et al. reported their experience at Henry Ford Medical Center between 1998 and 2004. Among their patients, 102 patients had no tissue diagnosis before the surgery and 27 ended up having benign pathology [9]. Large number of patients in their series had EUS ($n = 80$) or ERCP ($n = 68$) before the surgery. Despite the fact that they used EUS and ERCP frequently, the percentage of benign findings was similar to the other reports. They tried to combine several imaging, laboratory, and symptomatology findings to develop a scoring system that can predict malignant versus benign disease. They suggested that in the appropriate clinical setting, a combination of weight loss, jaundice, and increased

CA 19-9, often in combination with a biliary stricture or pancreatic mass should be strongly considered for surgery even if a preoperative tissue diagnosis is not present [8]. However, this criterion has not been validated by other studies.

Barnes et al. reviewed 510 pancreaticoduodenectomies performed at The Johns Hopkins Hospital during an 8-year period. One hundred and eight patients (21%) underwent surgery for benign disease, 83 (16%) of those underwent surgery for suspicion of malignancy [5]. In another report from the Johns Hopkins Hospital, Abraham et al. published a retrospective review of 442 patients who underwent the procedure between 1999 and 2001, in whom 40 patients (9.2%) were found to have some form of benign inflammatory condition of the pancreas or biliary tract [4]. van Gulik et al. described 220 patients who underwent Whipple and reported 6% benign findings. They suggested that at least 5% of benign finding is expected when performing Whipple procedure for a suspected malignant disease and given the grim prognosis of the pancreatic cancer this should not stop surgeons from performing the procedure on patients with clinically suspected malignancy but with no other confirming data [11].

In a report from Mayo Clinic, Smith et al. reviewed 484 patients who underwent Whipple procedure for suspected periampullary malignancy and found chronic inflammatory disease on final pathologic assessment in 24 patients (5%) [8]. Weber et al. reported a 4.5% incidence of pancreatitis on final pathologic review in 1,287 patients undergoing Whipple procedure at Memorial-Sloan Kettering [12]. Northwestern experience was published by Kennedy et al. They reported 162 patients undergoing Whipple surgery between 1993 and 2004, among them 21 patient (12.9%) had benign findings. In their experience, jaundice was more common in patients with malignant pathology but they were not able to find any other significant difference between patients with malignant or benign disease [13]. In their study, CT, MRI, and EUS suggested the presence of a discrete mass lesion in 67%, 71%, and 67% of patients, respectively, and they concluded that these findings confirm previous reports suggesting that these imaging tests can be highly accurate in predicting resectable versus unresectable disease in periampullary cancer but are less reliable in the differential diagnosis of pancreatic cancer and chronic pancreatitis [14].

In a series of more than 400 patients operated on for presumed pancreatic cancer, Patlas and colleagues [15] observed that 21 patients had pancreatitis and one had tuberculosis on final pathology or by clinical follow-up studies. All 22 patients were presented with painless jaundice and underwent CT scans and transabdominal ultrasounds, 18 had ERCP, and 9 had MRI. Ten had fine needle biopsies with no biopsy showing malignancy. A report from Duke University reported 494 patients who underwent Whipple procedure for suspected malignancy between 1992 and 2007 and showed that despite the use of aggressive preoperative work-up for pancreatic cancer, up to 7% of patients that undergo resection will have benign disease on postoperative pathologic examination. All of these patients had findings concerning for malignancy on both CT scanning and endosonography preoperatively [16]. In 2 more recent European studies, prevalence of benign disease in patients who underwent pancreatoduodenectomy for presumed malignancy reported to be 8.4% [17] and 15.6% [6].

In our report, despite the increasing use of EUS with FNA and ERCP with brushing, number of surgeries for benign pathology has been increased over the years. In these patients, findings of brush cytology and FNA have been invariably benign or nondiagnostic, but given the low negative predictive value of benign finding presence of mass on MRI/EUS, elevated CA 19-9, and high clinical suspicion for malignancy Whipple procedure was performed regardless of presurgical tissue diagnosis. One possible explanation for increased number of surgeries over time is that as the experience of surgeons with Whipple procedure has increased over the time and the morbidity from the procedure has decreased, more patients with negative work-up but high clinical suspicious have been selected for surgery.

Despite addition of EUS/FNA for examination of pancreatic masses, a highly sensitive and specific criteria for selecting patients for Whipple based on imaging, presurgical tissue pathology, and serologic data is still lacking and until such criteria is developed, about 10% of surgeries will be done for benign diseases that are being presumed malignant based on clinical judgment in combination with a spectrum of imaging findings. Given the lack of any definitive test to separate malignant from benign disease, this approach is reasonable since Whipple procedure is the only chance of increasing survival in pancreatic cancer. Further studies are required to formulate practical criteria to diagnose benign disease before surgery.

Acknowledgment

This work was independent and was not supported by any funding.

References

[1] R. H. Hawes, Q. Xiong, I. Waxman, K. J. Chang, D. B. Evans, and J. L. Abbruzzese, "A multispecialty approach to the diagnosis and management of pancreatic cancer," *The American Journal of Gastroenterology*, vol. 95, no. 1, pp. 17–31, 2000.

[2] A. B. Lowenfels, P. Maisonneuvi, G. Cavallini et al., "Pancreatitis and the risk of pancreatic cancer," *The New England Journal of Medicine*, vol. 328, no. 20, pp. 1433–1437, 1993.

[3] J. L. Cameron, T. S. Riall, J. Coleman, and K. A. Belcher, "One thousand consecutive pancreaticoduodenectomies," *Annals of Surgery*, vol. 244, no. 1, pp. 10–15, 2006.

[4] S. C. Abraham, R. E. Wilentz, C. J. Yeo et al., "Pancreaticoduodenectomy (Whipple resections) in patients without malignancy: are they all "chronic pancreatitis"?" *The American Journal of Surgical Pathology*, vol. 27, no. 1, pp. 110–120, 2003.

[5] S. A. Barnes, K. D. Lillemoe, H. S. Kaufman et al., "Pancreaticoduodenectomy for benign disease," *The American Journal of Surgery*, vol. 171, no. 1, pp. 131–135, 1996.

[6] T. M. Manzia, L. Toti, I. Lenci et al., "Benign disease and unexpected histologocal findings after pancreaticoduodenectomy: the role of endoscopic ultrasound fine needle aspiration," *Annals of the Royal College of Surgeons of England*, vol. 92, no. 4, pp. 295–301, 2010.

[7] A. R. Sasson, J. M. Gulizia, A. Galva, J. Anderson, and J. Thompson, "Pancreaticoduodenectomy for suspected malignancy: have advancements in radiographic imaging improved results?" *The American Journal of Surgery*, vol. 192, no. 6, pp. 888–893, 2006.

[8] C. D. Smith, K. E. Behrns, J. A. van Heerden, and M. G. Sarr, "Radical pancreatoduodenectomy for misdiagnosed pancreatic mass," *The British Journal of Surgery*, vol. 81, no. 4, pp. 585–589, 1994.

[9] D. A. Tessler, A. Catanzaro, V. Velanovich, S. Havstad, and S. Goel, "Predictors of cancer in patients with suspected pancreatic malignancy without a tissue diagnosis," *The American Journal of Surgery*, vol. 191, no. 2, pp. 191–197, 2006.

[10] J. S. Thompson, K. M. Murayama, J. A. Edney, and L. F. Rikkers, "Pancreaticoduodenectomy for suspected but unproven malignancy," *The American Journal of Surgery*, vol. 168, no. 6, pp. 571–573, 1994.

[11] T. M. van Gulik, J. W. A. J. Reeders, A. Bosma et al., "Incidence and clinical findings of benign, inflammatory disease in patients resected for presumed pancreatic head cancer," *Gastrointestinal Endoscopy*, vol. 46, no. 5, pp. 417–423, 1997.

[12] S. M. Weber, O. Cubukcu-Dimopulo, J. A. Palesty et al., "Lymphoplasmacytic sclerosing pancreatitis: inflammatory mimic of pancreatic carcinoma," *Journal of Gastrointestinal Surgery*, vol. 7, no. 1, pp. 129–139, 2003.

[13] T. Kennedy, L. Preczewski, S. J. Stocker et al., "Incidence of benign inflammatory disease in patients undergoing Whipple procedure for clinically suspected carcinoma: a single-institution experience," *The American Journal of Surgery*, vol. 191, no. 3, pp. 437–441, 2006.

[14] M. G. House, C. J. Yeo, J. L. Cameron et al., "Predicting resectability of periampullary cancer with three-dimensional computed tomography," *Journal of Gastrointestinal Surgery*, vol. 8, no. 3, pp. 280–288, 2004.

[15] M. Patlas, W. Deitel, B. Taylor, S. Gallinger, and S. R. Wilson, "Focal chronic pancreatitis mimicking pancreatic head carcinoma: are there suggestive features on ultrasound?" *Canadian Association of Radiologists Journal*, vol. 58, no. 1, pp. 15–21, 2007.

[16] S. G. de la Fuente, E. P. Ceppa, S. K. Reddy, B. M. Clary, D. S. Tyler, and T. N. Pappas, "Incidence of benign disease in patients that underwent resection for presumed pancreatic cancer diagnosed by endoscopic ultrasonography (EUS) and fine-needle aspiration (FNA)," *Journal of Gastrointestinal Surgery*, vol. 14, no. 7, pp. 1139–1142, 2010.

[17] M. J. van Heerde, K. Biermann, P. E. Zondervan et al., "Prevalence of autoimmune pancreatitis and other benign disorders in pancreatoduodenectomy for presumed malignancy of the pancreatic head," *Digestive Diseases and Sciences*, vol. 57, no. 9, pp. 2458–2465, 2012.

16

Postcolonoscopy Followup Recommendations: Comparison with and without Use of Polyp Pathology

Shiva K. Ratuapli, Suryakanth R. Gurudu, Mary A. Atia, Michael D. Crowell, Sarah B. Umar, M. Edwyn Harrison, Jonathan A. Leighton, and Francisco C. Ramirez

Division of Gastroenterology and Hepatology, Department of Medicine, Mayo Clinic Arizona, 13400 East Shea Boulevard, Scottsdale, AZ 85259, USA

Correspondence should be addressed to Francisco C. Ramirez; ramirez.francisco@mayo.edu

Academic Editor: Timothy A. Woodward

Background. Appropriate recommendations for a followup exam after an index colonoscopy are an important quality indicator. Lack of knowledge of polyp pathology at the time of colonoscopy may be one reason that followup recommendations are not made. *Aim.* To describe and compare the accuracy of followup recommendations made at colonoscopy based on the size and number of polyps with recommendations made at a later date based on actual polyp pathology. *Methods.* All patients who underwent screening and surveillance colonoscopy from March, 2012, to August, 2012, were included. Surveillance recommendations from the endoscopy reports were graded as "accurate" or "not accurate" based on the postpolypectomy surveillance guidelines established by US Multisociety Task Force on Colon Cancer. Polyp pathology was then used to regrade the surveillance recommendations. *Results.* Followup recommendations were accurate in 759/884 (86%) of the study colonoscopies, based upon size and number of polyps with the assumption that all polyps were adenomatous. After incorporating actual polyp pathology, 717/884 (81%) colonoscopies had accurate recommendations. *Conclusion.* In our practice, the knowledge of actual polyp pathology does not change the surveillance recommendations made at the time of colonoscopy in the majority of patients.

1. Introduction

Postpolypectomy surveillance constitutes 20% of the colonoscopies [1] performed, thereby contributing to a significant amount of health care expenditure [2, 3]. Prior to the development of postpolypectomy surveillance guidelines, which were based on the National Polyp Study in 1997, annual surveillance was a common practice. Since then, guidelines recommend the surveillance interval be based on risk of polyps found at index colonoscopy [4], rather than intense surveillance irrespective of polyp type.

In 2006, the US Multisociety Task Force on colorectal cancer (USMSTF) issued postpolypectomy surveillance guidelines [4] based on number of polyps, polyp size, and pathology as shown in Table 1. Subsequently in 2012, the USMSTF added surveillance recommendations for serrated lesions to the previous guidelines [5].

However several recent studies [6–8] have reported poor adherence to guidelines among gastroenterologists and primary care physicians. Lack of awareness of established guidelines [9] and intentional noncompliance due to personal preferences, as well as poor quality of bowel preparation [10] have been suggested as possible reasons for poor adherence to guidelines. Lack of polyp pathology at the time of colonoscopy, especially in an open access system, may be another reason that appropriate followup recommendations are not made.

Repeat surveillance colonoscopy earlier than recommended may increase healthcare costs, and delayed surveillance colonoscopy may lead to an interval cancer. Identifying and eliminating the factors that deter adherence to established guidelines are important. Decreasing or eliminating the need to rely on polyp pathology [11] may encourage

TABLE 1: 2006 USMSTF surveillance recommendations.

Baseline colonoscopy findings	Recommended surveillance interval (y)
No Polyps	10
Small (<10 mm) hyperplastic polyps	10
1-2 small (<10 mm) tubular adenomas	5–10
3–10 tubular adenomas	3
Any tubular adenoma ≥10 mm	3
>10 adenomas	<3

TABLE 2: Definitions of "accurate" and "not accurate" recommendations.

Number of Polyps	Accurate recommendations-marked "accurate" if following recommendations made	Inaccurate recommendations-marked "not accurate" if following recommendations made
	Screening	
No polyp	10 years, 5–10 years	5 years
1-2 polyps <10 mm	3–5 years, 5 years, 5–10 years	3 years
≥3 polyps	3 years, 3–5 years	<3 years
Any polyp >10 mm	3 years, 3–5 years	<3 years
	Surveillance	
No polyp	3–5 years, 5 years	3 years
1-2 polyps <10 mm	3–5 years, 5 years, 5–10 years	3 years
≥3 polyps	3 years, 3–5 years	<3 years

endoscopists to make more accurate recommendations at the time of the colonoscopy. There is a scarcity of clinical data on this subject. Therefore the aim of this study was to describe and compare the accuracy of the follow-up recommendations made using number, size and educated guess of pathology of polyps at the time of colonoscopy with recommendations based on actual polyp pathology.

2. Materials and Methods

The study was approved by the institutional review board of Mayo Clinic, as a quality improvement project. Endoscopy reports and electronic medical records of all the patients who underwent colonoscopies from March, 2012, to August, 2012, were reviewed. Only patients who underwent outpatient screening and surveillance colonoscopy were included in the study. Patients with poor bowel preparation, colonic malignancy, hereditary polyposis syndromes, incomplete exams, and large polyps requiring short term followup were excluded. Data on patient demographics, indication for procedure, quality of bowel preparation, polyp characteristics (number, size, and type of polyp) and anatomical location, and completion of colonoscopy were recorded. Information on whether surveillance recommendations were made at the time of colonoscopy as documented in the procedure report was also recorded.

All colonoscopies were performed either by an attending gastroenterologist or by fellows under direct supervision of the attending gastroenterologist. Complete colonoscopy was defined as intubating the cecum, identifying the appendiceal orifice and ileocecal valve. The quality of bowel preparation was rated by endoscopists based on five prespecified criteria as follows: "excellent," "good," "fair-adequate," "inadequate," or "poor."

The first step was to grade the initial recommendations taking into consideration the size and number of polyps and assuming that all removed polyps were adenomatous. Surveillance recommendations made by the endoscopists, based on the number and size of polyps at the time of colonoscopy were graded as "accurate" or "not accurate" based on the 2006 postpolypectomy surveillance guidelines issued by US Multisociety Task Force on colorectal cancer. The definitions of "accurate" and "not accurate" recommendations are listed in Table 2. For purposes of this study, the recommendations that gave a *range of time* but included the guideline recommendation were graded as accurate. The overall accuracy of surveillance recommendations was calculated by adding the accurate recommendations that gave a *range of time, that is, 3–5 years* and the accurate recommendations that gave a *specific time.* Early and late exams were defined as those that were recommended to be performed before and after the guideline recommended time, respectively. Patients with a *range of time* recommendations were categorized into two groups: (a) recommendations with a potential for early colonoscopy [i.e., for a correct recommendation of 5 years, 3–5 years; for a correct recommendation of 10 years: 5–10 years] (b) recommendations with potential for late colonoscopy [i.e., for a correct recommendation of 3 years, 3–5 years; for a correct recommendation of 5 years, 5–10 years] Polyp pathology was then reviewed, and adenomatous polyps were used to regrade the endoscopist's recommendations, using the same definitions for "accurate" and "not accurate" recommendations.

Standard high definition colonoscopes (Olympus America, Center Valley, PA) were used for all the procedures, most of which were performed under moderate sedation with choice of intravenous fentanyl, midazolam, or meperidine as per the preference of the performing endoscopist. Polyethylene glycol based bowel preparations were used in all of the patients.

3. Statistical Analysis

Data were entered manually and statistically assessed using IBM SPSS version 20.0 (SPSS Inc., Chicago, IL). Data distributions were evaluated using SPSS Explore and Descriptive functions along with stem-and-leaf plots and histograms. Frequency distributions were evaluated for all categorical variables. Summary statistics included point estimates and standard deviations for all continuous variables and number of patients and percentages for all categorical variables.

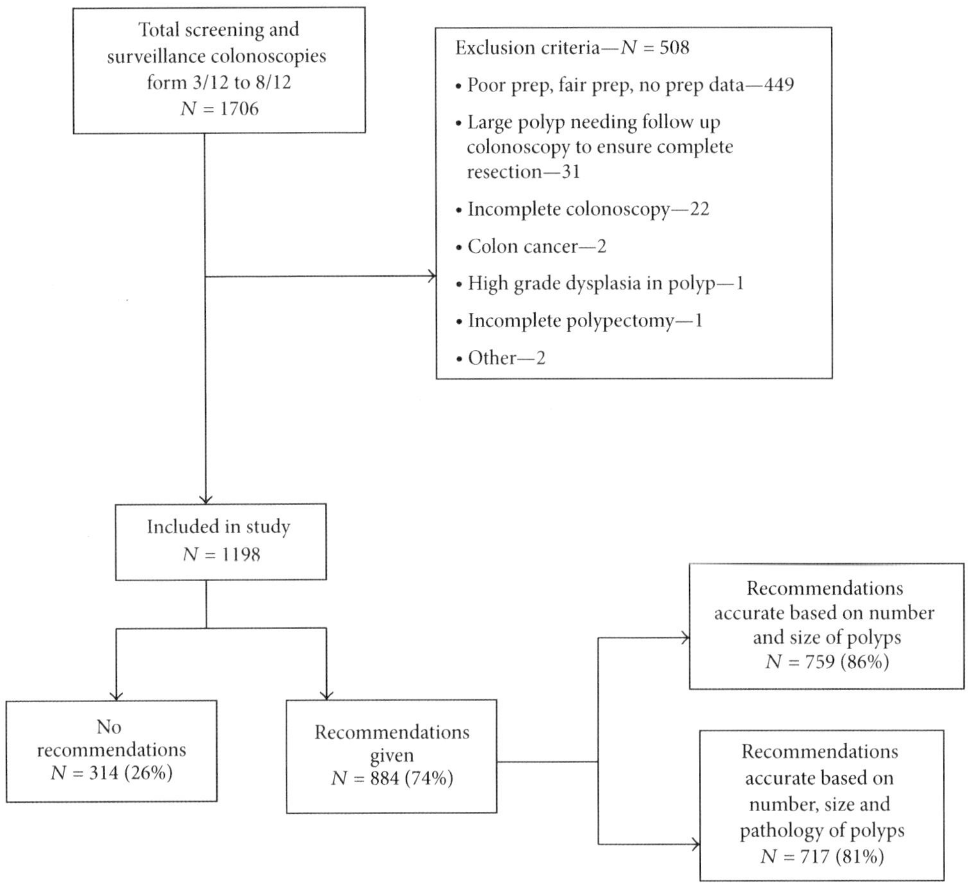

Figure 1: CONSORT diagram.

4. Results

4.1. Baseline Characteristics. Between March and August of 2012, a total of 1706 screening and surveillance colonoscopies were performed by 21 attending gastroenterologists and 7 gastroenterology fellows. After applying exclusion criteria, 1198 patients were included in the study as shown in Figure 1. Followup colonoscopy recommendations were not made in 26% (314) of the patients at the time of entering the endoscopic report. This group had a higher proportion of surveillance colonoscopies compared to the group where recommendations were given at the time of colonoscopy (Figure 2). The remaining 74% (884) patients were included in the final analysis. The mean age of the patients was 60 ± 9 years, and 48% (422) were women. The overall polyp and adenoma detection rate for this cohort of patients were 62% and 44%, respectively.

4.2. Accuracy of Surveillance Recommendations Based on Mode of Assessment. Accurate surveillance recommendations were made at the time of colonoscopy, based on number, size (and an educated guess of pathology) in 86% (759/884) of the patients. Based on actual pathology results, accurate recommendations were made in 81% (717/884) of the patients. Of these accurate recommendations, a *range of time* (e.g., 3–5 years for 5 years, 5–10 years for 10 years) was recommended instead of a *specific time*, in half of the patients, but this time range included the time recommended by the guidelines (Figure 3).

Subgroup analysis of the accuracy of recommendations at the time of the colonoscopy showed that the actual pathology decreased the proportion of accurate recommendations in screening but not surveillance colonoscopies as shown in Figure 4. Analysis of the inaccurate recommendations, using the two modes of assessment showed that the majority of these inaccurate recommendations were for an earlier interval than suggested by guidelines: 73% based on number and size of polyps, 92% based on number, size, and pathology of polyps (Figure 5). When polyp pathology was used to regrade the recommendations, the proportion of inaccurate recommendations was higher Figure 5.

5. Discussion

Our study suggests that actual polyp pathology does not change the initial surveillance interval recommendations at the time of colonoscopy in the majority of the patients. Knowing the polyp pathology changed recommendations in only 5% of our study patients. Our study results should increase the confidence and compliance in making appropriate followup surveillance interval recommendations at

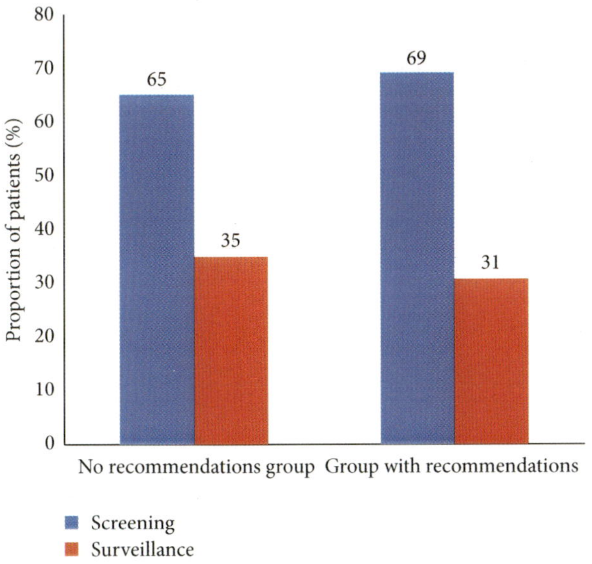

FIGURE 2: Distribution of screening and surveillance colonoscopies between the "no recommendations group" and "group with recommendations".

the time of the colonoscopy, rather than waiting for polyp pathology.

While confirming polyp pathology is important, it is not necessary for recommending the next interval colonoscopy. The hesitancy of making recommendations without pathology likely leads to low adherence among endoscopists in following current guidelines and/or amending the initial report. Similar to our study, three studies [12–14] have assessed accuracy of surveillance recommendations made at the time of colonoscopy. Gupta et al. [13] used the morphological features of polyps found during colonoscopies performed by 6 endoscopists, to predict future surveillance intervals, rather than the actual recommendations made by the endoscopist, and predicted correct surveillance interval in 83.2% of the 410 study patients. Similarly, Ignjatovic et al. [12] and Rex [14] used morphological characters of polyps during colonoscopy to predict surveillance intervals correctly in 98% and 94%, respectively. The accuracy rate of surveillance recommendations made without polyp pathology in our study (86%) was similar to that reported by Gupta et al. and lower than those reported by Ignjatovic et al. and Rex. Our study differs from the reported studies [12–14] in that we compared the original surveillance recommendations made by the performing colonoscopists from the initial endoscopy reports with the surveillance recommendations obtained by histopathological assessment of polyps. Additionally, our study included a larger number of study patients and a higher number of performing endoscopists, compared to the other studies.

Similar accuracy of surveillance recommendations with and without using polyp pathology, as seen in our study supports American Society of Gastrointestinal Endoscopy's PIVI (Preservation and Incorporation of Valuable Endoscopic Innovations) [11] to promote endoscopic technologies that aid in optical diagnosis of diminutive colon polyp histology. Our results could encourage endoscopists to either resect and discard or leave in place small diminutive polyps [13, 15], if high definition endoscopes with narrow band imaging were used in optical diagnosis of small polyps [16, 17].

The common cause for making inaccurate recommendations in our study was recommending an early colonoscopy than suggested by the guidelines. When polyp pathology was used to grade the accuracy of recommendations, 92% of the inaccurate recommendations were made for an earlier colonoscopy. An earlier than recommended followup colonoscopy exam can be considered detrimental for the healthcare system since it implies an unplanned and most likely unnecessary expense whereas a recommendation for late followup colonoscopy can be considered potentially detrimental for the patient since it would delay the diagnosis of significant colonic lesions arising from polyps.

There are other reasons that surveillance interval recommendations made after colonoscopy may not be accurate. As reported in other studies [9, 18–22], lack of awareness of guidelines or unwillingness of endoscopists to adhere to guidelines may be some of the reasons for not making accurate recommendations. Other possible reasons include the status of the bowel preparation at the time of colonoscopy, the endoscopist's level of comfort with current interval guidelines, unavailability of the patient's family history, and the lack of knowledge of the endoscopist's own adenoma detection rate in different segments of the colon. Additionally, we speculate that lack of confidence of the visual diagnosis of polyp pathology at the time of making recommendations may have led our endoscopists to recommend a colonoscopy early than necessary.

The limitation of this study is that it was retrospective in nature. Classifying recommendations that gave a *range of time* as accurate may not be ideal, as this may give the endoscopist or primary care provider enough room for interpretation leading more likely to opt for an earlier interval rather than the longer one. When grading the endoscopist's recommendation, all polyps were considered to be adenomatous, as it is not possible to know which polyps were thought to be hyperplastic or adenomatous by the endoscopist. However, it is reasonable to assume that the endoscopist would only remove polyps that had an appearance suspicious for adenomatous polyps. With this in mind, we assumed retrospectively that all polyps were considered adenomatous. Despite these limitations, our study was strengthened by its large sample size and inclusion of endoscopists with varied levels of experience, thereby increasing the generalizability of our results.

In conclusion, our study suggests that accurate surveillance guidelines can be recommended at the time of colonoscopy without knowing actual polyp pathology. In this cohort of patients, surveillance recommendations made at the time of colonoscopy based on number and size of polyps were accurate in 86% of patients and the surveillance interval after knowledge of polyp pathology did not change the recommendations in majority of patients. Periodic reviews of current guidelines, improvement of bowel preparation quality, and improvements in the endoscopic imaging technology and

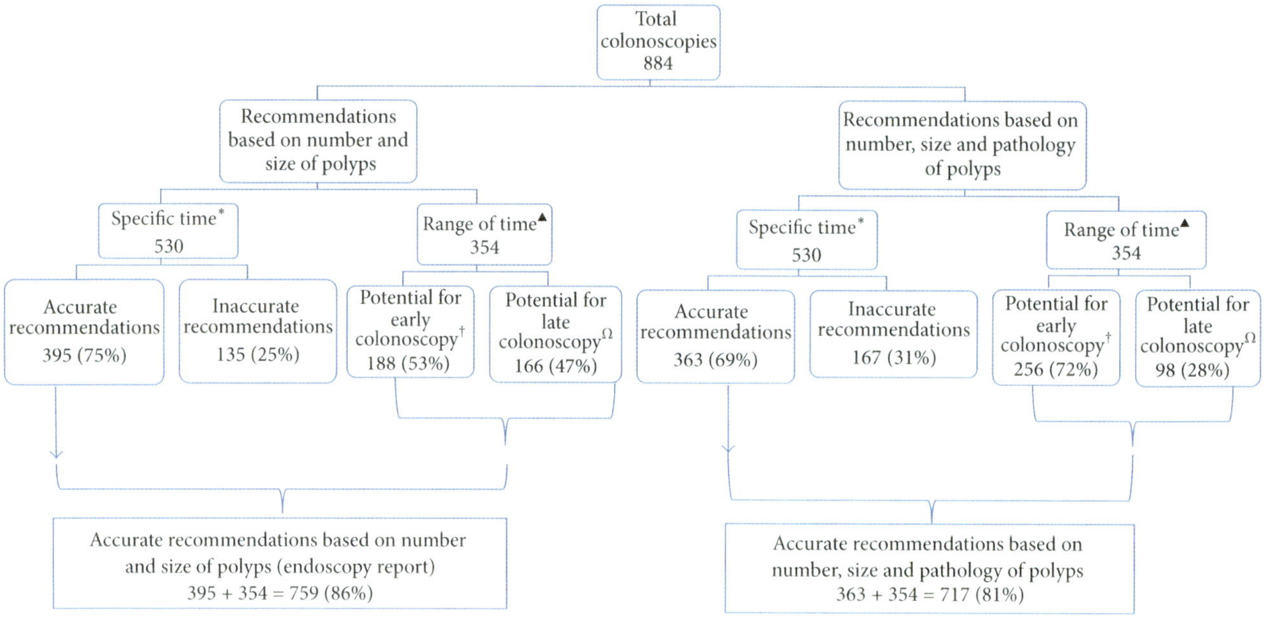

* Recommendations where Specific time was given (e.g., 3 yrs, 5 yrs, etc.)
▲ Recommendations where a range of time was given (e.g., 3–5 yrs, 5–10 yrs, etc.)
† Accurate recommendations but potential for earlier follow up colonoscopy (e.g., 3–5 yrs recommended for 5 yrs)
Ω Accurate recommendations but potential for late follow up colonoscopy (e.g., 3–5 yrs recommended for 3 yrs)

FIGURE 3: Accuracy of recommendations using two modes of assessment.

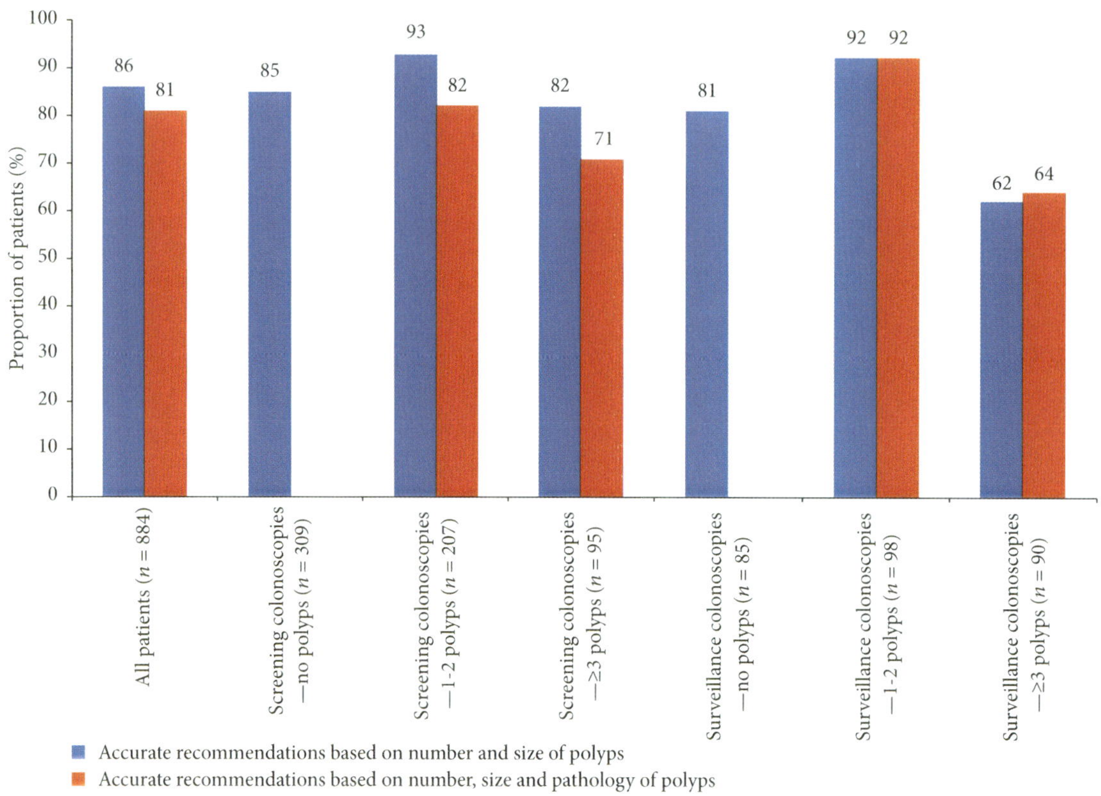

FIGURE 4: Accuracy of recommendations using two modes of assessment, in various subgroups.

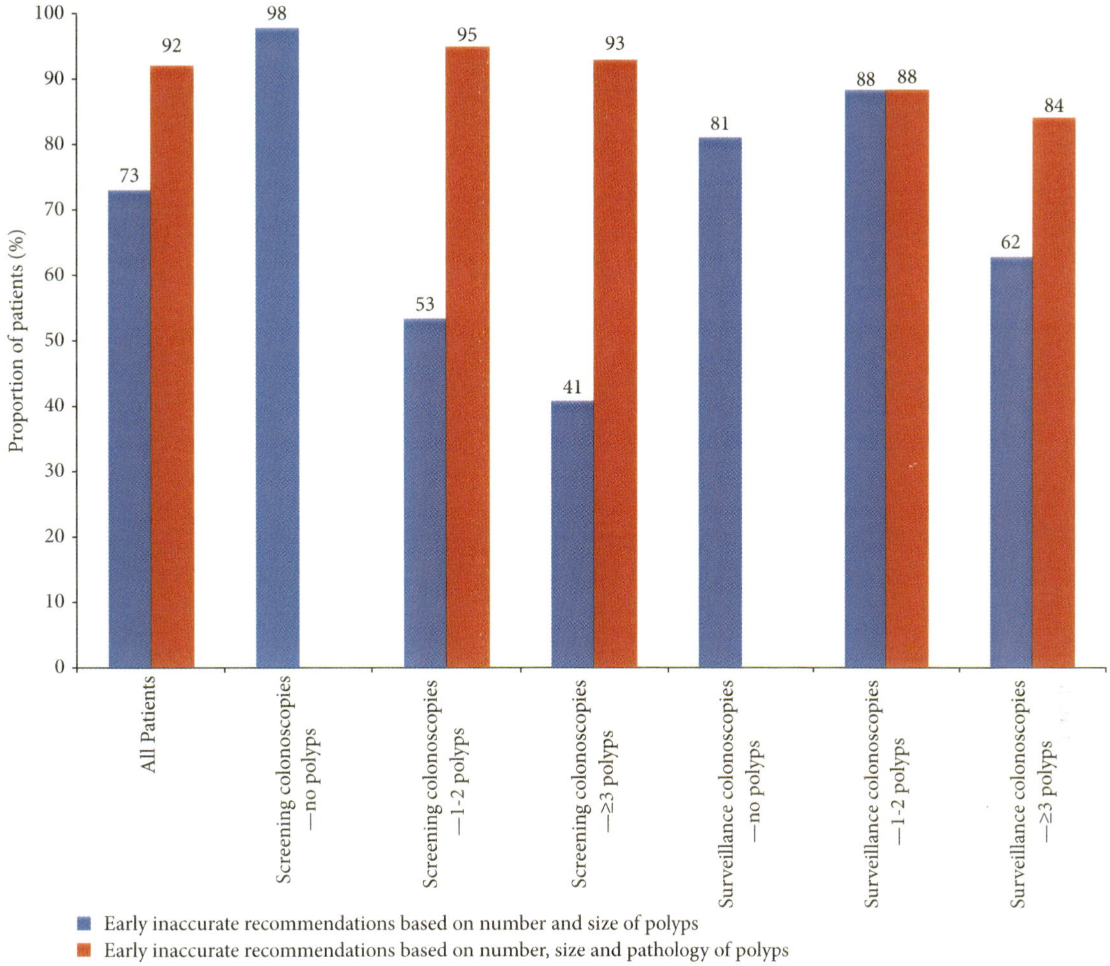

FIGURE 5: Distribution of inaccurate recommendations for an early colonoscopy using two modes of assessment in various subgroups.

awareness of individual endoscopist's polyp and adenoma detection rates in various colonic segments may improve the accuracy of interval recommendations based on visual diagnosis at the time of colonoscopy. Future studies should examine the effect of improving adherence to guidelines to see if an adequate accuracy may be achieved.

References

[1] D. A. Lieberman, P. L. de Garmo, D. E. Fleischer, G. M. Eisen, and M. Helfand, "Patterns of endoscopy use in the United States," *Gastroenterology*, vol. 118, no. 3, pp. 619–624, 2000.

[2] S. Vijan, J. Inadomi, R. A. Hayward, T. P. Hofer, and A. M. Fendrick, "Projections of demand and capacity for colonoscopy related to increasing rates of colorectal cancer screening in the United States," *Alimentary Pharmacology and Therapeutics*, vol. 20, no. 5, pp. 507–515, 2004.

[3] U. Ladabaum and K. Song, "Projected national impact of colorectal cancer screening on clinical and economic outcomes and health services demand," *Gastroenterology*, vol. 129, no. 4, pp. 1151–1162, 2005.

[4] S. J. Winawer, A. G. Zauber, R. H. Fletcher et al., "Guidelines for colonoscopy surveillance after polypectomy: a consensus update by the US Multi-Society Task Force on Colorectal Cancer and the American Cancer Society," *Gastroenterology*, vol. 130, no. 6, pp. 1872–1885, 2006.

[5] D. A. Lieberman, D. K. Rex, S. J. Winawer, F. M. Giardiello, D. A. Johnson, and T. R. Levin, "Guidelines for colonoscopy surveillance after screening and polypectomy: a consensus update by the us multi-society task force on colorectal cancer," *Gastroenterology*, vol. 143, no. 3, pp. 844–857, 2012.

[6] P. A. Mysliwiec, M. L. Brown, C. N. Klabunde, and D. F. Ransohoff, "Are physicians doing too much colonoscopy? A national survey of colorectal surveillance after polypectomy," *Annals of Internal Medicine*, vol. 141, no. 4, pp. 264–271, 2004.

[7] F. Radaelli, S. Paggi, A. Bortoli, and G. de Pretis, "Overutilization of post-polypectomy surveillance colonoscopy in clinical practice: a prospective, multicentre study," *Digestive and Liver Disease*, vol. 44, no. 9, pp. 748–753, 2012.

[8] G. C. Harewood, O. Rathore, S. Patchett, and F. Murray, "Assessment of adherence to published surveillance guidelines—opportunity to enhance efficiency of endoscopic practice," *Irish Medical Journal*, vol. 101, no. 8, pp. 248–250, 2008.

[9] S. D. Saini, R. S. Nayak, L. Kuhn, and P. Schoenfeld, "Why don't gastroenterologists follow colon polyp surveillance guidelines? Results of a national survey," *Journal of Clinical Gastroenterology*, vol. 43, no. 6, pp. 554–558, 2009.

[10] S. Ben-Horin, S. Bar-Meir, and B. Avidan, "The impact of colon cleanliness assessment on endoscopists' recommendations for follow-up colonoscopy," *American Journal of Gastroenterology*, vol. 102, no. 12, pp. 2680–2685, 2007.

[11] D. K. Rex, C. Kahi, M. O'Brien et al., "The American Society for Gastrointestinal Endoscopy PIVI (Preservation and Incorporation of Valuable Endoscopic Innovations) on real-time endoscopic assessment of the histology of diminutive colorectal polyps," *Gastrointestinal Endoscopy*, vol. 73, no. 3, pp. 419–422, 2011.

[12] A. Ignjatovic, J. E. East, N. Suzuki, M. Vance, T. Guenther, and B. P. Saunders, "Optical diagnosis of small colorectal polyps at routine colonoscopy (Detect InSpect ChAracterise Resect and Discard; DISCARD trial): a prospective cohort study," *The Lancet Oncology*, vol. 10, no. 12, pp. 1171–1178, 2009.

[13] N. Gupta, A. Bansal, D. Rao et al., "Accuracy of in vivo optical diagnosis of colon polyp histology by narrow-band imaging in predicting colonoscopy surveillance intervals," *Gastrointestinal Endoscopy*, vol. 75, no. 3, pp. 494–502, 2012.

[14] D. K. Rex, "Narrow-band imaging without optical magnification for histologic analysis of colorectal polyps," *Gastroenterology*, vol. 136, no. 4, pp. 1174–1181, 2009.

[15] D. G. Hewett, M. E. Huffman, and D. K. Rex, "Leaving distal colorectal hyperplastic polyps in place can be achieved with high accuracy by using narrow-band imaging: an observational study," *Gastrointestinal Endoscopy*, vol. 76, no. 2, pp. 374–380, 2012.

[16] A. Rastogi, K. Pondugula, A. Bansal et al., "Recognition of surface mucosal and vascular patterns of colon polyps by using narrow-band imaging: interobserver and intraobserver agreement and prediction of polyp histology," *Gastrointestinal Endoscopy*, vol. 69, no. 3, part 2, pp. 716–722, 2009.

[17] T. Yamada, S. Tamura, S. Onishi, and M. Hiroi, "A comparison of magnifying chromoendoscopy versus histopathology of forceps biopsy specimen in the diagnosis of minute flat adenoma of the colon," *Digestive Diseases and Sciences*, vol. 54, no. 9, pp. 2002–2008, 2009.

[18] B. J. John, S. Irukulla, G. Pilgrim, I. Swift, and A. M. Abulafi, "Surveillance colonoscopies for colorectal polyps—too often, too many! an Audit at a Large District General Hospital," *Colorectal Disease*, vol. 10, no. 9, pp. 898–900, 2008.

[19] A. H. Krist, R. M. Jones, S. H. Woolf et al., "Timing of repeat colonoscopy: disparity between guidelines and endoscopists' recommendation," *American Journal of Preventive Medicine*, vol. 33, no. 6, pp. 471–478, 2007.

[20] D. B. Nelson, "Appropriate use of surveillance colonoscopy after polypectomy," *Nature Clinical Practice Oncology*, vol. 2, no. 1, pp. 22–23, 2005.

[21] K. R. Yabroff, C. N. Klabunde, G. Yuan et al., "Are physicians' recommendations for colorectal cancer screening guideline-consistent?" *Journal of General Internal Medicine*, vol. 26, no. 2, pp. 177–184, 2011.

[22] I. Zbidi, R. Hazazi, Y. Niv, and S. Birkenfeld, "Colonosopy screening and surveillance of colorectal cancer and polyps: Physicians' knowledge," *Israel Medical Association Journal*, vol. 9, no. 12, pp. 862–865, 2007.

17

Spiral Enteroscopy Utilizing Capsule Location Index for Achieving High Diagnostic and Therapeutic Yield

Rohan Mandaliya,[1] Jason Korenblit,[2] Brendan O'Hare,[2] Anastasia Shnitser,[2] Ramalinga Kedika,[2] Rebecca Matro,[2] Dina Halegoua-De Marzio,[2] Anthony Infantolino,[2] and Mitchell Conn[2]

[1]*Department of Medicine, Thomas Jefferson University Hospital, 132 S 10th Street, Philadelphia, PA 19107, USA*
[2]*Division of Gastroenterology and Hepatology, Department of Medicine, Thomas Jefferson University Hospital, 132 S 10th Street, Philadelphia, PA 19107, USA*

Correspondence should be addressed to Mitchell Conn; mitchell.conn@jefferson.edu

Academic Editor: Lars Aabakken

Background and Aim. Spiral enteroscopy (SE) is a new small bowel endoscopic technique. Our aim is to review the diagnostic and therapeutic yield, safety of SE, and the predictive role of prior capsule endoscopy (CE) at an academic center. *Methods.* A retrospective review of patients undergoing SE after prior CE between 2008 and 2013 was performed. Capsule location index (CLI) was defined as the fraction of total small bowel transit time when the lesion was seen on CE. *Results.* A total of 174 SEs were performed: antegrade (147) and retrograde (27). Abnormalities on SE were detected in 65% patients. The procedure was safe in patients with surgically altered bowel anatomy ($n = 12$). The diagnostic yield of antegrade SE decreased with increasing CLI range. The diagnostic yield of retrograde SE decreased on decreasing CLI range. A CLI cutoff of 0.6 was derived that determined the initial route of SE. Vascular ectasias seen on CE were detected in 83% cases on SE; $p < 0.01$. *Conclusions.* SE is safe with a high diagnostic and therapeutic yield. CLI is predictive of the success of SE and determines the best route of SE. The type of small bowel pathology targeted by SE may affect its utility and yield.

1. Introduction

The advent of wireless capsule endoscopy has remarkably improved the endoscopic evaluation of the small bowel [1–3]. However, one of the major limitations of capsule endoscopy is that it is a purely diagnostic procedure. The introduction of double balloon enteroscopy in 2001, followed by single balloon enteroscopy, has allowed for the ability to perform diagnostic and therapeutic procedures deep into the small bowel [4–7]. More recently, spiral enteroscopy (SE) has been introduced for deep intubation of the small bowel. Double balloon enteroscopy and single balloon enteroscopy use a similar mechanism of advancement by sequential bowel pleating by a push-pull technique. In contrast, SE uses a plastic spiral tipped overtube coupled with an enteroscope that can be advanced as a unit by continuous rotation of the overtube. SE has not been studied in a large series and is still an emerging technique. Our institution has one of the largest experiences with this technique.

The most common indication for deep enteroscopy is small bowel pathology detected on prior capsule endoscopy. It has been a challenge to accurately detect lesions seen on capsule endoscopy via deep enteroscopy. Although SE has been initially shown as a safe and feasible means of deep small bowel intubation, its ability to detect lesions seen on capsule endoscopy has not been well reported. The time taken by the video capsule to traverse the small bowel varies from minutes to hours and may vary in different patients. This variation makes it difficult to predict the possible location of the lesion in the small bowel as well as the route most suitable for enteroscopy (antegrade or retrograde). Insertion of enteroscope via mouth is called antegrade approach while insertion of enteroscope via anus is called retrograde approach. We calculated an index called a capsule location index (CLI) that gives the location of the lesion in terms of the fraction of time of small bowel transit.

One of the aims of our study was to assess the safety as well as diagnostic and therapeutic yield of SE using either an antegrade or retrograde approach. In addition, we sought to determine if CLI is predictive of the success of SE and can help determine the best route of enteroscopy.

2. Materials and Methods

A retrospective analysis of patients who underwent capsule endoscopy and subsequent SE at Thomas Jefferson University Hospital between 2008 and 2013 was performed. The institutional review board of Thomas Jefferson University approved the study. The patients' electronic medical records, capsule endoscopy studies, and spiral enteroscopy reports were reviewed.

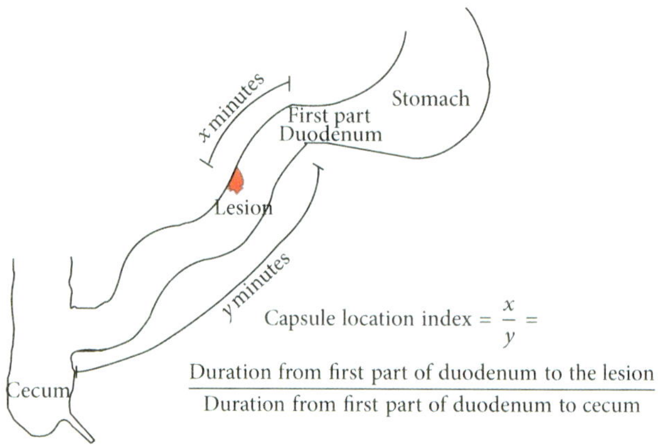

FIGURE 1: Schematic diagram for the calculation of Capsule Location Index.

2.1. Capsule Study. The PillCam SB (Given Imaging, USA) was used in all patients in this study. Patients underwent capsule endoscopy after a 12-hour fast with clear liquids allowed up to 4 hours before the test. Capsule endoscopy was evaluated by only one gastroenterologist expert in viewing capsule studies. Capsule endoscopy was considered positive if any lesion was detected in the small bowel. If two different lesions were seen, both the lesions were recorded and considered as two separate target lesions on spiral enteroscopy. The following information was recorded: the type of small bowel lesion found, time at the first duodenal image, time at which lesion is seen, time to reach the cecum, and small bowel transit time. CLI was derived to describe the location of the lesion as a time fraction of small bowel transit (Figure 1). It was calculated as the fraction of total small bowel transit time when the lesion was seen. Total small bowel transit time was defined as the time interval between the first duodenal image and the first cecal image:

$$\text{CLI} = \frac{\text{Duration from the first duodenal image to the lesion found}}{\text{Duration from the first duodenal image to cecum}}. \quad (1)$$

Not all the capsule endoscopies were complete to reach the cecum. Incomplete capsule endoscopies were defined as capsule not reaching the cecum within the recorded time. CLI could not be calculated in those studies.

2.2. Spiral Enteroscopy. A total of 174 SE procedures were performed in 148 patients. 19 patients had the procedure more than once either for inability to detect lesions or for persistent symptoms. Nine patients out of 19 had both antegrade and retrograde spiral procedures. For the sake of uniformity, each procedure was considered to be performed on a unique patient as the major outcome was to study the detection of lesion. Ninety-six percent (168/174) of all spiral enteroscopy procedures were performed by only one expert endoscopist who has been performing all forms of deep small bowel enteroscopy since 1990. The remaining six spiral enteroscopy procedures were performed by another expert endoscopist having expertise in double balloon enteroscopy. All procedures were carried out with the Olympus SIF-Q180 enteroscope (Spiral Medical, LLC, MA, USA) coupled with a spiral overtube. General anesthesia was used for all antegrade procedures and deep sedation was used for retrograde cases. Spiral enteroscopy was performed as previously described [8]. Examination of the small bowel and therapeutic maneuvers were performed during intubation and withdrawal of the enteroscope and overtube. The patients were followed up for any complications till discharge from the endoscopy unit as well as the next day via telephone call or inpatient follow-up. They were also asked to call the physician for any new symptoms.

Positive findings on SE were compared to the abnormal findings seen on capsule endoscopy. Studies in which SE identified the lesion seen on capsule endoscopy were considered positive. In cases where two different types of lesions were seen on capsule endoscopy, both the lesions were considered to be target lesions for SE. For cases in which multiple vascular ectasias were the target lesions on capsule endoscopy, detection by SE was considered positive if any vascular ectasias were detected on SE.

Inclusion criteria included patients of all ages who required deep enteroscopy for further evaluation of the lesions detected on capsule endoscopy, computed tomography (CT) scan, or CT enterography.

Exclusion criteria included patients with severe comorbidities precluding sedation and general anesthesia as well as patients with known esophageal varices and strictures precluding overtube insertion.

Data were recorded in an electronic database. Statistical analysis was performed using the SAS system, version 9.1 (SAS Institute Inc., Cary, NC). Chi-square test and Fisher's exact test were used for categorical variables. A p value of <0.05 was considered statistically significant.

3. Results

A total of 174 SE procedures were performed between 2008 and 2013. 147 were antegrade and 27 were retrograde SE.

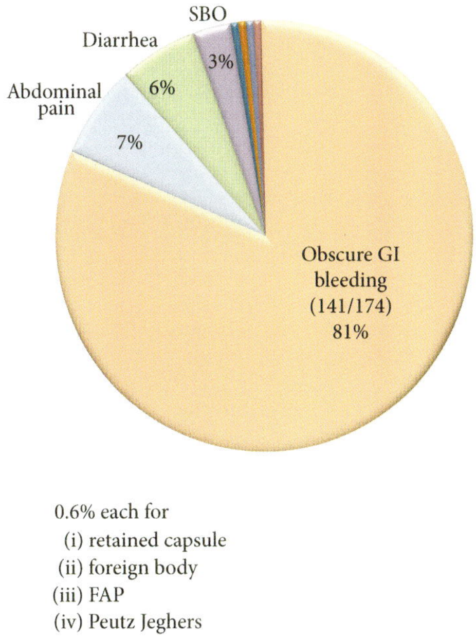

Figure 2: Overall indications of SE.

Table 1: Indications for SE based on capsule endoscopy findings.

Findings on capsule endoscopy	*N* (number of patients)
Vascular ectasia (VE)	35
Active bleeding	25
Mass/bulging	22
Blood	19
Ulcer	12
Polyp	11
Inflammation	8

Note. There were 16 patients with obscure GI bleeding who had prior capsule endoscopy not available for review.

Mean age of the patients was 66 (±14.6) years. 46% (81) were females and 54% (93) were males.

3.1. Indications of SE. The most common indication of SE was obscure GI bleeding (141, 81%). Figure 2 shows various indications of SE. Most SEs were performed due to abnormal prior capsule endoscopy. Table 1 provides the indications for SE based on the abnormality seen on capsule endoscopy. Vascular ectasia seen on the capsule endoscopy was the most common indication for SE with inflammation being the least common.

3.2. Yield of SE. SE yielded positive findings in 113/174 (65%) patients. Table 2 shows the various findings revealed on spiral enteroscopy. Vascular ectasias were the most common finding (60%). There were 5 patients with Dieulafoy's lesion in the small bowel. Two patients showed active jejunal diverticular bleeding.

3.3. Therapeutic Yield of SE. Endoscopic therapy was performed in 63% (109) of patients (Table 3). The most common therapy performed was argon plasma coagulation (APC), performed in 61% (66) of patients. Endoscopic clipping was successfully performed in 20 patients. Dilation of strictures as well as retrieval of endocapsule was also performed with SE.

Table 2: Findings on SE.

Findings	*N* (number of cases)
Vascular ectasia (VE)	60 (35%)
Inflammation	19 (11%)
Polyp	7 (4%)
Ulcer	7 (4%)
Mass	7 (4%)
Benign small bowel diverticula	6 (3.4%)
Dieulafoy's lesion	5 (2.8%)
Scalloping of the mucosa	5 (2.8%)
Small bowel diverticular bleeding	2 (1.1%)
Active bleeding of unknown cause	2 (1.1%)
Stricture	2 (1.1%)
Small bowel varices	1 (0.6%)

Ten patients had two findings on spiral enteroscopy.

Table 3: Various therapeutic maneuvers performed by SE.

Therapy performed	*N* (number of cases)
APC	66 (38%)
Biopsy	53 (31%)
Endoclip	20 (11.5%)
Polypectomy	7 (4%)
Dilatation of stricture	2 (1.1%)
Retrieval of endocapsule	1 (0.6%)

3.4. Safety of SE. SE was safe in patients with a history of surgically altered bowel anatomy. It was safe in seven patients having Roux-en-Y bypass and five patients having enteroenteral anastomosis. There were no major complications in all 174 patients. Four patients had minor complications. There were three patients with esophageal mucosal tears who were successfully treated conservatively or endoscopically with endoclips, while one patient had transient jejunal intussusception that resolved spontaneously during the procedure.

3.5. SE in relation to Prior Capsule Endoscopy. There were 132 prior positive capsule studies available to review. 115 out of 132 studies were complete (capsule reached the cecum within the recorded time) to calculate CLI.

The median time interval between capsule endoscopy and SE was one month. For active bleeding seen on capsule endoscopy, SE was performed within next 24 hours.

Almost half of the lesions were present in the first quarter of the small bowel transit time (0–0.25) (Figure 3).

3.6. Antegrade SE. The detection rate of lesions seen on complete capsule endoscopy by antegrade approach was 64.9% (76/117 lesions). Mean CLI was 0.22 in positive antegrade SE with a range of 0.00 to 0.72, while a negative antegrade

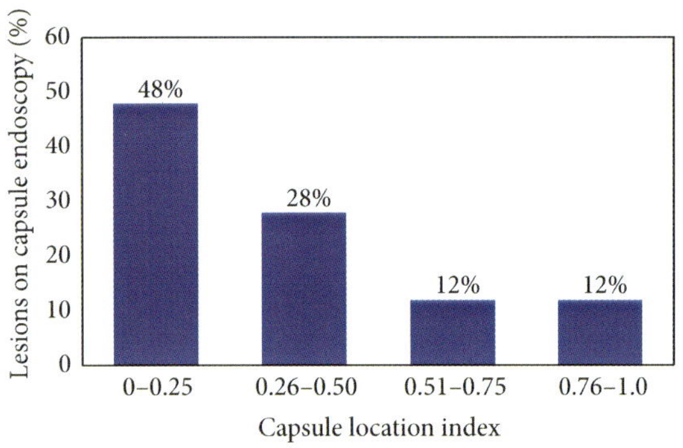

FIGURE 3: Distribution of lesions seen on capsule endoscopy with respect to capsule location index (CLI).

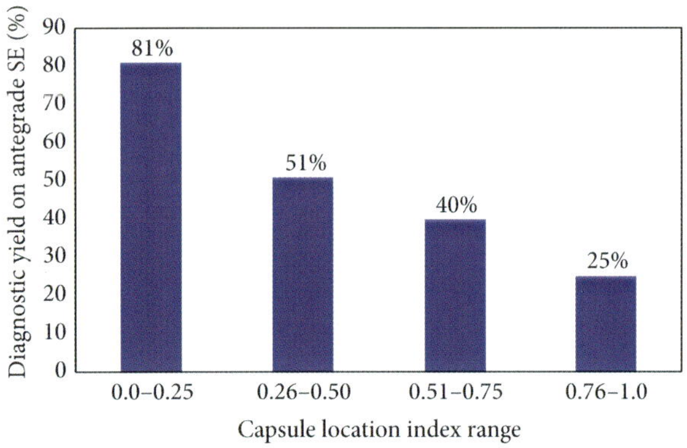

FIGURE 4: The diagnostic yield of antegrade SE with respect to CLI. Note that the yield decreases as the CLI range increases.

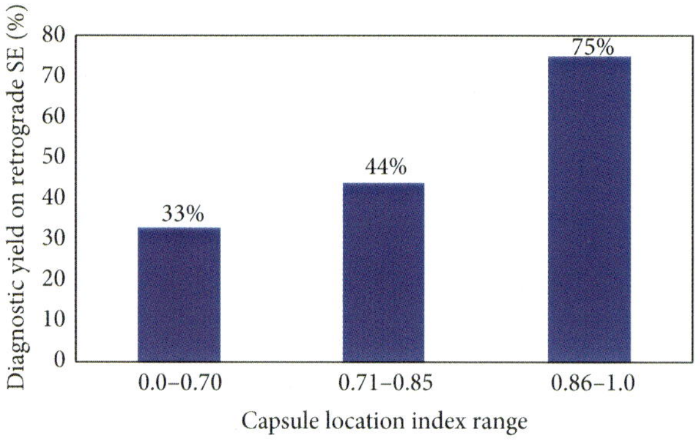

FIGURE 5: The diagnostic yield of retrograde SE with respect to CLI. Note that the yield decreases as the CLI range decreases.

TABLE 4: Detection rate of various lesions seen on capsule endoscopy by SE.

	Lesion on capsule	Corresponding SE	Detection rate
Vascular ectasia (VE)	35	29	83%
Blood	19	13	68%
Active bleeding	25	16	64%
Ulcer	12	7	58%
Inflammation	8	4	50%
Polyp	11	5	45%
Mass/bulging	22	7	32%

enteroscopy had a mean CLI of 0.40 with a range of 0.00 to 0.86. Figure 3 illustrates the decreasing diagnostic yield of antegrade SE at increasing range of CLI. There was significant difference in the diagnostic yield for lesion within CLI range (0.0–0.25), 81% (51/63) as compared to lesions within CLI range (0.26–1.0) 46% (25/54) ($p < 0.001$) (Figure 4).

3.7. Retrograde SE. The detection rate of lesion seen on capsule endoscopy by retrograde approach was 55% (11/20 lesions). Mean CLI was 0.88 for positive retrograde enteroscopy while negative retrograde enteroscopy had a mean CLI of 0.76. As shown in Figure 5, the diagnostic yield of retrograde SE decreases as the range of CLI decreases.

3.8. CLI Cut Offs. We sought to determine the capsule location index cutoffs in order to achieve a diagnostic yield of at least 70% in antegrade as well as retrograde SE, respectively, to be able to decide the initial route of enteroscopy.

Lesions within CLI of 0.6 were detected 70% of the times by initial antegrade approach. Diagnostic yield of 70% was achieved for CLI up to 0.6 versus 17% for lesions with CLI > 0.60, $p < 0.001$ (Fisher's test). Similarly, lesions with CLI ≥ 0.80 were detected 70% of the times by initial retrograde approach. There was diagnostic yield of 70% with lesions with CLI ≥ 0.80 versus 17% with CLI < 0.80, $p = 0.03$ (Fisher's test) (Figure 6). A CLI range of 0.61 to 0.79 had the lowest yield of 15% (2/13) by either approach (9 antegrade and 4 retrograde).

3.9. Yield of SE with respect to Various Lesions on CE. SE was able to detect lesions seen on capsule study at various rates based on the type of lesion (Table 4). Vascular ectasias seen on capsule study had the highest detection rate on spiral enteroscopy (83%), while mass/bulging had the lowest detection rate (32%). Active bleeding seen on capsule study was detected in 64% of cases with spiral enteroscopy. The overall detection rate of SE after capsule endoscopy was 62% (81/131).

4. Discussion

With the advent of capsule endoscopy, direct and painless evaluation of the entire small bowel became possible. Capsule endoscopy is considered to be superior to angiography, small bowel follow-through, and conventional push enteroscopy in detection of small bowel disease pathology especially in patients with bleeding [9]. However, one of the major limitations of capsule endoscopy is that it is a purely diagnostic procedure [10]. With the introduction of deep enteroscopy it is now possible to identify and treat lesions detected on capsule endoscopy. Spiral enteroscopy is the newest technique for deep small bowel intubation. Our institution has one of the

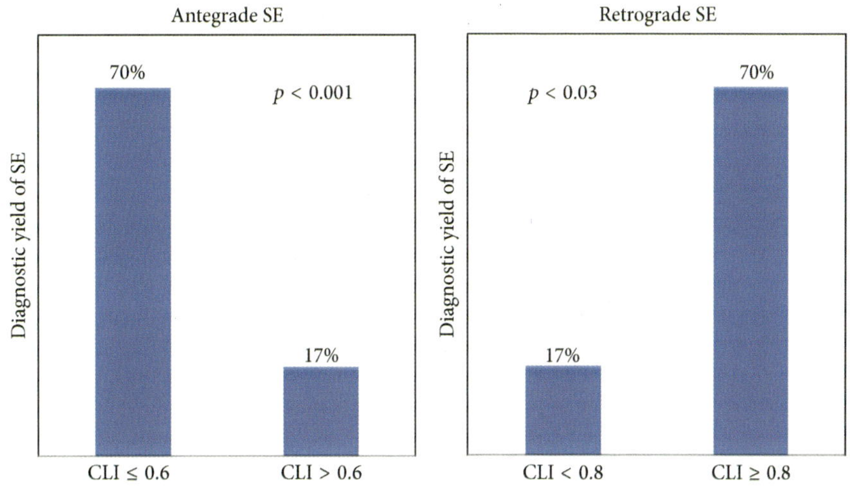

FIGURE 6: CLI cut offs for achieving 70% diagnostic yield on antegrade as well as retrograde approaches respectively.

largest experiences with SE. Preliminary data have shown SE to be a safe and well tolerated procedure [11].

Our results indicate that SE is a safe and effective deep enteroscopic technique. The diagnostic and therapeutic yields of the SE procedures in this study compare favorably with data previously published regarding balloon enteroscopy [12, 13]. The yield is also consistent with the recent preliminary data on SE [14]. In our study the most common indication for SE was obscure gastrointestinal bleeding and the most common finding was vascular ectasias (VE). It allows for endoscopic therapy such as argon plasma coagulation, clipping, biopsy, polypectomy, dilation of stricture, and injection of solution. We also successfully treated an active jejunal diverticular bleeding [15].

The procedure was well tolerated by the majority of the patients. It appears to be safe and therapeutic in patients with Roux-en-Y bypass and enteroenteral anastomosis. No major complications were noted. Esophageal mucosal tear occurred during withdrawal of the scope in three patients (2%). They were successfully treated. The utility of SE may be limited in patients with known esophageal pathology. The spiral enteroscopy technique may have an advantage over other deep enteroscopy techniques in terms of speed of advancement and stability while doing maneuvers and during withdrawal [11]. Endoscopic therapeutic procedures are easy to perform during SE. The configuration of the enteroscope and the overtube remains relatively straight, without significant loop formation which permits easy passage of the accessories [11]. In a study by Akerman et al., the rapidity of advancement of the enteroscope during spiral enteroscopy was superior to that of other deep small bowel intubation techniques with similar estimated depths of insertion [11].

SE like other deep enteroscopies may require both an antegrade and a retrograde study to investigate whole small bowel. The ability to select the best approach based on prior capsule endoscopy findings can improve success and minimize the need of multiple procedures and additional sedation. In a recent study evaluating the insertion route of push or pull enteroscopy, Gay used a % time index which was defined as lesion location as a percentage of the mouth to cecum time [16]. However, gastric emptying time varies in patients and we found that time to reach duodenum varies frequently. Li et al. used pylorus to cecum time to determine lesion location [10]. However, since pylorus is a sphincter, it may affect the passage of capsule. Since duodenum and cecum are stable landmarks we used small bowel transit time from the first part of duodenum to cecum to determine location of the lesion.

In our study, an antegrade approach CLI cutoff ≤ 0.25 revealed the highest yield of 81% and only a yield of 46% for the lesions with CLI > 0.25. CLI within 0.6 had a 70% diagnostic yield with initial antegrade approach. Initial antegrade approach should be considered for lesions with CLI up to 0.6. For retrograde approach, a CLI of $\geq$0.8 had a diagnostic yield of 70%. Initial retrograde approach should be considered for lesions with CLI $\geq$0.8. Lesions with CLI between 0.61 and 0.79 remain a challenge, as they were successfully detected only 15% of the time by either approach. This may guide us in informing the patients about the low likelihood of detection of a lesion before going for long standing enteroscopy procedure requiring general anesthesia. They may require a more invasive/surgical procedure.

For those cases in which capsule endoscopy is incomplete, antegrade SE should be the first procedure of choice if a pathologic lesion was seen on capsule endoscopy. A repeat capsule endoscopy could be considered with or without endoscope placement if gastric emptying time contributed to the incomplete study.

Our study has somewhat similar results to the study by Li et al. which utilized double balloon enteroscopy. Some minor differences are as follows: the cutoff of retrograde approach derived in their study was 0.6 compared to 0.8 in our study. We believe that, for lesions with CLI between 0.6 and 0.8, initial approach should be individualized based on the presentation of the patient and informing the patient about the low chances of lesion to be detected by either approach. The prior study excluded patients with positive capsule studies showing submucosal tumor but with subsequent negative balloon enteroscopy via either approach which may affect the yield of the enteroscopy procedure. In comparison, we included all the patients with positive capsule endoscopy with subsequent negative spiral enteroscopy. We included 22 capsule studies showing submucosal tumor, with lowest yield on spiral enteroscopy (7/22, 32%). It is important to note that there is a false positive rate for capsule endoscopy which is difficult to confirm. One other note is that there were higher cases of obscure gastrointestinal bleeding in our study compared to Li et al. study (81% versus 67%). Since bleeding is often self-limited and the lesion may heal in time, it might have led to some differences in the diagnostic yield.

Vascular ectasias were the most common finding on capsule endoscopy and SE. 83% of the vascular ectasias seen by capsule endoscopy were reached by SE. Similarly, active bleeding was also easily detected on SE (64% of studies). This shows that capsule endoscopy may be indicated as an initial test in patients with obscure active gastrointestinal bleeding followed by SE, as angiographic embolization may not be a preferred option in small bowel bleeding source due to risk of ischemia.

Other findings such as ulcer, mass/bulging, polyp, and inflammation often are single and may be missed during enteroscopy. These lesions may also be nonspecific, transient, and overdiagnosed during capsule endoscopy. One factor may be the time interval between capsule study and enteroscopy. Most of the cases in our study had a median interval of 1 month. It may be possible that lesions such as ulcer or inflammation may have healed over time. This delay may lead to lower detection rate of these types of lesions on spiral enteroscopy.

In a recent study, Buscaglia et al. evaluated the diagnostic yield of SE performed for evaluation of abnormal capsule findings on smaller group of patients (56 patients) and included only antegrade approach. Findings on capsule study were detected by SE in 30/56 (53.6%) cases, comparable to our detection rate of 62% [17]. Their main focus was to determine the yield of SE and not to predict the route of enteroscopy or success of enteroscopy.

The strengths of the study are as follows. (1) There are a large number of patients compared to previous two studies [10, 17]. (2) Almost all the procedures were performed by a single expert endoscopist. This decreases the variability in performance and detection rates. The major limitation of the study is its retrospective nature. Also as mentioned earlier, the time interval between capsule endoscopy and spiral enteroscopy may affect the detection rate of the lesions by spiral enteroscopy.

In conclusion from this large volume retrospective study, SE is safe with a high diagnostic and therapeutic yield. CLI is predictive of the success of SE and determines the best route of SE. Lesions within a location index of 0.6 should be approached first with antegrade route while those with a location index ≥ 0.8 should be initially approached by retrograde route. The type of small bowel pathology targeted by SE may affect its utility and yield.

Authors' Contribution

Rohan Mandaliya contributed to study concept and design; acquisition of data; analysis and interpretation of data; statistical analysis; graphical representation of the results; and drafting of the paper. Jason Korenblit contributed to assisting in and performing the spiral enteroscopy; preparing reports of the procedure; and critical revision of the paper for important intellectual content. Brendan O'Hare contributed to assisting in and performing the spiral enteroscopy; preparing reports of procedure; and critical revision of the paper for important intellectual content. Anastasia Shnitser contributed to assisting in and performing the spiral enteroscopy; preparing reports of the procedure; and critical revision of the paper for important intellectual content. Ramalinga Kedika contributed to assisting in and performing the spiral enteroscopy; preparing reports of the procedure; and critical revision of the paper for important intellectual content. Rebecca Matro contributed to assisting in and performing the spiral enteroscopy; preparing reports of the procedure; and critical revision of the paper for important intellectual content. Dina Halegoua-De Marzio contributed to assisting in and performing the spiral enteroscopy; preparing reports of the procedure; and critical revision of the paper for important intellectual content. Anthony Infantolino contributed to study concept and design; editing the paper; and critical revision of the paper for important intellectual content. Mitchell Conn contributed to study concept and design; analysis and interpretation of the data; editing the paper, critical revision of the paper for important intellectual content; statistical analysis; administrative, technical, or material support; study supervision.

Acknowledgment

This study was supported by Thomas Jefferson University.

References

[1] G. Iddan, G. Meron, A. Glukhovsky, and P. Swain, "Wireless capsule endoscopy," *Nature*, vol. 405, no. 6785, pp. 417–418, 2000.

[2] G. D. Meron, "The development of the swallowable video capsule (M2A)," *Gastrointestinal Endoscopy*, vol. 52, no. 6, pp. 817–819, 2000.

[3] G. G. Ginsberg, A. N. Barkun, J. J. Bosco et al., "Wireless capsule endoscopy," *Gastrointestinal Endoscopy*, vol. 56, no. 5, pp. 621–624, 2002.

[4] H. Yamamoto, Y. Sekine, Y. Sato et al., "Total enteroscopy with a nonsurgical steerable double-balloon method," *Gastrointestinal Endoscopy*, vol. 53, no. 2, pp. 216–220, 2001.

[5] S. A. Gross and M. E. Stark, "Initial experience with double-balloon enteroscopy at a U.S. center," *Gastrointestinal Endoscopy*, vol. 67, no. 6, pp. 890–897, 2008.

[6] T. Tsujikawa, Y. Saitoh, A. Andoh et al., "Novel single-balloon enteroscopy for diagnosis and treatment of the small intestine: preliminary experiences," *Endoscopy*, vol. 40, no. 1, pp. 11–15, 2008.

[7] D. Hartmann, A. Eickhoff, R. Tamm, and J. F. Riemann, "Balloon-assisted enteroscopy using a single-balloon technique," *Endoscopy*, vol. 39, supplement 1, article E276, 2007.

[8] J. R. Judah, D. Collins, J. K. Gaidos, W. Hou, C. E. Forsmark, and P. V. Draganov, "Prospective evaluation of gastroenterologist-guided, nurse-administered standard sedation for spiral deep small bowel enteroscopy," *Digestive Diseases and Sciences*, vol. 55, no. 9, pp. 2584–2591, 2010.

[9] M. Pennazio, C. Spada, R. Eliakim et al., "Small-bowel capsule endoscopy and device-assisted enteroscopy for diagnosis and treatment of small-bowel disorders: European Society of Gastrointestinal Endoscopy (ESGE) clinical guideline," *Endoscopy*, vol. 47, no. 4, pp. 352–376, 2015.

[10] X. Li, H. Chen, J. Dai, Y. Gao, and Z. Ge, "Predictive role of capsule endoscopy on the insertion route of double-balloon enteroscopy," *Endoscopy*, vol. 41, no. 9, pp. 762–766, 2009.

[11] P. A. Akerman, D. Agrawal, D. Cantero, and J. Pangtay, "Spiral enteroscopy with the new DSB overtube: a novel technique for deep peroral small-bowel intubation," *Endoscopy*, vol. 40, no. 12, pp. 974–978, 2008.

[12] B. R. Upchurch, M. R. Sanaka, A. R. Lopez, and J. J. Vargo, "The clinical utility of single-balloon enteroscopy: a single-center experience of 172 procedures," *Gastrointestinal Endoscopy*, vol. 71, no. 7, pp. 1218–1223, 2010.

[13] C. W. Teshima and G. May, "Small bowel enteroscopy," *Canadian Journal of Gastroenterology*, vol. 26, no. 5, pp. 269–275, 2012.

[14] D. Morgan, B. Upchurch, P. Draganov et al., "Spiral enteroscopy: prospective U.S. Multicenter study in patients with small-bowel disorders," *Gastrointestinal Endoscopy*, vol. 72, no. 5, pp. 992–998, 2010.

[15] R. Mandaliya and M. Conn, "Massive jejunal diverticular bleeding successfully treated with spirus enteroscopy," *The American Journal of Gastroenterology*, vol. 109, pp. S627–S627, 2014.

[16] G. Gay, M. Delvaux, and I. Fassler, "Outcome of capsule endoscopy in determining indication and route for push-and-pull enteroscopy," *Endoscopy*, vol. 38, no. 1, pp. 49–58, 2006.

[17] J. M. Buscaglia, R. Richards, M. N. Wilkinson et al., "Diagnostic yield of spiral enteroscopy when performed for the evaluation of abnormal capsule endoscopy findings," *Journal of Clinical Gastroenterology*, vol. 45, no. 4, pp. 342–346, 2011.

Colonoscopy Practice in Lagos, Nigeria: A Report of an Audit

C. A. Onyekwere,[1] J. N. Odiagah,[2] O. O. Ogunleye,[3] C. Chibututu,[4] and O. A. Lesi[5]

[1] *Gastroenterology Unit, Department of Medicine, Lagos State University College of Medicine/Teaching Hospital, P.O. Box 203 Satelitte Town, Lagos, Nigeria*
[2] *Gastroenterology Unit, Department of Medicine, Lagos State University Teaching Hospital, PMB 21266, Ikeja, Lagos, Nigeria*
[3] *Clinical Pharmacology Unit, Department of Medicine, Lagos State University College of Medicine/Teaching Hospital, PMB 21266, Ikeja, Lagos, Nigeria*
[4] *Cornell Health Centre, Surulere, Lagos, Nigeria*
[5] *Department of Medicine, University of Lagos College of Medicine/Teaching Hospital, Private Mail Bag 12003, Lagos, Nigeria*

Correspondence should be addressed to C. A. Onyekwere; ifymobi@yahoo.com

Academic Editor: P. J. O'Dwyer

Background. Colonoscopy effectiveness depends on the quality of the examination. Community-based report of quality of colonoscopy practice in a developing country will help in determining standard and also serve as a stimulus for improvement in service. *Aim.* To review the quality of colonoscopy practice and document pattern of colonic disease including polyp detection rate in Lagos, Nigeria. *Method.* A protocol that captured the patients' demographics, indication, and some quality indices of colonoscopy was developed and sent to all the identified colonoscopy units in Lagos to complete for all procedures performed between January 2011 and June 2012. All data were collated and analyzed. The quality indices studied were compared with guideline standard. *Results.* Twelve colonoscopy centers were identified but only nine centers responded. The gastroenterologist/endoscopists were physicians (3) and surgeons (5). Six hundred and seven colonoscopy procedures were performed during this period (M : F = 333 : 179) while the sex was not disclosed in 95 subjects. The examination indications were lower GI bleeding (24.2%), altered bowel habits (9.2%), lower abdominal pain (9.1%), screening for CRC (4.3%) and unspecified (46.8%). Conscious sedation was generally used while bowel preparation (good in 81.4%) was done with low residue diet and stimulant laxatives. Caecal intubation rate was 81.2%. Common endoscopic findings were haemorrhoids (43.2%), polyps/masses (13.4%), diverticulosis (11.1%), and no abnormality (23.4%). Polyp was detected in 6.8% of cases. *Conclusion.* Colonoscopy utilization is low, and the quality of practice is suboptimal; although limited resources could partly explain this, however it is not clear if the low rate of polyp detection is due to missed lesions or low population incidence.

1. Introduction

Colorectal cancer (CRC) is a common malignancy especially in the Western countries and the third leading cause of cancer death [1]. Recent reports indicate that it is also not uncommon in sub-Saharan Africa including Nigeria [2]. Early detection of colorectal cancer (CRC) has been shown to improve disease outcome [3]. Colonoscopy is the gold standard for colorectal cancer (CRC) screening [4]. There is therefore the need to ensure proper conduct of this procedure. Colonoscopy effectiveness ultimately depends on many variables related to the quality of the examination, which tends to be widely variable in clinical practice [5]. Many quality indices have been studied to optimise endoscopy procedure from the perspective of both the patient and the physician, including caecal intubation rate, adenoma detection rate, withdrawal time and quality of colonoscopy reporting. The later emphasises amongst others the documentation of caecal landmark as well. One clinical relevance of this is the occurrence of interval CRC, a marker of poor quality colonoscopy. Interval CRC is defined as that which occurs within a specified period of time after a colonoscopy (usually 5 years) [6]. Most interval CRCs occur because adenomas or actual CRC is missed during a colonoscopy. Several guidelines have been developed to enhance the quality of colonoscopy including the American Society for Gastrointestinal Endoscopy guideline [7] and the position statement of the European Society for Gastrointestinal Endoscopy [8]. Three aspects of quality are addressed by the American Society for Gastrointestinal Endoscopy (ASGE) guideline [7]: (1) risk stratification before the procedure, (2) the procedure itself, and (3) the post procedure including complications and surveillance strategy.

Colonoscopy is highly underutilized and even where used is underreported in sub-Saharan Africa; an earlier report [9] had indicated low level of practice of CRC screening. The few African reports [10, 11] showed indications and findings in relatively small study population with a number of them revealing advanced presentation of most cases of CRC in line with observed pattern in regions of low CRC screening [12, 13]. Also a report [14] of colonoscopy outcome from a tertiary hospital in Jos in Northern Nigeria showed polyp detection rate of 6%, a figure much less than that from Western countries. Most western reports indicate that a much higher rate and inability to detect adenomatous polyps in a minimum of 25% in men and 15% in females above fifty years of age during screening colonoscopy is adjudged to be poor quality performance [7]. But no report exists about compliance with quality indices amongst those performing colonoscopy in Nigeria sub-Saharan Africa. There is therefore a need to document colonoscopy outcomes in our population including our polyp detection rate which could serve as a quality indicator for future assessment of colonoscopy performance. The society of gastroenterology and hepatology in Nigeria is made up of health professional drawn from several disciplines whose interest is to foster the course of gastroenterology and is affiliated to the World Gastroenterology Organisation. This report will also serve to sensitize gastroenterology practitioners on need to improve on colonoscopy performance.

2. Aim

The aim of this paper is to review the quality of practice of colonoscopy in Lagos, Nigeria, and document our pattern of colonic disease including polyp detection rate.

3. Method

This was a retrospective study and complied with all ethical protocols as contained in the Helsinki declaration. All patients undergoing colonoscopy were meant to sign written consent. A protocol that captured the following quality indicators (quality/completeness of reporting, bowel preparation, caecal intubation, polyp detection, and complication) was developed and used to ascertain the extent of compliance in various colonoscopy units in Lagos between January 2011 and June 2012. Also the demographics, indications, and the colonoscopy findings of the patients were to be recorded. A total of 12 colonoscopy centres were identified and contacted on phone about the survey. The protocol was sent to them to complete and return. They were either to record data of all patients seen in a centre during the study period in a form of cumulative data spread sheet or to fill out each patients' information on a form as they deem more convenient. Further calls and visits were made to them to clarify any issues about the protocols and to retrieve the completed forms from them physically where they were unable to send data by electronic transfer.

The bowel preparation was graded as good, fair, or poor as reported by the performing colonoscopist in line with the ASGE guideline in which good refers to a clear fluid in the colon, and fair refers to small residual semisolid faeces. According to the guideline the minimum caecal intubation rate is 90 for all colonoscopy procedures while the minimum recommended adenoma detection rate is 25 for men and 15 for women above 50 years. All data were collated and analysed using SPSS statistical package. Subjects' age distribution and quality of bowel preparation were presented as chart while colonoscopy indication and findings were presented in frequency tables. The quality indices studied were compared with guideline standard.

4. Results

A total of 12 colonoscopy centres were identified but we were only able to evaluate nine centres (one public and eight private) that responded. Eight centres returned in a form of cumulative data sheet while one had individual forms for each patient. Three (3) of the endoscopists were gastroenterology physicians, and five (5) were general surgeons.

The data of one centre (which had 152 cases) could not be analysed because of the form in which the data were submitted and so was not included in this report.

Six hundred and seven colonoscopy procedures were performed during this period (333 males, 179 females while the sex was not disclosed in 95 subjects).

4.1. Subjects Demographics. Patients were aged between 17 and 89 years (mean:51.21 years); however the age was unreported in 42.7% of cases. Of 348 cases that had their ages reported, 54% were more than or equal to 50 years while the median age group was from 50–59 years. Fifty-five percent of them were males, while 29.5% were females; sex was unreported in 15.7% of cases (Figure 1).

4.2. Indications for Colonoscopy. The indications for colonoscopy examination are shown in Table 1. The commonest indications were lower gastrointestinal bleeding (24.2%), altered bowel habits (9.2%), lower abdominal pain (9.1%), screening for colorectal cancer (4.3%), unspecified (46.8%).

4.3. Premedication and Bowel Preparation. Premedication involved use of benzodiazepines, opioid analgesics, and antispasmodics. Bowel preparation for the subjects that had colonoscopy consisted of ingestion of only low residue diet for some days prior to examination and use of stimulant laxatives which included Epsom salt, Castor oil, and Picolax prior to examination. The quality of bowel preparation graded as from good to poor is shown in Figure 2 with good bowel preparation in 81% of them.

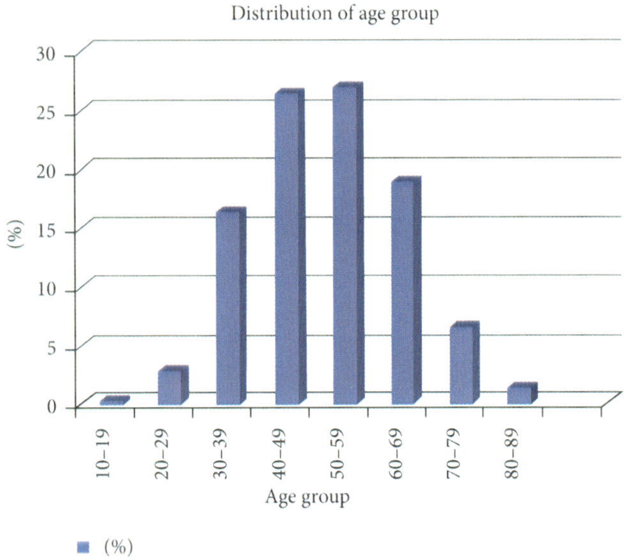

Figure 1: Age distribution according to decades of subjects undergoing colonoscopy.

Table 1: Clinical indications for colonoscopy amongst those disclosed.

Clinical indication	Frequency	Percentage
Lower GI bleeding	141	23.2
Abdominal pain	55	9.1
Colorectal cancer screening	26	4.3
Constipation	24	4.0
Others	18	3.0
Diarrhoea	13	2.1
Altered bowel habits	13	2.1
Anal pain	11	1.8
Anaemia	6	1.0
History of polyps/masses	5	0.8
Metastatic liver disease	4	0.7
Haematochezia + diarrhea	3	0.5
Haematochezia + constipation	3	0.5
Epigastric pain	1	0.2
Total	284	100.0

Total valid number = 284.

4.4. Caecal Intubation Rate. The caecal intubation rate 81.2% (the proportion of patients in whom there was insertion of the colonoscopy tip into the caecal caput) reflects a complete examination; permitting examination of the medial aspect of the caecum proximal to the ileocaecal valve is shown in Table 2.

4.5. Colonoscopy Findings. The findings are as shown in Table 3. The commonest findings were vascular lesions comprising mainly haemorrhoids (43.2%), polyps/masses (13.4%), diverticulosis (11.1%), and no abnormality (23.4%). The polyp detection rate was 6.8% (40). Of these 40, 25 were males, 11 females, while sex undisclosed in 11. Two-thirds of those having polyps were 50 years and above while the remaining third were less than 50 years old. Commonly affected locations with lesions were the anus (37.7%), rectum (3%), and sigmoid colon (3%).

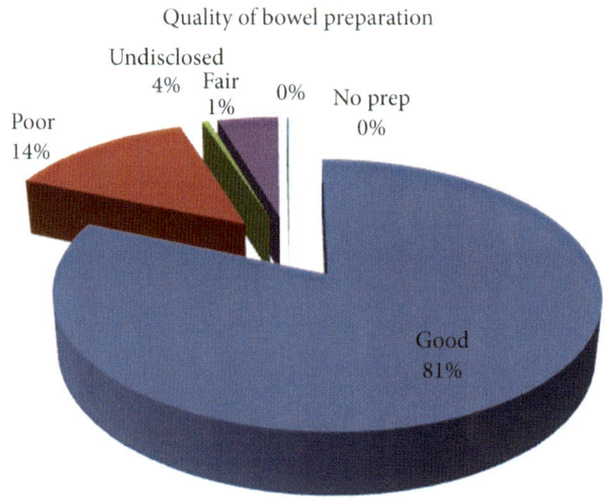

Figure 2

Table 2: Ceacal intubation rate.

Ceacal intubation	Frequency	Percentage
Undisclosed	18	3
Yes	493	81.2
No	96	15.8
Total	607	100

4.6. Complications of Procedure. No complications were reported.

5. Discussion

Our data over an eighteen month period appear low when compared with reports [5, 15] from the developed countries including the Western nations. Chen et al. had analysed over 10 000 subjects in his assessment of the role of the endoscopist versus age and sex in predicting adenoma detection at colonoscopy examination. Similarly Baxter et al. studied the relationship between endoscopist characteristics determined from administrative data and occurrence of interval CRC in over 14 000 patients undergoing colonoscopy during a five-year period. The present finding is a reflection of low level of colonoscopy practice as had been reported earlier [10, 11]. High cost of colonoscopy services, low infrastructure, and awareness amongst other factors may be partly responsible. The scope of health insurance coverage is low and generally most people pay for their health bills (colonoscopy inclusive) off pocket.

One observation here is the preponderance of private health establishment in the study. There are two sides to healthcare facilities in Lagos; the government owned and the private sector led. The government hospitals have three levels of care: primary, secondary, and tertiary. There are

TABLE 3: (a) Endoscopic findings. (b) Site of colonoscopy abnormalities in the patients.

(a)

Types of endoscopic findings	Frequency	%
Normal	55	9.1
DD and vascular	142	23.4
Ulcerative and vascular	4	0.7
Mass and colitis	3	0.5
Colitis and vascular	4	0.7
Melanosis coli and haemorrhoids	2	0.3
Megacolon	3	0.5
Upper GI	5	0.8
Adhesion/obstruction	2	0.3
Extrinsic compression	1	0.2
Perianal abscess	1	0.2
Ulcerative lesion	8	1.3
No colonic haustrations	1	0.2
Natal cleft intertrigo	1	0.2
Anal cushions	1	0.2
Long sigmoid	1	0.2
DD and ulcerations	1	0.2
Spastic colon	1	0.2
Mass/inflammation/haemorrhoids	3	0.5
Mass/DD/haemorrhoids	1	0.2
Ulceration and colitis	1	0.2
Masses/growth	57	9.4
Diverticulosis	39	6.4
Erosive colitis	18	3.0
Vascular lesions/haemorrhoids	213	35.1
Masses and diverticulosis	4	0.7
Masses and vascular	13	2.1
Total	607	100.0

*The polyp detection rate was 6.8%. DD: diverticular disease.

(b)

Location	Frequency	%
None	255	42.0
Ceacum	3	0.5
Ascending colon	7	1.2
Transverse colon	6	1.0
Descending colon	5	0.8
Sigmoid	18	3.0
Rectum	18	3.0
Anus	229	37.7
Pancolitis	12	2.0
Multiple locations	54	8.9

two tertiary hospitals in Lagos, one of which participated in this study while the second is just commencing colonoscopy service. The other government hospitals at other levels of care do not offer colonoscopy services; hence the option available to those requiring the service is the private sector hospitals. However no difference is observed in the data between the solitary government hospital and the private ones.

Also there is an evident low level of colonoscopy reporting amongst the practitioners with a lot of the variables including age and sex not recorded. Lack of appropriate software for reporting colonoscopy may contribute to this. There is a slight male predominance amongst the study subjects and the indications for examination though similar to earlier report differed in more cases of rectal bleeding in this report [9, 14]. There is a low rate of CRC screening using colonoscopy in our environment, even though the mean age of the majority of subjects was over fifty years. This could contribute to late presentation of most cases of CRC as previous reports [12, 16] had indicated.

Bowel preparation relied on having the subjects on low residue diet as well as use of stimulant purgatives which are known to cause abdominal discomfort including cramping and bloating from gas which could affect patience tolerance of the procedure and ultimately affect completeness of the examination. Although generally the quality of preparation was fair, this could be better with the use of more modern proprietary formulations using polyethylene glycol.

The caecal intubation rate (82%) is slightly below the recommended ASGE average. Although reasons for incomplete examination were not investigated, this could be related to patients' tolerance and calmness during examination which may be influenced by the type of bowel preparation and premedication as earlier reported. Brahmania et al. [17] in their study of maximizing completion rate of incomplete colonoscopy amongst gastroenterologist in a Vancouver Hospital noted reasons for incomplete colonoscopy to include; poor bowel preparation, pain or inadequate sedation, structural anomaly including tortuous colon, diverticular disease, and obstructing mass lesion. Most of the examinations in the present study were done using conscious sedatives as opposed to use of deep sedation with agents like propofol in developed countries. This fact had been alluded to by Nwokediuko and Obienu in a recent report [18]. It may also be a reflection of the level of expertise of the examiners. The low volume of colonoscopy performed may ultimately affect the level of skill and expertise as has been previously reported [19, 20].

The colonic pathology observed is similar to earlier reports from Africa [9, 14] including the polyp detection rate (6.8%) which is much lower than that in Western literature. This may reflect the population incidence or an underestimation due to missed lesion resulting from inadequate bowel preparation and lower caecal intubation rate. Polyp prevalence has been reported to vary with age and sex as our report shows a male predominance and older age (>50 years), while some reports have noted geographical differences in polyp detection though such differences were ascribed to environmental factors including diet rather than race [21]. There are no published population-based data on the prevalence of polyp in our setting, although an earlier study [22] had noted a higher polyp detection rates in the white population. Also low incidence of colon cancer reported in our population has been attributed to a number of factors including dietary and rarity of predisposing colonic lesion polyps inclusive [2]. Further studies are required to validate this low polyp detection rate.

We were limited in not having histological data to confirm the nature of the observed colonic pathology and so unable to further classify the polyps and comment on the adenoma detection rate. The risks of the patients for CRC as well as withdrawal time during colonoscopy performance were not equally assessed as these have been shown to influence colonoscopy outcome.

Overall our colonoscopy practice is yet to attain the standard set in Western guideline; similar findings or worse (caecal intubation rate between 56 and 76%) were recorded in UK [23] over a decade ago but this improved with better training and infrastructure. It is our believe that this type of audit is going to be a regular exercise by the Society of Gastroenterology and Hepatology in Nigeria (Lagos chapter) to encourage an improvement in our endoscopy service.

6. Conclusion

There are too few colonoscopy centres in Lagos, with low volume of procedures and generally poor reporting of procedures. There is a low rate of CRC screening using colonoscopy in our environment. The observed caecal intubation rate is less than 90% recommended by most guidelines. There is also a low rate of polyp detection, when compared to international standards (US). It is not clear whether this is due to missed lesions (as a result of low rates of good bowel preparation and low caecal intubation rates) or due to a low incidence of polyps in our setting, as no prior population-based data are available.

7. Limitations of the Study

This retrospective analysis relied on data submitted by the endoscopists, so one cannot rule out underreporting. Our sample size appears small but this is a reflection of the level of practice of colonoscopy in our setting.

The data of each colonoscopist were not individually assessed, but a general analysis was done to assess the overall reporting, performance and, outcome of colonoscopy in Lagos, Nigeria.

Acknowledgments

The authors express their gratitude to the following for their contribution in this study: Professor Akande, Professor Ogunbiyi, Dr. Anomneze, Dr. Coker, Dr. Ajayi, Dr. Sebanjo, Dr. Oluyemi, Dr. A Pascal, and Dr. J Ojukwu. This paper is on behalf of the Society of Gastroenterology and Hepatology in Nigeria (SOGHIN) Lagos Chapter.

References

[1] World Gastroenterology Organization, *International Digestive Cancer Alliance Practice Guidelines Colorectal Cancer Screening*, World Gastroenterology Organization, Munich, Germany, 2007.

[2] F. B. Abdulkareem, F. A. Faduyile, A. O. Daramola et al., "Malignant gastrointestinal tumours in South Western Nigeria: a histopathologic analysis of 713 cases," *West African Journal of Medicine*, vol. 28, no. 3, pp. 173–177, 2009.

[3] K. R. Douglas, "Colorectal cancer screening," *ASGE Clinical Update*, vol. 14, no. 4, pp. 1–4, 2007.

[4] Multi-Disciplinary Taskforce, New consensus colorectal cancer screening guidelines, *Gastroenterology*, May 2008.

[5] S. Chen and D. K. Rex, "Endoscopist is comparable to age and gender as predictor of adenomas at colonoscopy," *The American Journal of Gastroenterology*, vol. 100, p. S393, 2005.

[6] A. Pabby, R. E. Schoen, J. L. Weissfeld et al., "Analysis of colorectal cancer occurrence during surveillance colonoscopy in the dietary Polyp Prevention Trial," *Gastrointestinal Endoscopy*, vol. 61, no. 3, pp. 385–391, 2005.

[7] D. K. Rex, J. L. Petrini, T. H. Baron et al., "Quality indicators for colonoscopy," *American Journal of Gastroenterology*, vol. 101, no. 4, pp. 873–885, 2006.

[8] B. Rembacken, J. F. Hassan, A. Riemann et al., "Quality in screening colonoscopy: position statement of the European Society of GastrointestinalEndoscopy (ESGE)," *Endoscopy*, vol. 44, no. 10, pp. 957–968, 2012.

[9] E. O. Ogutu, F. A. Okoth, and G. N. Lule, "Colonoscopic findings in Kenyan African patients," *East African Medical Journal*, vol. 75, no. 9, pp. 540–543, 1998.

[10] A. O. Arigbabu and W. O. Odesanmi, "Colonoscopy. First experience in Nigeria," *Diseases of the Colon and Rectum*, vol. 28, no. 10, pp. 728–731, 1985.

[11] C. A. Onyekwere, A. O. Ogbera, F. B. Abdulkareem, and J. Ashindoitiang, "Colorectal carcinoma screening in Lagos, Nigeria, are we doing it right?" *Gastroenterology Research*, vol. 2, pp. 38–42, 2009.

[12] A. O. Tade, "Right sided colon cancer at Olabisi Onabanjo University Shagamu South West Nigeria; a ten year review," *Nigerian Medical Practitioner*, vol. 49, pp. 82–84, 2006.

[13] J. P. Keating, P. Pater, S. Lolohea, and J. K. Wickremesekera, "The epidemiology of colorectal cancer: what can we learn from the New Zealand Cancer Registry?" *New Zealand Medical Journal*, vol. 116, article U437, 2003.

[14] O. I. Bashiru and M. A. Misauno, "Colonoscopy in a tertiary hospital in Nigeria," *Journal of Medicine in the Tropics*, vol. 13, pp. 72–74, 2011.

[15] N. N. Baxter, R. Sutradhar, S. S. Forbes, L. F. Paszat, R. Saskin, and L. Rabeneck, "Analysis of administrative data finds endoscopist quality measures associated with postcolonoscopy colorectal cancer," *Gastroenterology*, vol. 140, no. 1, pp. 65–72, 2011.

[16] A. A. Adesanya and J. T. da Rocha-Afodu, "Colorectal cancer in Lagos: a critical review of 100 cases," *The Nigerian Postgraduate Medical Journal*, vol. 7, no. 3, pp. 129–136, 2000.

[17] M. Brahmania, J. Park, S. Svarta, J. Tong, R. Kwok, and R. Enns, "Incomplete colonoscopy: maximizing completion rates of gastroenterologists," *Canadian Journal of Gastroenterology*, vol. 26, no. 9, pp. 589–592, 2012.

[18] S. C. Nwokediuko and O. Obienu, "Sedation practices for routine diagnostic upper gastrointestinal endoscopy," *World Journal of Gastroenterology*, vol. 4, no. 6, pp. 260–265, 2012.

[19] J. B. Marshall and J. S. Barthel, "The frequency of total colonoscopy and terminal ileal intubation in the 1990s," *Gastrointestinal Endoscopy*, vol. 39, no. 4, pp. 518–520, 1993.

[20] W. Atkin, P. Rogers, C. Cardwell et al., "Wide variation in adenoma detection rates at screening flexible sigmoidoscopy," *Gastroenterology*, vol. 126, no. 5, pp. 1247–1256, 2004.

[21] J. V. Ashley, C. W. Betsy, W. G. Eugene, A. T. Cynthia, L. R. Cheryl, and A. T. Patricia, "Dietary polyamine intake and risks of colorectal adenomatous polyps," *The American Journal of Clinical Nutrition*, vol. 96, no. 1, pp. 1333–1141, 2012.

[22] G. S. Cooper, A. Chak, and S. Koroukian, "The polyp detection rate of colonoscopy: a national study of medicare beneficiaries," *American Journal of Medicine*, vol. 118, no. 12, pp. 1413.e11–1413.e14, 2005.

[23] C. J. A. Bowles, R. Leicester, C. Romaya, E. Swarbrick, C. B. Williams, and O. Epstein, "A prospective study of colonoscopy practice in the UK today: are we adequately prepared for national colorectal cancer screening tomorrow?" *Gut*, vol. 53, no. 2, pp. 277–283, 2004.

19

Transpancreatic Precut Sphincterotomy for Biliary Access: The Relation of Sphincterotomy Size to Immediate Success Rate of Biliary Cannulation

Lien-Fu Lin

Division of Gastroenterology, Department of Internal Medicine, Tungs' Taichung Metroharbor Hospital, Section 8, No. 699 Taiwan Boulevard, Wuqi District, Taichung 435, Taiwan

Correspondence should be addressed to Lien-Fu Lin; aucardla@yahoo.com.tw

Academic Editor: Everson Artifon

Background. Transpancreatic precut sphincterotomy (TPS) is an option for difficult common bile duct (CBD) access, and the reports are few, with immediate success rate varying from 60 to 96%. The description of relation between the size of TPS and the immediate success rate of CBD cannulation was not found in the literature. *The Aim of the Study.* To evaluate the relation of large TPS to immediate success rate of CBD cannulation. *Methods.* A retrospective analysis was performed in prospectively collected data of 20 patients. TPS was performed with traction papillotome in the main pancreatic duct (MPD) directing towards 11 o'clock. Needle knife (NK) was used to enlarge TPS in five patients, and the other 15 cases had large TPS from the beginning of sphincterotomy. Prophylactic pancreatic stent was inserted in 18 cases, with diclofenac given in 12 cases. *Results.* The immediate success rate of CBD cannulation was 90% and with an eventual success rate of 100%. The failure in one immediate CBD cannulation with large TPS was due to atypical location of CBD orifice, and the other failed immediate CBD cannulation was due to inadequate size of TPS. Complications included 3 cases of post-TPS bleeding and 3 cases of mild pancreatitis. *Conclusion.* TPS is an effective procedure in patients with difficult biliary access and can have high immediate success rate with large TPS.

1. Introduction

The initial success rate of selective CBD cannulation was reported to be 70% after a standard cannulation using guide wire and papillotome with the criteria of 5 attempts of cannulation [1]. Using double-guide wire (DGW) technique, the success rate varies from 47 to 73% with the pancreatitis rate of 14–38% [1–3]. Transpancreatic precut sphincterotomy (TPS) can be an alternative technique because the access is already in the MPD. The reports of TPS are few when compared to needle knife precut sphincterotomy, and detailed description of the size of TPS in relation to immediate successful CBD cannulation was not emphasized in the literature. The immediate success rate of TPS for biliary access varies from 60 to 96% [4, 5]. Diclofenac rectally administered and prophylactic pancreatic stent (PS) placement can reduce the incidence of postendoscopic retrograde cholangiopancreatography pancreatitis (PEP) [6]. We evaluate the primary outcome of immediate success rate of CBD cannulation with large TPS and secondary outcome of the complications with this new technique in our hospital.

2. Materials and Methods

Between January 2012 and October 2013, a retrospective analysis of prospectively collected data of 20 cases of TPS with inaccessible bile duct was conducted. There were 13 male and 7 female patients with a mean age of 54 ± 16 (25–82) years. The procedure was performed by a single operator who has experience on ERCP and endoscopicsphincterotomy

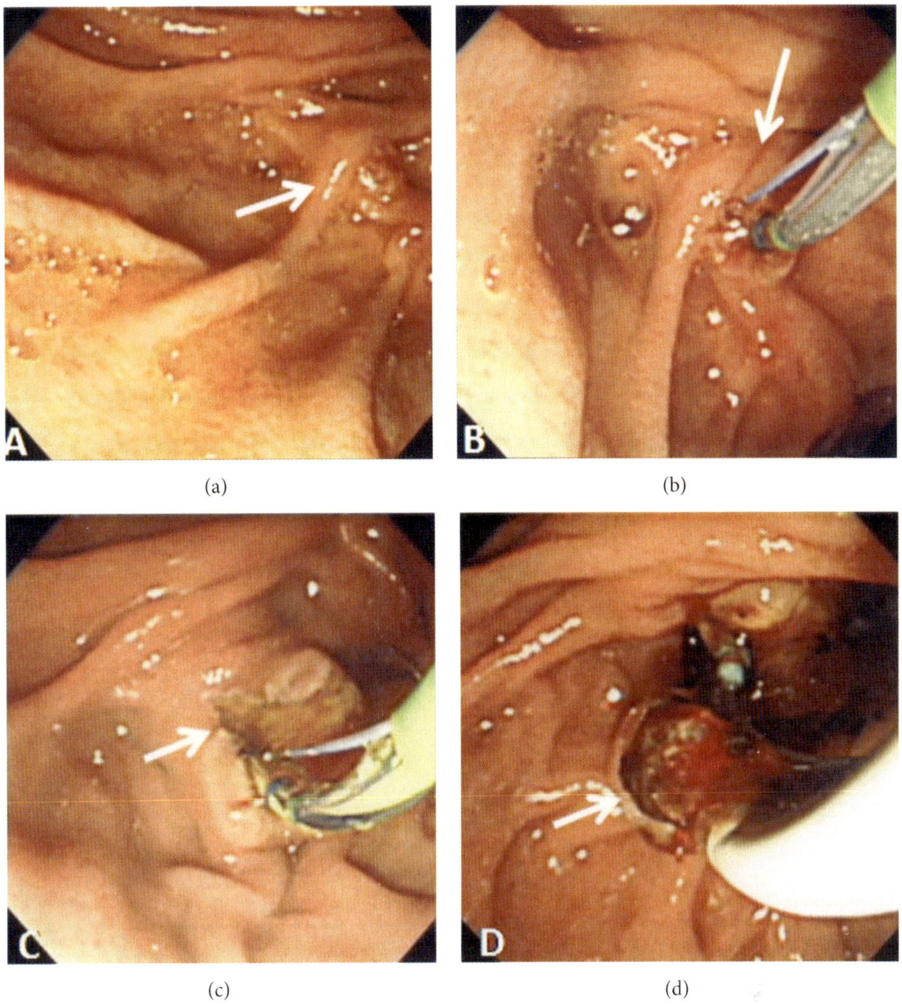

FIGURE 1: (a) Deviated papilla (arrow), (b) transpancreatic precut sphincterotomy in 11 o'clock direction (arrow), (c) CBD orifice (arrow) located left to the pancreatic duct occupied by sphincterotome, and (d) CBD stone extracted (arrow).

(EST) for more than 1000 cases. A total of 112 cases of endoscopic retrograde cholangiopancreatography (ERCP) were performed during that period when TPS was started as a precut technique. The inclusion criteria were (1) failed selective deep CBD cannulation after 20 minutes and (2) successful access in the MPD. The exclusion criteria were (1) post-Billroth II gastrectomy cases and (2) failed access to the MPD. After access to the MPD, TPS was performed with the traction sphincterotome directing towards 11 o'clock, and CBD orifice is usually located left to the pancreatic duct after TPS (Figures 1 and 2). Needle knife was required to extend the TPS over the pancreatic stent (Figure 3) to get biliary access due to inadequate sphincterotomy in 5 cases. Large TPS incision up to superior margin of the papilla was performed in the other 15 cases (Figure 4). Pancreatic stent (PS) was placed either before or after the complete biliary procedure. The PS was removed after 4-5 days when there were no post-TPS bleeding and no spontaneous passage of the pancreatic stent. Diclofenac was given in patients who had balloon dilatation of the papilla or contrast injection into main pancreatic duct. Written consents were obtained from all of the patients. After TPS, serum amylase was tested on the next day and repeated on the 3rd day if the amylase level was elevated 3 times above the normal limit.

The instruments and current setting used were (1) duodenoscope (TJF 240, Olympus Optical Co., Ltd., Tokyo, Japan), (2) sphincterotome (Olympus KD-431Q-0720), (3) Boston Scientific Microvasive Jag wire, (4) Wilson Cook Zimmon pancreatic stent 5Fr-4 cm, (5) Wilson Cook Huibregtse HPC-3 needle knife, (6) electrosurgical generator (Olympus PSD 60), and (7) current setting (Endocut setting output of 120Watts and effect 2).

The definitions were as follows: (1) inaccessible bile duct was defined as failure after 20 minutes of CBD cannulation [7, 8], (2) complications of pancreatitis and bleeding were defined according to the criteria used by Cotton et al. [9], and (3) large incision sphincterotomy was defined as incision up to superior margin of the bulging papilla [4].

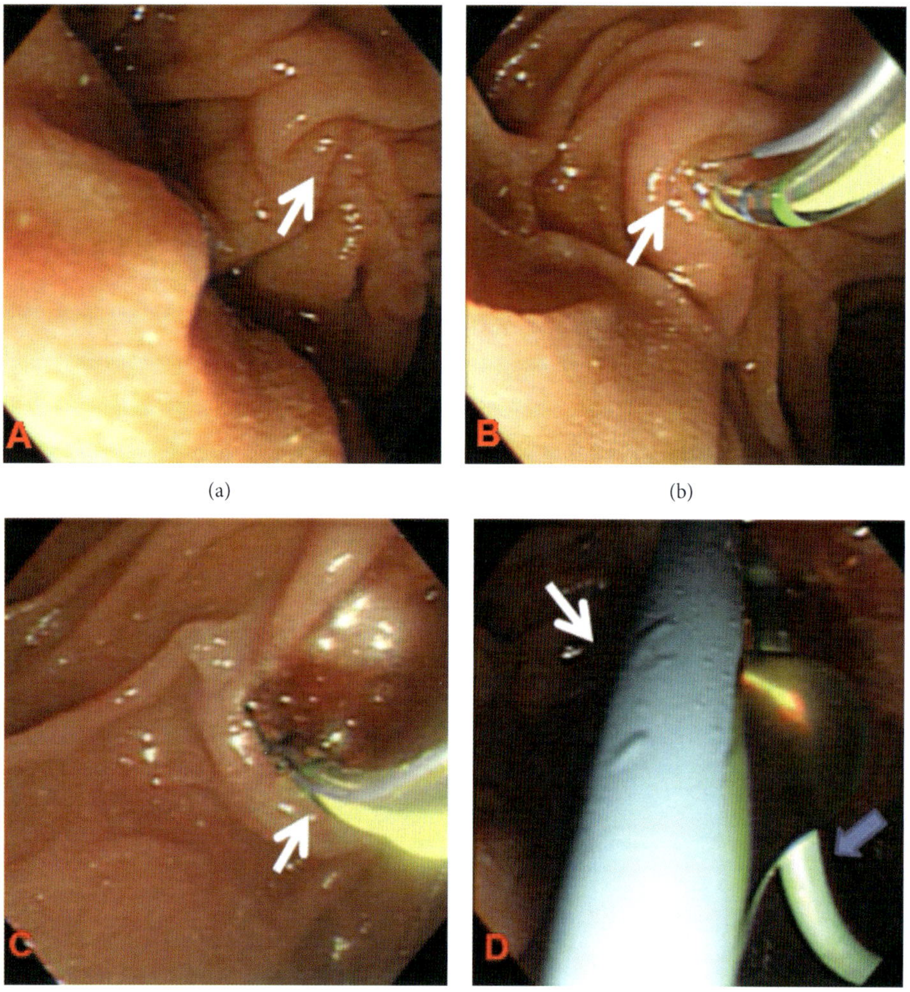

(a) (b) (c) (d)

Figure 2: (a) Long papilla (arrow), (b) transpancreatic precut sphincterotomy in 11 o'clock direction (arrow), (c) CBD cannulation by sphincterotome (arrow), and (d) postbiliary and pancreatic stenting (white and blue arrows).

3. Results

The results were shown in Table 1. The etiologies were 14 cases of common bile duct stone, 3 pancreatic head cancers, 1 bile leak, 1 biliary dilatation, and 1 chronic pancreatitis. The reasons for difficult selective CBD cannulation were periampullary diverticulum, long, and/or deviated papilla. Three cases had undergone trial of CBD cannulation with DGW technique but failed to get biliary access. Five cases needed additional needle knife sphincterotome to enlarge the TPS incision. All cases of large TPS incision had successful initial CBD cannulation except one owing to atypical location of CBD orifice (Figure 5). The immediate success rate of CBD cannulation after TPS was 90% and the eventual success rate was 100%. The other failed immediate CBD cannulation was due to inadequate size of TPS.

One massive delayed bleeding required surgery with uneventful recovery after failed endoscopic hemostasis and transarterial embolization. This severe bleeding case had undergone large TPS incision. One mild immediate bleeding was treated with endoscopic local epinephrine injection and clipping. The other mild repeated bleeding was managed endoscopically as well. Three cases of mild pancreatitis recovered within 2 days, though they had received prophylactic pancreatic stenting, and 2 cases had diclofenac given rectally. There was no perforation complication.

4. Discussion

Techniques for difficult deep CBD cannulation include guide wire technique, DGW technique, and precut access. The success rate of CBD cannulation is not high in DGW technique ranging from 47 to 73% but the pancreatitis rate can be as high as 38% [1, 2]. Our unpublished success rate with DGW technique was 60% with a mild pancreatitis of 6%. Precut technique can have needle knife precut (free hand cutting at the papillary orifice or cutting the papilla over a pancreatic stent), needle knife fistulotomy above papillary orifice, and transpancreatic precut sphincterotomy (TPS) using traction papillotome [10].

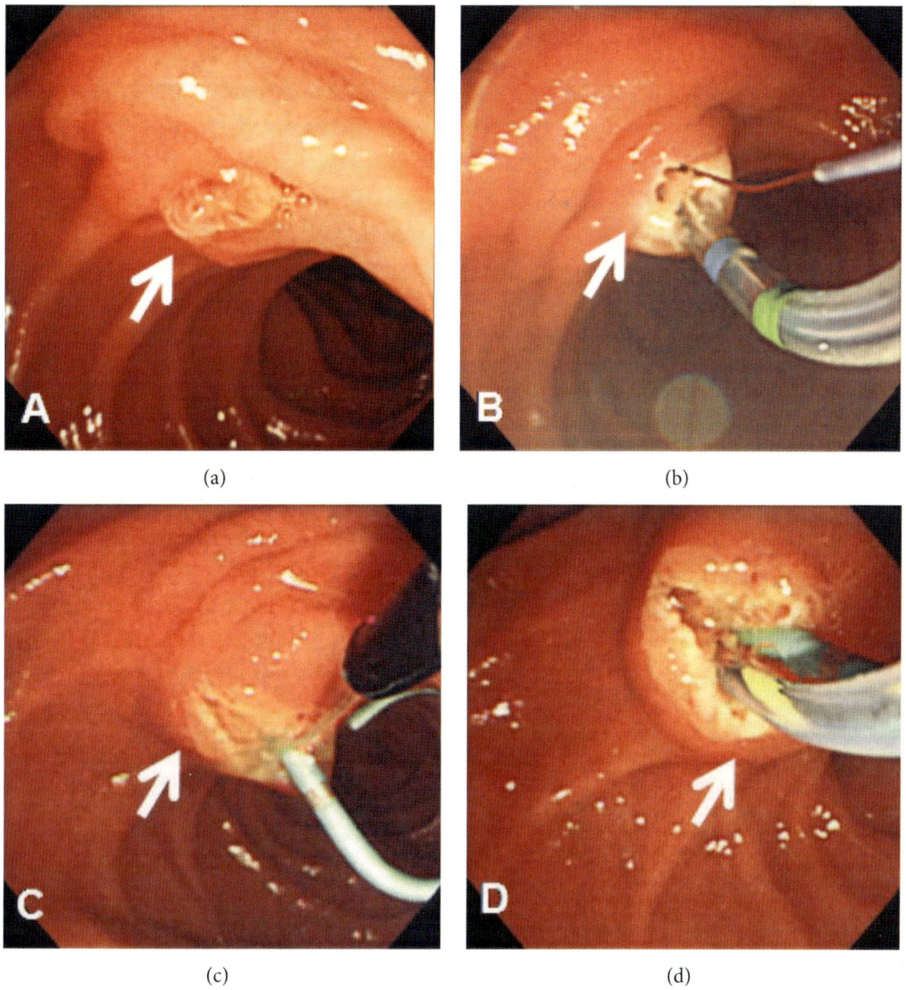

FIGURE 3: (a) Papilla (arrow), (b) transpancreatic precut sphincterotomy in 11 o'clock direction (arrow) with inadequate incision, (c) needle knife used to enlarge the incision (arrow), and (d) CBD cannulation (arrow).

TPS was first described by Goff et al. [11], and very few reports about comparison between TPS with needle knife sphincterotomy can be found [12]. TPS was reported to have a higher success rate and less complication compared with standard needle knife precut [13] and also a safe, effective procedure in patients with difficult bile duct access where classical sphincterotomy or needle knife procedures fail [14]. But on the other hand, Wang et al. conducted a multicenter prospective trial of TPS with needle knife precut sphincterotomy and concluded that there is no significant difference in success rate and complications [15].

The immediate success rate of TPS varies from 60 to 96% [4, 5]. No specific emphasis on or description about the size of TPS with the immediate success rate could be found in the literature. Although Goff reported a size of 5–7 mm of TPS achieving a success rate of 96%, but an initial success rate of only 60% was described by Akashi et al. with medium and large TPS [4]. Kapetanos et al. described an initial success rate of 75% without mentioning the exact length of TPS [16]. High initial success rate of 97% with large TPS was achieved by Halttunen et al. [17], and Kahaleh et al. also reported 85% success rate with large TPS [18]. Out of 20 cases of TPS in our hospital, 14 cases of large TPS incision at first attempt resulted in immediate successful CBD cannulation and faster procedure because no additional needle knife enlargement was needed. One large TPS that failed to get the biliary access was attributed to the atypical location of CBD orifice. Therefore, the key to a higher successful immediate biliary access is to incise a large TPS at the first attempt. The reason of requiring additional needle knife for extension of TPS in 5 cases was due to inadequate incision of TPS. Our immediate success rate of CBD cannulation was 90%, and eventual success rate was 100%.

The incidence of post-TPS bleeding varies from 3.7 to 5% [7, 16], our post-TPS bleeding was 15% which was a little higher and may be due to a small number of cases. Massive post-TPS bleeding was not reported in the literature. Severe postsphincterotomy bleeding was presumed to result from incision through an aberrant retroduodenal artery [19, 20], and the length of incision is not an important predictor of

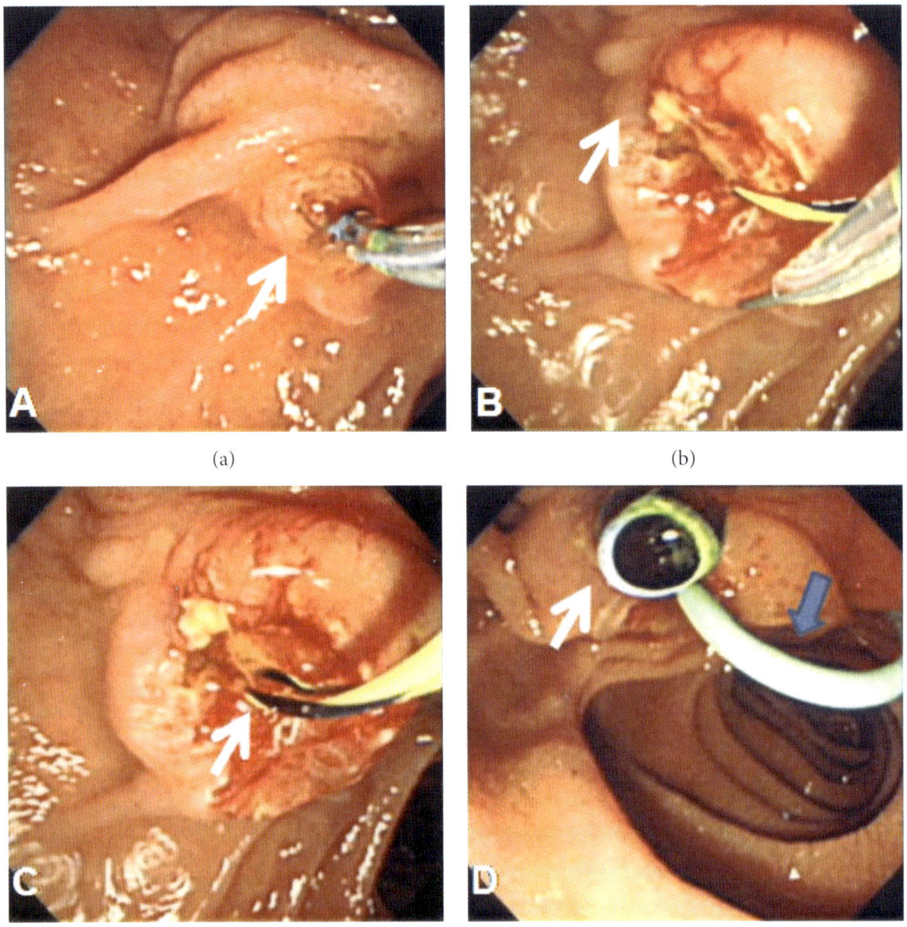

(a) (b) (c) (d)

Figure 4: (a) Transpancreatic precut sphincterotomy in 11 o'clock direction (arrow), (b) large incision sphincterotomy (arrow), (c) successful CBD cannulation (arrow), and (d) postbiliary and pancreatic stenting (white and blue arrows).

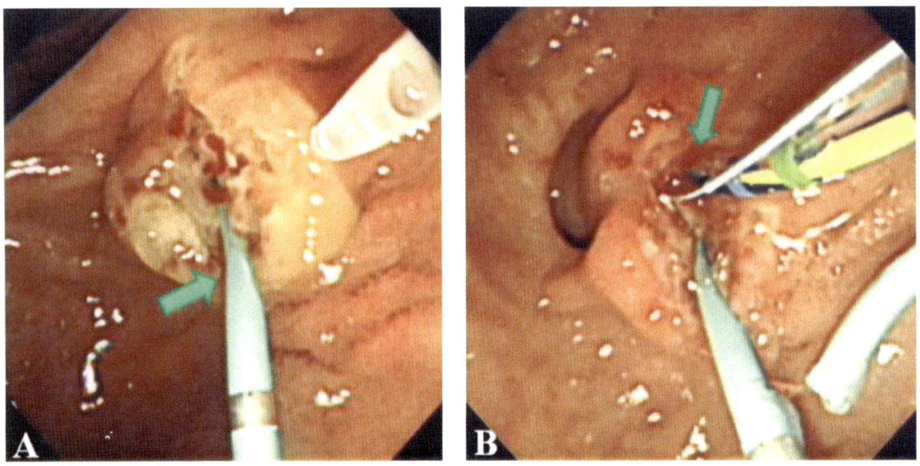

(a) (b)

Figure 5: (a) Posttranspancreatic precut sphincterotomy with pancreatic stenting (arrow) and (b) CBD orifice located on the right side of pancreatic duct (arrow).

Table 1

No.	Age	Sex	Diagnosis	Papilla	DGW	NKS	Success	Bleeding	P stent	Voren	Panreatitis
1	49	M	Pan cancer	Long	—	—	Yes	1 mild	Yes	—	—
2	47	F	CBDS	Long	—	—	Yes	No	Yes	100	—
3	44	M	Bile leak	Long	—	—	Yes	1 massive#	Yes	—	—
4	45	F	CBDS	Long, deviated	Yes	—	Yes	No	Yes	—	—
5	45	M	CBDS	Long, deviated	—	Yes	Yes	1 mild	Yes	—	Mild
6	32	F	CBDS	Deviated	Yes	Yes	Yes	No	Yes	—	—
7	77	M	CBDS	Long	—	Yes	Yes*	No	Yes	75	—
8	39	M	CCP	Long	—	—	Yes	No	Yes	100	—
9	25	M	CBDS	Deviated	—	Yes	Yes	No	Yes	100	—
10	72	M	CBDS	Long	Yes	—	Yes	No	Yes	75	—
11	56	F	CBDS	Long, deviated	—	—	Yes	No	Yes	—	—
12	56	F	CBDS	Long, deviated	—	—	Yes	No	Yes	100	Mild
13	58	M	CBDS	Deviated	—	—	Yes	No	Yes	75	—
14	56	M	Pan ccncer	Deviated	—	—	Yes	No	0	—	—
15	82	M	CBDS	PAD	—	Yes	Yes	No	Yes	50	—
16	70	F	BD (pap bx)	Long, deviated	—	—	Yes	No	Yes	75	Mild
17	73	M	Pan cancer	Deviated	—	—	Yes	No	0	—	—
18	70	M	CBDS	Long, deviated	—	—	Yes	No	Yes	100	—
19	64	M	CBDS	Deviated	—	—	Yes	No	Yes	100	—
20	29	F	CBDS	PAD	—	—	Yes*	No	Yes	100	—

DWG: double guide wire technique, NK: needle knife, P: pancreatic, Diclo: diclofenac, CBDS: common bile duct stone, BD: bile duct dilatation, Pap: papillary, PAD: periampullary diverticulum, *Second attempt of CBD cannulation, #massive delayed TPS bleeding ended with surgery after failed endoscopic hemostasis and transarterial emboiization.
Long papilla: >2 cm and with difficult selective CBD cannulation.
Deviated papilla: difficult to adjust the papillary orifice in an en-face position.
Lower dose of diclofenac was given in older patients with mildly elevated renal function.

bleeding [21]. The cause of massive post-TPS (initial large TPS) bleeding in our series was attributed to have incised a larger branch of gastroduodenal artery after reviewing the angiography. More cases of TPS are needed for evaluation for post-TPS bleeding.

The incidence of pancreatitis without prophylactic stenting after TPS ranged from 5.5 to 21% [4, 7, 13] and reduced to 3.5% if prophylactic pancreatic stenting was performed [5]. We had 3 cases (15%) of mild pancreatitis, but all of them recovered in 2 days. All 3 cases had prophylactic pancreatic stenting done, and two had received diclofenac administration. The cause of pancreatitis in our series could be due to contrast injection into MPD or deep GW placement in the MPD. Severe post-TPS pancreatitis can occur without pancreatic stenting [3, 13]; therefore, pancreatic stenting is necessary in TPS procedure [6].

The advantages of large TPS are (1) definite complete unroofing of the papilla that makes CBD cannulation easier enabling a higher immediate success rate of biliary access and (2) probably low incidence of perforation which has been reported in two studies [5, 18]. The other credits of TPS are less technically demanding and easier to control the depth of cutting [13]. The limitations in this study are (1) small number of cases and (2) nonrandomized study for median or large TSP incision for comparison of immediate CBD cannulation success rate.

5. Conclusion

TPS is an effective procedure in patients with difficult biliary access and can have high immediate success rate with large sized TPS.

References

[1] A. Herreros de Tejada, J. L. Calleja, G. Díaz et al., "Double-guidewire technique for difficult bile duct cannulation: a multicenter randomized, controlled trial," *Gastrointestinal Endoscopy*, vol. 70, no. 4, pp. 700–709, 2009.

[2] K. Ito, N. Fujita, Y. Noda et al., "Pancreatic guidewire placement for achieving selective biliary cannulation during endoscopic retrograde cholangio-pancreatography," *World Journal of Gastroenterology*, vol. 14, no. 36, pp. 5595–5600, 2008.

[3] Y. W. Yoo, S. W. Cha, W. C. Lee et al., "Double guidewire technique vs transpancreatic precut sphincterotomy in difficult biliary cannulation," *World Journal of Gastroenterology*, vol. 19, no. 1, pp. 108–114, 2013.

[4] R. Akashi, T. Kiyozumi, K. Jinnouchi, M. Yoshida, Y. Adachi, and K. Sagara, "Pancreatic sphincter precutting to gain selective access to the common bile duct: a series of 172 patients," *Endoscopy*, vol. 36, no. 5, pp. 405–410, 2004.

[5] J. S. Goff, "Long-term experience with the transpancreatic sphincter pre-cut approach to biliary sphincterotomy," *Gastrointestinal Endoscopy*, vol. 50, no. 5, pp. 642–645, 1999.

[6] J.-M. Dumonceau, A. Andriulli, J. Deviere et al., "European Society of Gastrointestinal Endoscopy (ESGE) Guideline: prophylaxis of post-ERCP pancreatitis," *Endoscopy*, vol. 42, no. 6, pp. 503–515, 2010.

[7] H. Miyatani and Y. Yoshida, "Endoscopic needle knife precut papillotomy for inaccessible bile duct following failed pancreatic duct access," *Clinical Medicine*, vol. 2009, no. 2, pp. 1–5, 2009.

[8] K. W. Yoon, C. H. Park, S. Y. Park et al., "Guidewire cannulation increases the success rate of needle-knife fistulotomy for difficult bile duct access," *Journal of Gastroenterology and Hepatology*, vol. 25, no. 1, pp. 14–18, 2010.

[9] P. B. Cotton, G. Lehman, J. Vennes et al., "Endoscopic sphincterotomy complications and their management: an attempt at consensus," *Gastrointestinal Endoscopy*, vol. 37, no. 3, pp. 383–393, 1991.

[10] M. L. Freeman and N. M. Guda, "ERCP cannulation: a review of reported techniques," *Gastrointestinal Endoscopy*, vol. 61, no. 1, pp. 112–125, 2005.

[11] J. S. Goff, "Common bile duct pre-cut sphincterotomy: transpancreatic sphincter approach," *Gastrointestinal Endoscopy*, vol. 41, no. 5, pp. 502–505, 1995.

[12] T. DaVee, J. A. Garcia, and T. H. Baron, "Precut sphincterotomy for selective biliary duct cannulation during endoscopic retrograde cholangiopancreatography," *Annals of Gastroenterology*, vol. 25, pp. 1–12, 2012.

[13] M. F. Catalano, J. D. Linder, and J. E. Geenen, "Endoscopic transpancreatic papillary septotomy for inaccessible obstructed bile ducts: comparison with standard pre-cut papillotomy," *Gastrointestinal Endoscopy*, vol. 60, no. 4, pp. 557–561, 2004.

[14] A. Weber, T. Roesch, S. Pointner et al., "Transpancreatic precut sphincterotomy for cannulation of inaccessible common bile duct: a safe and successful technique," *Pancreas*, vol. 36, no. 2, pp. 187–191, 2008.

[15] P. Wang, W. Zhang, F. Liu et al., "Success and complication rates of two precut techniques, transpancreatic sphincterotomy and needle-knife sphincterotomy for bile duct cannulation," *Journal of Gastrointestinal Surgery*, vol. 14, no. 4, pp. 697–704, 2010.

[16] D. Kapetanos, G. Kokozidis, D. Christodoulou et al., "Case series of transpancreatic septotomy as precutting technique for difficult bile duct cannulation," *Endoscopy*, vol. 39, no. 9, pp. 802–806, 2007.

[17] J. Halttunen, I. Keränen, M. Udd, and L. Kylänpää, "Pancreatic sphincterotomy versus needle knife precut in difficult biliary cannulation," *Surgical Endoscopy and Other Interventional Techniques*, vol. 23, no. 4, pp. 745–749, 2009.

[18] M. Kahaleh, J. Tokar, T. Mullick, S. J. Bickston, and P. Yeaton, "Prospective evaluation of pancreatic sphincterotomy as a precut technique for biliary cannulation," *Clinical Gastroenterology and Hepatology*, vol. 2, no. 11, pp. 971–977, 2004.

[19] J. W. C. Leung, F. K. L. Chan, J. J. Y. Sung, and S. C. S. Chung, "Endoscopic sphincterotomy-induced hemorrhage: a study of risk factors and the role of epinephrine injection," *Gastrointestinal Endoscopy*, vol. 42, no. 6, pp. 550–554, 1995.

[20] J. E. Geenen and J. A. LoGuidice, "Endoscopic sphincterotomy for diseases of the biliary tree," *Advances in surgery*, vol. 14, pp. 31–51, 1980.

[21] M. L. Freeman, D. B. Nelson, S. Sherman et al., "Complications of endoscopic biliary sphincterotomy," *The New England Journal of Medicine*, vol. 335, no. 13, pp. 909–918, 1996.

Efficacy, Safety, and Long-Term Follow-Up Results of EUS-Guided Transmural Drainage for Pancreatic Pseudocyst

Shin Kato, Akio Katanuma, Hiroyuki Maguchi, Kuniyuki Takahashi, Manabu Osanai, Kei Yane, Toshifumi Kim, Maki Kaneko, Ryo Takaki, Kazuyuki Matsumoto, Tomoaki Matsumori, Katsushige Gon, and Akiko Tomonari

Center for Gastroenterology, Teine-Keijinkai Hospital, Sapporo 006-8555, Japan

Correspondence should be addressed to Shin Kato; shinchan1231@gmail.com

Academic Editor: Charles Melbern Wilcox

Background and Aim. EUS-guided transmural drainage (EUS-GTD) is now considered a minimally invasive and effective alternative to surgery for drainage of symptomatic pancreatic pseudocysts. However, the technique is rather difficult, and sometimes serious complications occur to patients undergoing this procedure. We retrospectively evaluated efficacy, safety, and long-term follow-up results of EUS-GTD for pancreatic pseudocyst. *Methods.* Sixty-seven patients with pancreatic pseudocyst who underwent EUS-GTD from April 2000 to March 2011 were enrolled. We retrospectively evaluated (1) technical success, (2) clinical success, (3) adverse event of procedure, and (4) long-term follow-up results. *Results.* Total technical success rate was 88%. Ninety-one percent of external drainage, 79% of internal drainage, and 66% of puncture and aspiration only achieved clinical success. There was only one case with an adverse event, perforation (1.5%). The case required emergency operation. Total recurrence rate was 23.9%. Median follow-up period was 33.9 months. The recurrence rates in the cases of stent remaining, spontaneously dislodged, removed on schedule, external tube removal, and aspiration only were 10.0%, 12.5%, 42.9%, 50%, and 0%, respectively. *Conclusion.* EUS-GTD is a relatively safe and effective therapeutic method. However, further analysis should be done by larger series to determine the method of EUS-GTD for pancreatic pseudocyst.

1. Introduction

Endoscopic ultrasonography guided transmural drainage (EUS-GTD) is now a widely reported and established procedure for drainage of symptomatic pancreatic pseudocyst. The technical success rate of this procedure has been reported to be more than 90% on the other hand, complication rate is less than 5% [1–5]. Severe adverse events such as bleeding or perforation sometimes occur, but in general, EUS-GTD has been recognized as a relatively safe and effective therapeutic method and is performed as a common procedure in many institutes. However, some factors including the long-term outcome, appropriate period of stenting, and timing of removing the stent have not been determined yet.

2. Patients and Methods

Patient characteristics are described in Table 1. Sixty-seven patients with pancreatic pseudocyst who underwent EUS-GTD from April 2000 to March 2011 were enrolled. Indications of EUS-GTD at our center are as follows: symptomatic pancreatic cysts, infection or hemorrhage, rapid increase in size, and no communication with MPD. In this study, 3 cases after acute pancreatitis (type 1) had walled off necrosis. Abdominal computed tomography and transabdominal ultrasonography had been taken in all cases before EUS-GTD.

All procedures were performed using curved linear array EUS (GF UCT-240, GF UCT-260 Olympus Medical Systems, Tokyo, Japan). The used needles are EchoTip Ultra 19G (Cook Medical Inc., Winston Salem, NC, USA), GW, Visiglide 0.025 inch (Olympus Medical Systems), Jagwire 0.035 inch (Boston Scientific Japan, Tokyo, Japan), dilation catheter, Needlecut 3V (Olympus Medical Systems), and Soehendra biliary dilation catheter (Cook Medical Inc.). We used Pigtail nasobiliary catheter (6,7 Fr, Olympus Medical Systems. 7.5 Fr, Boston

Table 1: Clinical characteristics of the patients.

Gender M : F	50 : 17
Median age, yr (range)	56 (31~85)
Median cyst size, diameter in mm (range)	72 (19–186)
Cyst location	
Head	23
Body and tail	44
Classification	
Type I*: acute pancreatitis	15
Type II: acute exacerbation of chronic pancreatitis	14
Type III: retention cyst	26
Type IV: pancreatic fistula after pancreatic surgery	12

*3 cases in type I had walled off necrosis.

Scientific Japan) for external drainage and 7 Fr double pigtail catheter (Olympus Medical Systems) for internal drainage.

We evaluated (1) technical success rate of initial drainage, (2) Clinical Success rate, (3) adverse event of procedure, and (4) long-term follow-up results after EUS-GTD.

3. Technique of EUS-GTD

All procedures were performed in the fluoroscopy unit under given intravenous sedative agent. Following steps were used to perform EUS-GTD.

The cystic lesion of pancreas was examined with ultrasonographically, and doppler assessment of gastric or duodenal wall was performed to confirm the absence blood vessels at the puncture site. Then, pancreatic pseudocyst was punctured with EchoTip 19G needle (Figure 1(a)) and the GW was passed through the needle into the lumen of the cyst. The position of GW was confirmed by ultrasonography and fluoroscopy (Figure 1(b)). After placing the GW, electrocautery was applied with NeedleCut3V, and dilation was achieved with a Soehendra biliary dilation catheter (Figure 1(c)). After dilatation, 2nd GW was inserted through Soehendra biliary dilation catheter, and plastic stent and drainage tube were placed under the guidance of GW. 7Fr double pigtail stent was used for internal drainage and 6Fr ENBD pigtail catheter for external drainage (Figures 1(d) and 1(e)).

We mainly chose external drainage. However, in cases where patients were likely to remove the tube by themselves or there was no infected fluid in the cyst, we chose internal drainage. In some cases with pseudocyst with small size and no infected fluid, we performed only puncture and aspiration. From April 2010, we inserted both internal and external drainage tube at one procedure session.

4. Results

4.1. Technical Success. Total technical success rate was 88.1% (59/67) (Table 2). Technical success rates of transgastric approach and transduodenal approach were 88.3% and 75.0%, respectively. Depending on the procedure, the success rates of external drainage, internal drainage, both internal

Table 2: Technical success rate of initial drainage.

Access route	Stomach	88.3% (53/59)
	Duodenum	75% (6/8)
Success rate of procedure	External drainage	83.7% (36/43)
	Internal drainage	95% (19/20)
	Internal and external drainage	100% (3/3)
	Puncture and aspiration only	100% (1/1)
Total*		88.1% (59/67)

*The rate was defined as the cases that the procedures accomplished as planned successfully. Failed 8 cases had puncture and aspiration later.

Table 3: Clinical success rate.

Initial drainage	Rate
External drainage	91.7% (33/36)
Internal drainage	78.9% (15/19)
Internal and external drainage	66.7% (2/3)
Puncture and aspiration only	66.7% (6/9)*
Total	83.4% (56/67)

*8 cases (internal or external drainage failed) were included.

external drainage, and punctured and aspiration only were 83.7%, 95%, 100%, and 100%, respectively. Reasons for technical failure were difficulty in advancing the GW or its displacement in 2 cases, difficulty in achieving dilation in 4 cases, and difficulty with drainage tube placement in 2 cases. In these failed cases, we performed puncture and aspiration only.

4.2. Clinical Success. In our series, clinical success was defined as cases in which initial EUS-GTD contributed to cyst shrinking over 10 mm or improvement of clinical symptoms. Table 3 shows that clinical success rate of external drainage was 91.7% (33/36), internal drainage was 78.9%, both internal and external drainage was 66.7% (2/3), and puncture and aspiration only was also 66.7% (6/9). Total clinical success rate was 83.4% (56/67). In the failed 3 cases of external drainage, 1 case had additional multiple stenting which contributed to cyst shrinking, and 2 cases had operation. The failed 4 cases of internal drainage had added external tube drainage and all cases achieved cyst shrinking consequently. The failed 1 case of external and internal drainage had additional multiple stenting which was effective. In the failed 3 cases of puncture and aspiration only, each case had either operation, ESWL, or EPS (Table 4). 92.5% of the cases (62/67) achieved improvement by EUS-GTD.

4.3. Adverse Event of Procedure. The rate of adverse event was 1.5% (1/67). There was one case with perforation in our series. The perforation case had a type III pancreatic cyst (Figure 2(a)). Perforation occurred during balloon dilatation for multiple stents placement. After balloon dilatation, we recognized leakage of contrast medium and advancing of the GW into the abdominal cavity (Figures 2(b) and 2(c)). This case required surgical operation (Figure 2(d)).

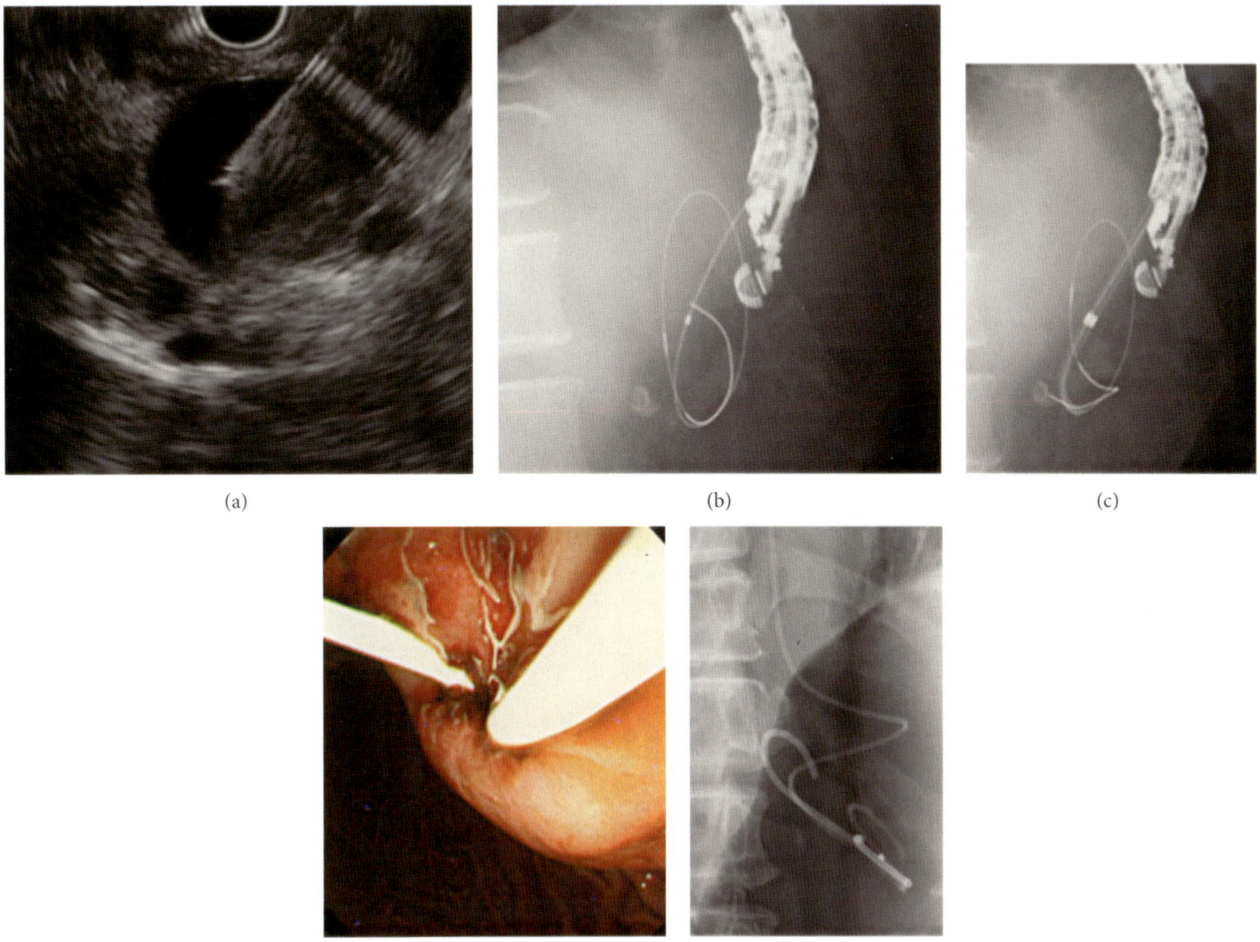

FIGURE 1: (a) Pancreatic pseudocyst was punctured with EchoTip 19 G needle. (b) Fluoroscopy image showed that the guide wire was passed through the needle into the lumen of cyst. (c) After electrocautery, Soehendra dilation catheter was inserted into the lumen for dilatation. (d) and (e) 7 Fr double pigtail stent and 6 Fr ENBD pigtail catheter were placed.

TABLE 4: Management of failed cases in initial drainage.

Initial drainage	Failed cases	Additional therapy	
External drainage ($n = 36$)	3	Multiple stents	1
		Repuncture* → operation	1
		Operation	1
Internal drainage ($n = 19$)	4	Add external drainage	4
External and internal drainage ($n = 3$)	1	Multiple stents	1
Puncture and aspiration only ($n = 9$)	3	ESWL	1
		EPS	1
		Operation**	1

ESWL: extracorporeal shock wave lithotripsy. EPS: endoscopic pancreatic stent. *CT guided—cyst drainage. **Operation for an adverse event caused by EUS-CD procedure.

4.4. Long-Term Follow-Up Results (Table 5). In the 46 cases which finally achieved clinical improvement by EUS-GTD and were observed for more than 1 year, overall recurrence rate was 23.9% (11/46). Median follow-up period of the above cases was 33.9 months. Final stent conditions were as follows: 40 cases had internal drainage (ID), 4 cases had external tube removal (stent free), and 2 cases had only puncture and aspiration. Stent was still remaining in 10 cases of ID and 1 of them had recurrences (10%). In 16 cases of ID, stent was dislodged spontaneously, and 2 of them had recurrences (12.5%). In 14 cases of ID, stents were removed on schedule and 6 of them had recurrence (42.9%). 2 cases of aspiration only and external drainage tube removal had recurrences (20%).

We also analyzed the factors of recurrence by comparing recurrence group ($n = 11$) and nonrecurrence group ($n = 35$) (Table 6, Fischers test, P value <.05 was considered statistically significant); however, no factors were significant to determining recurrences.

5. Discussion

The technical success rate of EUS-GTD has been reported to be more than 90% in several studies [1–5]. In our series, the

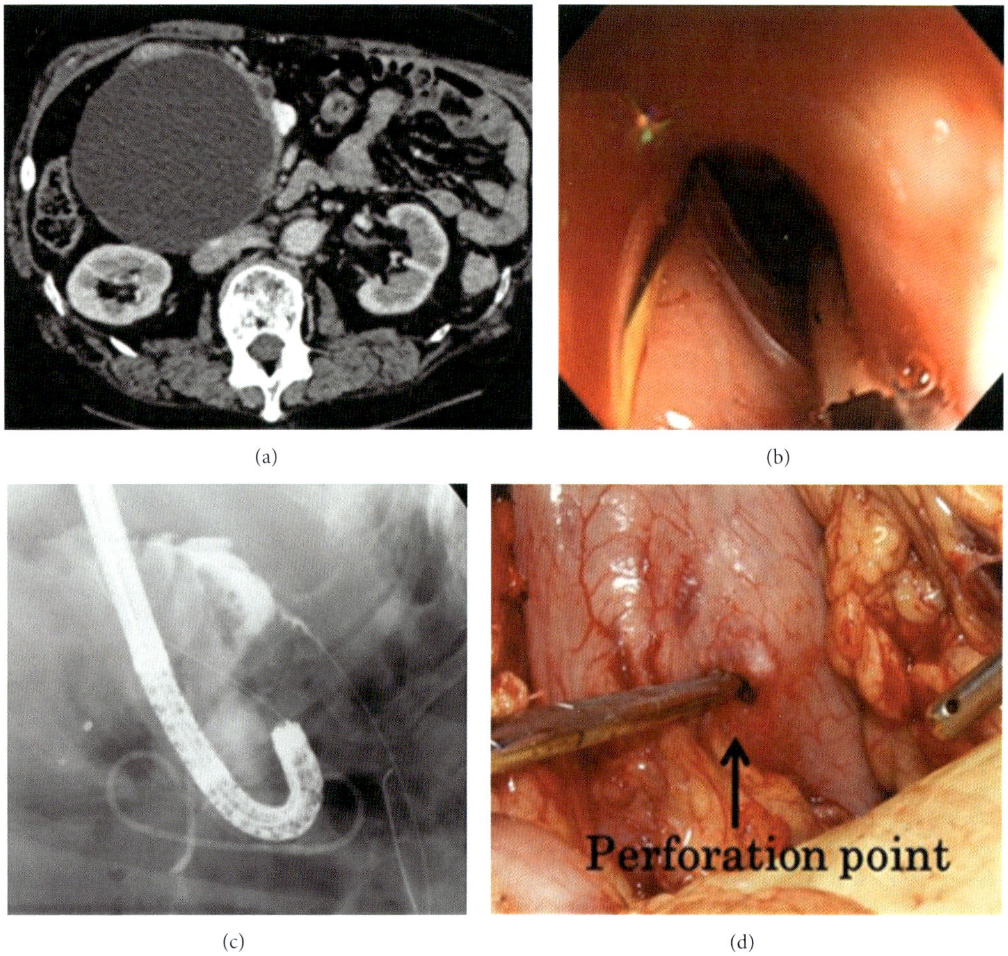

Figure 2: (a) Type III pancreatic pseudocyst. (b) The edge of omentum was observed through the hole dilated by balloon. (c) Leakage of contrast medium and advancing of the guide wire into the abdominal cavity were observed. (d) Perforation point was clearly confirmed by operation.

Table 5: Recurrence rate and stent condition.

Recurrence rate 23.9% (11/46)		n = 46	
Final drainage	Stent condition*		Recurrence
Internal drainage (n = 40)	Still remaining	10	1 (10%)
Single stent (n = 34)	Spontaneous dislodged	16	2 (12.5%)
Multiple stent (n = 6)	Scheduled removal	14	6 (42.9%)
Puncture and aspiration only (n = 2)	Stent-free	2	0 (0%)
External tube removal (n = 4)	Stent-free	4	2 (50%)

*The duration of internal drainage: 0.5~97.1 (median 20) months.

technical success rate was 88.1%. The technical success rate of external drainage was slightly low (83.7%), but the rates of internal drainage and both internal and external drainage were relatively high (95% and 100%, resp.). Clinical success rate was 83.4%, and by adding extra EUS-GTD procedure, 92.5% of the cases achieved clinical improvement. Our result also supported that EUS-GTD is an effective procedure for pancreatic pseudocyst.

It is stated in previous studies that some cases with walled off necrosis after acute pancreatitis need not only tube drainage but also debridement. The success rate of EUS drainage for pancreatic abscess or necrosis was lower compared with clear fluid pancreatic pseudocyst [6]. One of the recent studies also reported that multiple transluminal gateway technique for EUS guided drainage was clearly effective for walled off necrosis of pancreas [7]. In our series, 3 cases had walled off necrosis; however, all improved by only conservative external drainage without debridement.

Severe adverse events such as perforation and bleeding sometimes occur in EUS-GTD. The rate of adverse event was reported to be less than 5% [5]. Our series also had 1 case with perforation and that case needed operation. In our case, perforation occurred when balloon dilatation was performed. Balloon dilatation method has been thought to be a safer method compared to using electrocautery [8]. However, if the

Table 6: Evaluation of factors for recurrence.

	Recurrence (11)	Non-recurrence (35)	P value
Patients characteristics			
Male	9	29	0.7064
Age < 50	4	15	0.9756
Age ≥ 70	4	8	0.6197
Location of cyst, Ph	3	11	0.9089
Diameter of cyst ≥ 10 cm	2	6	0.7064
Infection	5	14	0.7485
Procedure			
Internal tube drainage	9	31	0.9466
External tube removal	2	2	0.4685
Puncture, aspiration only	0	2	0.9706
Stent remaining	1	9	0.4551
Initial clinical failure	2	1	0.2732
Multiple stenting	1	5	0.9744

cyst wall of pancreas and gastric wall are not adhered to each other, the risk of perforation is clearly increased. Pancreatic cyst of our perforation case was type III, and this seemed to be the main cause of perforation. In our institute, first step drainage for type III cyst is endoscopic transpapillary drainage except in cases with severe clinical symptoms such as cyst infection or abdominal pain. In 14 cases out of 26 type III cysts, we performed transpapillary drainage (ENPD) first, but the procedure was not effective. In 3 cases, we failed to place ENPD and performed transmural drainage only. There were 9 cases in which transmural drainage was directly performed due to severe cyst infection or remarkable abdominal pain. EUS-GTD was performed directly in the case with perforation due to cyst infection.

Since the rate of adverse events in our series is low (1.5%), it can be said that EUS-GTD is a relatively safe procedure for pancreatic pseudocyst drainage. Although EUS-GTD is a safe and effective therapy method for drainage of pancreatic pseudocyst, prospective studies which compare EUS-GTD to surgery to evaluate the long-term outcome are required [9].

We had chosen external drainage mainly and in some cases, we chose internal drainage. Recently, we insert both internal and external drainage tube in one session of procedure. Several current studies recommended insertion of both internal and external drainage tube by using double guidewire technique [10, 11]. There is no prospective study comparing efficacy between both internal and external tube placement at once or external tube or internal tube only. In our series, it was necessary to replace external drainage tube to internal drainage tube in 26 cases and to replace internal drainage tube to external drainage tube in 1 case. Since recannulating the pseudocyst is sometimes cumbersome, the combination placement of internal and external drainage tube using double guidewire technique will be an effective and reasonable method for pancreatic pseudocyst drainage.

Total recurrence rate in our study was 23.9%. The current another study also reported that recurrence rate of fluid collection was 13.4% [12]. The reasons for recurrence may include not only stent condition but also any background of pancreas condition. We also analyzed several factors for recurrences; however, no particular factors were significant in our series. The result was not shown to be significant. The reason for this may be that this was a single center study, and was performed retrospectively. A larger prospective series study is required for detecting the factors for recurrence.

6. Conclusion

EUS-GTD is a relatively safe and effective therapeutic method. Therefore, EUS-GTD can be the first choice for therapy of pancreatic pseudocyst. However, further analysis should be done by a larger series to check the efficacy and safety and to determine the method of EUS-GTD for pancreatic pseudocyst.

References

[1] S. Varadarajulu, C. M. Wilcox, A. Tamhane, M. A. Eloubeidi, J. Blakely, and C. L. Canon, "Role of EUS in drainage of peripancreatic fluid collections not amenable for endoscopic transmural drainage," *Gastrointestinal Endoscopy*, vol. 66, no. 6, pp. 1107–1119, 2007.

[2] M. Krüger, A. S. Schneider, M. P. Manns, and P. N. Meier, "Endoscopic management of pancreatic pseudocysts or abscesses after an EUS-guided 1-step procedure for initial access," *Gastrointestinal Endoscopy*, vol. 63, no. 3, pp. 409–416, 2006.

[3] C. V. Lopes, C. Pesenti, E. Bories, F. Caillol, and M. Giovannini, "Endoscopic-ultrasound-guided endoscopic transmural drainage of pancreatic pseudocysts and abscesses," *Scandinavian Journal of Gastroenterology*, vol. 42, no. 4, pp. 524–529, 2007.

[4] M. R. Antillon, R. J. Shah, G. Stiegmann, and Y. K. Chen, "Single-step EUS-guided transmural drainage of simple and complicated pancreatic pseudocysts," *Gastrointestinal Endoscopy*, vol. 63, no. 6, pp. 797–803, 2006.

[5] S. Varadarajulu, "EUS followed by endoscopic pancreatic pseudocyst drainage or all-in-one procedure: a review of basic techniques (with video)," *Gastrointestinal Endoscopy*, vol. 69, no. 2, pp. S176–S181, 2009.

[6] R. Sadik, E. Kalaitzakis, A. Thune, J. Hansen, and C. Jönson, "Eus-guided drainage is more successful in pancreatic pseudocysts compared with abscesses," *World Journal of Gastroenterology*, vol. 17, no. 4, pp. 499–505, 2011.

[7] S. Varadarajulu, M. A. Phadnis, J. D. Christein, and C. M. Wilcox, "Multiple transluminal gateway technique for EUS-guided drainage of symptomatic walled-off pancreatic necrosis," *Gastrointestinal Endoscopy*, vol. 74, no. 1, pp. 74–80, 2011.

[8] S. Varadarajulu, A. Tamhane, and J. Blakely, "Graded dilation technique for EUS-guided drainage of peripancreatic fluid collections: an assessment of outcomes and complications and technical proficiency (with video)," *Gastrointestinal Endoscopy*, vol. 68, no. 4, pp. 656–666, 2008.

[9] S. Seewald, T. L. Ang, M. Kida, K. Y. K. Teng, and N. Soehendra, "EUS 2008 Working Group document: evaluation of EUS-guided drainage of pancreatic-fluid collections (with video),"

Gastrointestinal Endoscopy, vol. 69, no. 2, supplement, pp. S13–S21, 2009.

[10] T. Itoi, F. Itokawa, T. Tsuchiya, T. Kawai, and F. Moriyasu, "Eus-guided pancreatic pseudocyst drainage: simultaneous placement of stents and nasocystic catheter using double-guidewire technique," *Digestive Endoscopy*, vol. 21, supplement s1, pp. S53–S56, 2009.

[11] R. Puri, S. R. Mishra, R. B. Thandassery et al., "Outcome and complication of endoscopic ultrasound guided pancreatic pseudocyst drainage using combined endoprosthesis and naso-cystic drain," *Journal of Gastroenterology and Hepatology*, vol. 27, no. 4, pp. 722–727, 2012.

[12] S. Seewald, T. L. Ang, H. Richter et al., "Long term results after endoscopic drainage and necrosectomy of symptomatic pancreatic fluid collection," *Digestive Endoscopy*, vol. 24, pp. 36–41, 2011.

21

Multicenter Randomized Trial of 10-French versus 11.5-French Plastic Stents for Malignant Biliary Obstruction

Mihir S. Wagh,[1] Mario de Bellis,[2] Evan L. Fogel,[2] James T. Frakes,[3] John F. Johanson,[3] Tahir Qaseem,[4] Douglas A. Howell,[4] Glen A. Lehman,[2] and Stuart Sherman[2]

[1] *Division of Gastroenterology, University of Florida, 1600 SW Archer Road, HD 602, Gainesville, FL 32610, USA*
[2] *Division of Gastroenterology/Hepatology, Indiana University Medical Center, Indianapolis, IN 46202, USA*
[3] *Rockford GE Associates, Rockford, IL 61107, USA*
[4] *Division of Gastroenterology, Maine Medical Center, Portland, ME 04102, USA*

Correspondence should be addressed to Mihir S. Wagh; mihir.wagh@medicine.ufl.edu

Academic Editor: Tony C. K. Tham

Background. There is little prospective data on whether bigger plastic stents are better for patients with malignant biliary obstruction with jaundice. *Goals*. Multicenter prospective study to compare technical success, clinical response, stent occlusion, and patient survival in patients with malignant biliary obstruction randomized to 10-French or 11.5-French plastic stent. *Study*. Patients with malignant biliary obstruction were randomized to 10-French or 11.5-French biliary stents. Patients were prospectively assessed for stent occlusion, stent-related interventions, hospital stay, and change in bilirubin. Main outcome measurements included technical success, clinical response, rates of stent occlusion, and survival. *Results*. 234 patients (47 hilar and 187 common bile duct strictures) were randomized. Outcomes were similar for the 10-French and 11.5-French groups (technical success 99.1% versus 97.4%, $P = 0.37$). Overall, median stent survival was 213 days, but there was no statistically significant difference in stent survival between 10-French and 11.5-French stents (149 versus 258 days, $P = 0.16$). Stent survival was significantly longer when placed for common bile duct versus hilar strictures (231 versus 115 days, $P = 0.049$). *Conclusions*. The theoretical advantage of improved bile flow for the 11.5-French stent does not translate into more prolonged patency, better clinical response, and longer patient survival than the 10-French stent.

1. Introduction

The majority of patients presenting with symptoms of malignant biliary obstruction are considered unsuitable for surgery because of locally advanced or metastatic disease or poor performance status. Palliative biliary stenting at ERCP is frequently the only planned therapy. Endoscopic biliary stenting was first described by Soehendra and Reynders-Frederix [1] in 1980 and since then has become the preferred method to relieve jaundice and improve quality of life for patients with advanced malignant biliary obstruction [2–5]. Several studies have shown that this technique is associated with fewer complications and lower costs than surgical bypass or percutaneous drainage [6–10].

The major limitation to long-term biliary stenting is stent occlusion which particularly affects plastic stents whose average patency is 4 months for the 10 French (Fr) polyethylene stents [11, 12]. The most commonly used plastic stent is the straight polyethylene stent with distal and proximal end holes and an adjacent side hole at its tip [13].

The most cost effective strategy to prolong stent patency is the use of larger stent diameter. However, while in some studies stent patency was significantly longer for large-diameter plastic stent rather than small diameter stents, other investigators found no prolongation of stent patency and noted more complications when larger stents were used [14–19]. Another approach to prolong stent patency has been the use of expandable metal stents whose large diameter (30 Fr) ensures a long term patency rate which is about twice as long as the 10 Fr plastic biliary stent [20–27]. Though recent studies have shown the increasing role of expandable metal stents for initial biliary decompression of patients with malignant biliary obstruction, and despite the improved patency of metal stents, plastic stents are still widely used all over the world for treatment of malignant bile duct obstruction being especially cost effective in patients with estimated survival of less than 4 months and in countries, with low-cost ERCP. Thus while expandable metal stents may be the near standard in wealthy countries it is not that way in many other countries.

Given all the above, the standard polyethylene plastic stent is still often the first choice for endoscopic biliary stenting of patients with established or suspected malignant biliary obstruction (though expandable metal stents may be initially placed in these patients). The question of whether "bigger is better" still has not been answered. It remains controversial whether the potential advantage of improved bile flow for the 11.5 Fr stent is clinically significant and outweighs the disadvantage of using these more cumbersome stents. We conducted a multicenter prospective randomized study that compared the 10 Fr and 11.5 Fr polyethylene (plastic) biliary stents in patients with suspected or proven malignant biliary obstruction.

2. Methods

Patients with suspected or proven malignant biliary obstruction who were unresectable or inoperable and were undergoing ERCP were candidates for the study. This was a multicenter randomized trial conducted at 3 institutions: Indiana University Medical Center, Maine Medical Center, and Rockford GE Group. Approval for the study from the Institutional Review Board of each institution was obtained. A written and informed consent for the procedure with details about the stenting procedure and the two different plastic biliary stents used was obtained in writing from all patients.

2.1. Exclusion Criteria. Patients were excluded from the study if (a) they had previously undergone biliary stenting, (b) surgery was planned, (c) a guidewire could not be passed through the stricture, (d) they had an expected survival of <3 months, or (e) there was impending duodenal obstruction. This study compared the ability to place a 10 Fr versus 11.5 Fr biliary stent, and hence patients in whom a guidewire could not be passed above the stricture were excluded as neither type of stent could be placed in these cases. Also, patients with expected survival of <3 months were excluded to allow assessment of stent occlusion which would not be possible if the patient expired within 3 months.

2.2. Procedure/Technique. After cannulation of the main bile duct, a cholangiogram was obtained to define the location and the extent of the biliary stricture. A guidewire was then passed through the stricture and, after securing access to the proximal biliary tree with the wire, more complete intrahepatic filling was obtained when felt clinically necessary. A biliary sphincterotomy was performed at the discretion of the endoscopist performing the procedure. The biliary stricture was then sampled for tissue and/or dilated at the discretion of the endoscopist. The patient was randomized to a 10 Fr or an 11.5 Fr plastic biliary stent following guidewire advancement upstream to the stricture using random computer-generated numbers and sealed opaque envelopes. The biliary stent chosen was placed using standard techniques. Hilar and common bile duct (CBD) strictures were randomized separately. Patients with hilar strictures had only one stent placed on the more obstructed/dilated side and based on pre-ERCP radiographic findings of intrahepatic duct dilation and hepatic lobe atrophy. Efforts were made to avoid contrast filling and manipulation of liver segments that were not going to be stented. Stents were not changed prophylactically. When a patient developed signs and symptoms suggestive of stent occlusion, the stent was changed on an emergent basis. Stent occlusion was confirmed by the 10 cm water column test [28].

2.3. Follow-Up. Patients were followed till death or first stent-related intervention by telephone interview or clinic visit at 1- to 2-month intervals after stent placement to assess for symptoms of stent occlusion and to determine the clinical response rate. The 10 Fr and 11.5 Fr stent groups were compared for technical success rate of stent deployment, clinical response rates, rates of stent occlusion, number of stent-related interventions and hospital days, and patient survival. Stent obstruction from various causes (occlusion, migration, or tumor overgrowth) was separately assessed as well.

2.4. Statistical Analysis. The statistical analysis was performed using the log rank test, the Wilcoxon test, and the chi-square test. Pearson's chi-square test was used to compare categorical variables between the groups, and Fisher's exact test was used when cell frequencies were low. For continuous variables, a two-sample t-test or Wilcoxon's test was used to compare the groups after checking the assumption of normality and homoscedasticity. Regression analysis using baseline bilirubin as a covariate was used to reassess the effect of stent on bilirubin change. The interaction between stent group and baseline bilirubin was tested but was not significant. Diagnostics for model lack of fit and presence of outliers suggested 3 outliers and influential points. The regression model was run with and without the outliers. Statistical analyses were performed using the statistical software package SAS version 9.1 (SAS Institute, Cary, NC). Estimates of patient survival and stent survival were analyzed by the Kaplan-Meier method. Patients who died before a reintervention was required (i.e., stent exchange) were censored from the analyses of stent survival. In all the analysis performed a P value less than 0.05 was considered statistically significant.

Our prior experience indicated a median stent survival of 5 months for the 10 Fr stent. The estimated number of patients to gain 83% power (P-sided alpha = 0.05) to detect a 50% increase in the median stent survival to 7.5 months was 100 patients in each group.

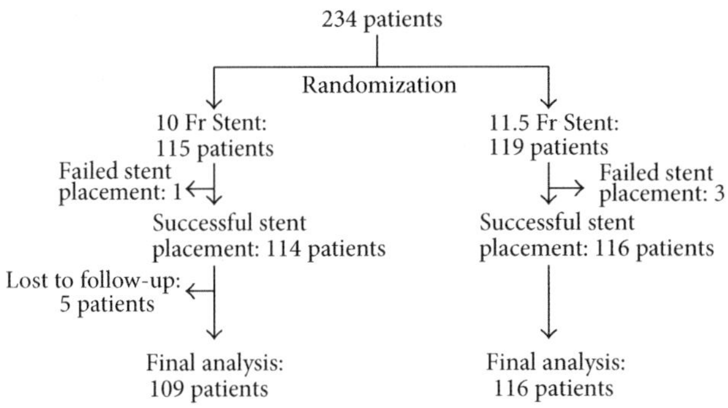

Figure 1

3. Results

During a 3-year period 234 patients with suspected or proven malignant obstructive jaundice underwent ERCP for biliary decompression and were randomized to a 10 Fr or an 11.5 Fr plastic biliary stent (Figure 1). 115 patients received a 10 Fr stent and 119 were stented with an 11.5 Fr stent. There were 133 males and 101 females (median age 68 years). 80% (187) of patients had a common bile duct stricture and 20% (47) a hilar stricture. Tumor types included pancreatic cancer (56%), cholangiocarcinoma (22%), metastatic tumors (13%), gallbladder cancer (4%), and other (5%). The two stent groups were similar with regard to the age, gender, stricture location, and stent diameter placed at center (Table 1).

Stents were successfully placed in 114/115 patients (99.1%) in the 10 Fr group and 116/119 patients (97.4%) in the 11.5 Fr stent group ($P = 0.37$). Placement of 11.5 Fr biliary stents did not require larger biliary sphincterotomies or more aggressive dilation of the stricture. Five patients, who received a 10 Fr stent, were lost to follow-up. Therefore, the final analysis of the data was performed on a total of 225 patients (109 with 10 Fr stent and 116 with 11.5 Fr stent). The median follow-up was 143 days for the 10 Fr stent group and 159 days for the 11.5 Fr stent group.

In the 225 patients stented, median overall stent survival was 213 days with 83 reinterventions (events) performed for stent exchange. However, stent survival was not significantly influenced by the stent size. The median patency for the 11.5 Fr stents was 258 days, while the 10 Fr stents stayed patent for 149 days ($P = 0.16$). When stent survival was related to the location of the stricture, it was found that the overall median stent patency was significantly longer for a CBD stricture (231 days) than for a hilar stricture (115 days, $P = 0.049$). There was a trend toward an increased stent survival for 11.5 Fr stents (311 days) compared to 10 Fr stents (149 days) placed for CBD strictures ($P = 0.071$), but this difference did not reach statistical significance. No statistically significant difference in stent survival was found between 11.5 Fr and 10 Fr stents when stent survival was examined for a hilar stricture location ($P = 0.93$).

Table 2 shows the outcomes in both groups. The decrease in total bilirubin from baseline was 10.6 mg/dL in the 11.5 Fr group and 8.7 mg/dL in the 10 Fr group ($P = 0.03$). However, the baseline bilirubin prior to stent placement was 12.8 mg/dL and 10.8 mg/dL in the two groups, respectively ($P = 0.03$). To make valid comparisons between the 2 groups, the effect of stenting was reassessed and tested after adjusting for baseline bilirubin in a regression model. The model suggested a better fit for the data, with no stent effect. The bilirubin decrease (10.6 mg/dL in the 11.5 Fr group and 8.7 mg/dL in the 10 Fr group) was no longer significant ($P = 0.077$) after adjusting for the difference in baseline bilirubin. Stent-related hospital days to treat complications (i.e., cholangitis), stent-related interventions, frequency of death before stent occlusion, and patient survival were similar for the two groups. Stent obstruction occurred in 77 patients (38 (32%) in the 11.5 Fr group and 39 (34%) in the 10 Fr group) (Tables 2 and 3). More than one cause for stent obstruction (occlusion, migration, and tumor overgrowth) was seen in some patients.

Table 4 shows that there was no significant difference in stent obstruction when comparing 11.5 Fr and 10 Fr stents placed for CBD obstruction (27% versus 30%, $P = 0.64$)

Table 1: Demographic data: frequencies by stent size.

Variable	10 Fr ($n = 115$)	11.5 Fr ($n = 119$)	P value
Age			0.736
65	36.5% (42)	38.7% (46)	
>65	63.5% (73)	61.3% (73)	
Center			0.740
IU	60.9% (70)	62.2% (74)	
MMC	31.3% (36)	27.7% (33)	
RGC	7.8% (9)	10.1% (12)	
Gender			0.924
Female	43.5% (50)	42.9% (51)	
Male	56.5% (65)	57.1% (68)	
Stricture location			0.974
CBD	80% (92)	79.8% (95)	
Hilar	20% (23)	20.2% (24)	

IU: Indiana University; MMC: Main Medical Center; RGC: Rockford GE Associates.
CBD: common bile duct.

Table 2: Outcomes in patients stented with 10 Fr and 11.5 Fr stents.

	10 Fr ($n = 115$)	11.5 Fr ($n = 119$)	P value
Technical success	99.1% (114/115)	97.4% (116/119)	0.37
Baseline bilirubin (mg/dL)	10.7 ± 6.8	12.8 ± 7.6	0.03
Bilirubin decrease (mg/dL)	8.7 ± 6.1*	10.6 ± 6.9*	0.077*
Days to stent failure	149	258	0.16
Stent-related hosp. days (Mean)	1.6 ± 3.5	1.9 ± 3.8	0.50
Stent-related interventions (mean)	0.74 ± 1.5	0.82 ± 1.5	0.66
Median patient survival days	151	206	0.20

* After adjusting for difference in baseline bilirubin.

TABLE 3: Total complications by stent size.

Complication	10 Fr (n = 115)		11.5 Fr (n = 119)	
	Number (%) of patients	Median time to complication (Days)	Number (%) of patients	Median time to complication (Days)
Death	95 (83%)	120	95 (80%)	170
Death before occlusion	66 (57%)	82.5	66 (55%)	114.5
Stent obstruction (all causes)	39 (34%)	107	38 (32%)	147
Stent occlusion	35 (30%)	110	36 (30%)	147
Stent migration	5 (4%)	61	5 (4%)	56
Tumor overgrowth	1 (1%)	14	3 (3%)	74

TABLE 4: Stent obstruction by stricture location.

Stricture location	10 Fr	11.5 Fr	P value
Common duct	28/92 (30%)	26/95 (27%)	0.64
Hilar	11/23 (48%)	12/24 (50%)	0.88
Total	39/115 (34%)	38/119 (32%)	0.75

TABLE 5: Incidence of early (≤30 days) complications.

Complication	10 Fr n = 115	11.5 Fr n = 119	P value
Death	7 (6%)	13 (11%)	0.19
Stent occlusion	6 (5%)	4 (3%)	0.48
Stent migration	2 (2%)	2 (2%)	0.97
Tumor overgrowth	1 (0.9%)	0 (0%)	0.31
Other	1 (0.9%)	4 (3%)	0.19

and when comparing these two stents placed for hilar lesions (50% versus 48%, P = 0.88).

The incidence of early (<30 days) stent complications was similar for the two groups (Table 5) but this study was not powered to detect this. There were 13 early (<30 days) deaths (11%) in the 11.5 Fr stent group and 7 (6%) in the 10 Fr stent group (P = 0.19). Stent occlusion occurred in 4 (3%) patients with 11.5 Fr stents and in 6 (5%) patients with 10 Fr stents (P = 0.48). Stent migration rate was 2% in each of the two groups. There was no difference in rates of tumor overgrowth.

4. Discussion

Patients with malignant biliary obstruction often have an unresectable tumor and/or are unfit for surgery. These patients require palliation of the obstructive jaundice and can be managed by surgery, endoscopy, or interventional radiology [6–10]. Since the initial report [1], endoscopic stenting has become the preferred method for palliation of patients with malignant obstructive jaundice and has been shown to improve the quality of life of these patients [4, 5, 29]. A recent meta-analysis concluded that both surgery and endoscopic stenting are effective for the palliation of malignant obstructive jaundice [30]. Patients undergoing endoscopic stenting have lower 30-day mortality and less early complications than surgical bypass but require repeat ERCP to exchange the plastic stent for occlusion [7–10, 30]. Ten-French plastic stents usually become obstructed after 4 months [11, 12].

Stent occlusion is an important clinical problem that has been studied extensively in an attempt to improve stent patency. Since deposition of sludge in the stent is not preventable, the simplest and most effective approach to prolonging stent survival is to use large diameter stents. Rey and colleagues noted that by increasing the internal stent diameter by 0.2 mm the rate of the bile flow increased 300% [31]. Zimmon and Clemett reported good palliation of obstructive jaundice with single/multiple 5 Fr stents, but 38 episodes of cholangitis occurred in 22 patients (among the 162 patients stented) [32]. High rates of cholangitis (40%) were reported by Kiil and colleagues who used single 7 Fr stents for biliary decompression [33]. These stents had a relatively low patency rate with stent occlusion occurring at a median of 49 days after the initial placement. Insertion of multiple small-diameter stents as suggested by Zimmon and Clemett may improve the overall patency rate [32]. However, the flow capacity of two 5 Fr stents is nearly 10 times lower than that of a single 10 Fr stent [14]. These authors calculated that the flow capacity of a 10 Fr stent (103 mL/min) is 270% greater than that of an 8 Fr stent (41 mL/min) and recommended the use of at least a 10 Fr stent for endoscopic palliation of malignant biliary obstruction. Maillot and colleagues obtained similar results in a porcine model [34]. Siegel and colleagues reported that the patency rate of 12 Fr stents was longer than that of 10 Fr stents (190 versus 150 days) and recommended routine use of these large stents [15]. However, three retrospective studies failed to confirm that stents larger than 10 Fr have any significant advantage in the palliative treatment of patients with malignant biliary strictures compared with the 10 Fr stent [17, 18, 35, 36].

The question whether bigger is definitively better for a plastic stent has clinical importance since the plastic stent often is the first choice for the palliation of patients with malignant biliary obstruction, despite the introduction of metal stents into clinical practice [20, 21, 23, 26, 27]. Despite the improved patency of metal stents, plastic stents are still widely used for treatment of malignant bile duct obstruction, being especially cost effective in patients with estimated survival of less than 4 months and in countries with low-cost ERCP. Thus while expandable metal stents may be the near standard in wealthy countries it is not that way in many other countries.

In this multicenter prospective randomized trial we evaluated the patency rates for 10 Fr and 11.5 Fr stents placed at ERCP to drain patients with malignant biliary obstruction. To our knowledge, this is the first prospective randomized trial addressed to answer the question whether bigger is better for plastic biliary stents. In our study, the technical success rate of stent placement, stent occlusion rate, stent-related interventions and hospital days, and the patients' survival were not statistically different for the 10 Fr and 11.5 Fr stent groups (Table 2).

Clinical response rate to stenting as assessed by reduction in bilirubin was different in the two groups. The decrease in total bilirubin from baseline was 10.6 mg/dL in the 11.5 Fr group and 8.7 mg/dL in the 10 Fr group ($P = 0.03$). However, there was a difference in the baseline bilirubin prior to stent placement in each group. After adjusting for this difference in baseline bilirubin, the decrease in bilirubin (10.6 mg/dL in the 11.5 Fr group and 8.7 mg/dL in the 10 Fr group) was no longer significant ($P = 0.077$). Also, from a practical standpoint, the numerical bilirubin value may not be very important in patient management as long as biliary stenting is able to alleviate jaundice. Hence the minimal difference in reduction in bilirubin after placement of 11.5 Fr or 10 Fr stents may not have much clinical significance.

Our data on stent patency are similar to those reported by Kadakia and Starnes [17] although we found a slight trend toward stent survival for the 11.5 Fr stent. Matsuda et al. reported no significant difference in median stent survival for 10 Fr and 11.5/12 Fr stents [18]. Dowsett and colleagues reported no significant difference in stent survival between 10 Fr and 12 Fr stents [35]. However, the 12 Fr stents were more difficult to insert with a technical success rate of only 51% when compared to 98% for 10 Fr stents. In our study, the success rate of stent insertion was 99.1% for 10 Fr and 97.4% for 11.5 Fr stents ($P = 0.37$). Similar results were reported by Kadakia and Starnes who successfully placed a 10 Fr stent in 85% of cases and an 11.5 Fr stent in 79%. We noted that 11.5 Fr stents were somewhat more difficult to advance through the stricture although the time to stent placement was not measured.

In our study, a trend for improved patency rates was seen for the 11.5 Fr stent for common bile duct strictures. The 11.5 Fr stents had a median survival of 258 days while the 10 Fr stents stayed patent for a median of 149 days. However, this marked numerical difference was not statistically significant ($P = 0.071$), and there was no reduction in the number of stent-related interventions and hospital days for stent dysfunction. Although the sample size was small, there was no improvement or trend toward improvement in the stent patency rates for 11.5 Fr stents placed for hilar strictures (median patency of 112 days versus 115 days, respectively, for the 11.5 Fr and 10 Fr stents. $P = 0.93$). Stents placed for hilar obstruction in our series occluded faster than stents placed for more distal obstruction. Similarly, Dowsett et al. reported that stent changes were more frequent in high than in low (below cystic duct insertion) (30% versus 20%) common duct obstruction [35]. This is probably related to the longer stents required for proximal strictures and the slower flow dynamics [14].

The incidence of early (<30 days) stent complications was similar for the two groups, but this study was not powered to detect this. Similarly, there was no statistically significant difference in complication rates ($P = 0.87$) between 10 Fr and 11.5 Fr stent groups in the series reported by Kadakia and Starnes [17].

5. Conclusion

Our data suggests that the theoretical advantages of improved bile flow and long-term stent patency for the 11.5 Fr plastic stent are not seen clinically. However, the 11.5 Fr stent may be more effective than the 10 Fr stent in providing longer periods of drainage in common bile duct obstruction. This finding did not translate into a reduction in stent-related interventions or stent-related hospital days. There appears to be no advantage to decompressing a malignant biliary stricture with the more difficult-to-place 11.5 Fr stent.

Acknowledgment

This study was supported by a research grant from the American College of Gastroenterology.

References

[1] N. Soehendra and V. Reynders-Frederix, "Palliative bile duct drainage-a new endoscopic method of introducing a transpapillary drain," *Endoscopy*, vol. 12, no. 1, pp. 8–11, 1980.

[2] K. L. Cheung and E. C. S. Lai, "Endoscopic stenting for malignant biliary obstruction," *Archives of Surgery*, vol. 130, no. 2, pp. 204–207, 1995.

[3] J. H. Siegel and H. Snady, "The significance of endoscopically placed prostheses in the management of biliary obstruction due to carcinoma of the pancreas: results of nonoperative decompression in 277 patients," *American Journal of Gastroenterology*, vol. 81, no. 8, pp. 634–641, 1986.

[4] A. B. Ballinger, M. McHugh, S. M. Catnach, E. M. Alstead, and M. L. Clark, "Symptom relief and quality of life after stenting for malignant bile duct obstruction," *Gut*, vol. 35, no. 4, pp. 467–470, 1994.

[5] N. S. Abraham, J. S. Barkun, and A. N. Barkun, "Palliation of malignant biliary obstruction: a prospective trial examining impact on quality of life," *Gastrointestinal Endoscopy*, vol. 56, no. 6, pp. 835–841, 2002.

[6] A. G. Speer, P. B. Cotton, and R. C. G. Russell, "Randomised trial of endoscopic versus percutaneous stent insertion in malignant obstructive jaundice," *The Lancet*, vol. 2, no. 8550, pp. 57–62, 1987.

[7] G. V. Raikar, M. M. Melin, A. Ress et al., "Cost-effective analysis of surgical palliation versus endoscopic stenting in the management of unresectable pancreatic cancer," *Annals of Surgical Oncology*, vol. 3, no. 5, pp. 470–475, 1996.

[8] A. C. Smith, J. F. Dowsett, R. C. G. Russell, A. R. W. Hatfield, and P. B. Cotton, "Randomised trial of endoscopic stenting

versus surgical bypass in malignant low bileduct obstruction," *The Lancet*, vol. 344, no. 8938, pp. 1655–1660, 1994.

[9] H. A. Shepherd, G. Royle, A. P. R. Ross, A. Diba, M. Arthur, and D. Colin-Jones, "Endoscopic biliary endoprosthesis in the palliation of malignant obstruction of the distal common bile duct: a randomized trial," *British Journal of Surgery*, vol. 75, no. 12, pp. 1166–1168, 1988.

[10] J. R. Andersen, S. M. Sorensen, A. Kruse, M. Rokkjaer, and P. Matzen, "Randomised trial of endoscopic endoprosthesis versus operative bypass in malignant obstructive jaundice," *Gut*, vol. 30, no. 8, pp. 1132–1135, 1989.

[11] E. D. Libby and J. W. Leung, "Prevention of biliary stent clogging: a clinical review," *American Journal of Gastroenterology*, vol. 91, no. 7, pp. 1301–1308, 1996.

[12] W. Van Steenbergen, "Treatment of malignant biliary stenosis: which stent to use?" *Acta Gastro-Enterologica Belgica*, vol. 64, no. 4, pp. 309–313, 2001.

[13] D. Scheeres, W. O'Brien, L. Ponsky, and J. Ponsky, "Endoscopic stent configuration and bile flow rates in a variable diameter bile duct model," *Surgical Endoscopy*, vol. 4, no. 2, pp. 91–93, 1990.

[14] A. G. Speer, P. B. Cotton, and K. D. MacRae, "Endoscopic management of malignant biliary obstruction: stents of 10 French gauge are preferable to stents of 8 French gauge," *Gastrointestinal Endoscopy*, vol. 34, no. 5, pp. 412–417, 1988.

[15] J. H. Siegel, W. Pullano, B. Kodsi, A. Cooperman, and W. Ramsey, "Optimal palliation of malignant bile duct obstruction: experience with endoscopic 12 French prostheses," *Endoscopy*, vol. 20, no. 4, pp. 137–141, 1988.

[16] F. M. Pedersen, "Endoscopic management of malignant biliary obstruction. Is stent size of 10 French gauge better than 7 French gauge?" *Scandinavian Journal of Gastroenterology*, vol. 28, no. 2, pp. 185–189, 1993.

[17] S. C. Kadakia and E. Starnes, "Comparison of 10 French gauge stent with 11.5 French gauge stent in patients with biliary tract diseases," *Gastrointestinal Endoscopy*, vol. 38, no. 4, pp. 454–459, 1992.

[18] Y. Matsuda, K. Shimakura, and T. Akamatsu, "Factors affecting the patency of stents in malignant biliary obstructive disease: univariate and multivariate analysis," *American Journal of Gastroenterology*, vol. 86, no. 7, pp. 843–849, 1991.

[19] J. C. Pereira-Lima, R. Jakobs, M. Maier, C. Benz, B. Kohler, and J. F. Riemann, "Endoscopic biliary stenting for the palliation of pancreatic cancer: results, survival predictive factors, and comparison of 10-French with 11.5-French gauge stents," *American Journal of Gastroenterology*, vol. 91, no. 10, pp. 2179–2184, 1996.

[20] P. H. P. Davids, A. K. Groen, E. A. J. Rauws, G. N. J. Tytgat, and K. Huibregtse, "Randomised trial of self-expanding metal stents versus polyethylene stents for distal malignant biliary obstruction," *The Lancet*, vol. 340, no. 8834-8835, pp. 1488–1492, 1992.

[21] K. Knyrim, H. J. Wagner, J. Pausch, and N. Vakil, "A prospective, randomized, controlled trial of metal stents for malignant obstruction of the common bile duct," *Endoscopy*, vol. 25, no. 3, pp. 207–212, 1993.

[22] D. L. Carr-Locke, T. J. Ball, P. J. Connors et al., "Multicenter, randomized, controlled trial of metal stents for malignant obstruction of the common bile duct," *Gastrointestinal Endoscopy A*, vol. 39, p. 310, 1993.

[23] A. Schmassmann, E. Von Gunten, J. Knuchel, U. Scheurer, H. F. Fehr, and F. Halter, "Wallstents versus plastic stents in malignant biliary obstruction: effects of stent patency of the first and second stent on patient compliance and survival," *American Journal of Gastroenterology*, vol. 91, no. 4, pp. 654–659, 1996.

[24] F. Prat, O. Chapat, B. Ducot et al., "A randomized trial of endoscopic drainage methods for inoperable malignant strictures of the common bile duct," *Gastrointestinal Endoscopy*, vol. 47, no. 1, pp. 1–7, 1998.

[25] M. Kaassis, J. Boyer, R. Dumas et al., "Plastic or metal stents for malignant stricture of the common bile duct? Results of a randomized prospective study," *Gastrointestinal Endoscopy*, vol. 57, no. 2, pp. 178–182, 2003.

[26] D. O. Faigel, "Preventing biliary stent occlusion," *Gastrointestinal Endoscopy*, vol. 51, no. 1, pp. 104–106, 2000.

[27] K. G. Yeoh, M. J. Zimmerman, J. T. Cunningham, and P. B. Cotton, "Comparative costs of metal versus plastic biliary stent strategies for malignant obstructive jaundice by decision analysis," *Gastrointestinal Endoscopy*, vol. 49, no. 4, pp. 466–471, 1999.

[28] S. O. Ikenberry, S. Sherman, R. H. Hawes, M. Smith, and G. A. Lehman, "The occlusion rate of pancreatic stents," *Gastrointestinal Endoscopy*, vol. 40, no. 5, pp. 611–613, 1994.

[29] S. Sherman, G. Lehman, D. Earle et al., "Endoscopic palliation of malignant bile duct obstruction: improvement in quality of life," *Gastrointestinal Endoscopy*, vol. 43, no. 4, p. 321, 1996.

[30] M. C. Taylor, R. S. McLeod, and B. Langer, "Biliary stenting versus bypass surgery for the palliation of malignant distal bile duct obstruction: a meta-analysis," *Liver Transplantation*, vol. 6, no. 3, pp. 302–308, 2000.

[31] J. F. Rey, P. Maupetit, and M. Greff, "Experimental study of biliary endoprosthesis efficiency," *Endoscopy*, vol. 17, no. 4, pp. 145–148, 1985.

[32] D. S. Zimmon and R. C. Clemett, "Experience with 5 French biliary and pancreatic endoscopic stents," *Gastrointestinal Endoscopy AB*, vol. 30, p. 168, 1985.

[33] J. Kiil, A. Kruse, and M. Rokkjaer, "Endoscopic biliary drainage," *British Journal of Surgery*, vol. 74, no. 12, pp. 1087–1090, 1987.

[34] N. Maillot, P. Aucher, S. Robert et al., "Polyethylene stent blockage: a porcine model," *Gastrointestinal Endoscopy*, vol. 51, no. 1, pp. 12–18, 2000.

[35] J. F. Dowsett, S. J. Williams, A. R. W. Hatfield et al., "Does stent diameter matter in the endoscopic palliation of malignant biliary obstruction? A randomised trial of 10 Fr versus 12 Fr endoprostheses," *Gastroenterology A*, vol. 96, p. 128, 1989.

[36] J. T. Frakes, J. F. Johanson, and J. J. Stake, "Optimal timing for stent replacement in malignant biliary tract obstruction," *Gastrointestinal Endoscopy*, vol. 39, no. 2, pp. 164–167, 1993.

Long-Term Endoscopic Follow-Up of Patients with Chronic Radiation Proctopathy after Brachytherapy for Prostate Cancer

Masahiro Ohtani,[1] Hiroyuki Suto,[1] Takuto Nosaka,[1] Yasushi Saito,[1] Yoshihiko Ozaki,[1] Ryoko Hayama,[1] Tatsushi Naito,[1] Kazuto Takahashi,[1] Kazuya Ofuji,[1] Hidetaka Matsuda,[1] Katsushi Hiramatsu,[1] Tomoyuki Nemoto,[1] Hiroki Shioura,[2] Hirohiko Kimura,[2] Yoshitaka Aoki,[3] Osamu Yokoyama,[3] and Yasunari Nakamoto[1]

[1]*Second Department of Internal Medicine, Faculty of Medical Sciences, University of Fukui, 23-3 Matsuokashimoaizuki, Eiheiji-cho, Yoshida-gun, Fukui 910-1193, Japan*
[2]*Department of Radiology, Faculty of Medical Sciences, University of Fukui, Fukui 910-1193, Japan*
[3]*Department of Urology, Faculty of Medical Sciences, University of Fukui, Fukui 910-1193, Japan*

Correspondence should be addressed to Yasunari Nakamoto; nakamoto-med2@med.u-fukui.ac.jp

Academic Editor: Patrick J. O'Dwyer

Background. Chronic radiation proctopathy (CRP) is late toxicity and associated with morbidity. *Aim*. To investigate the predictors of prognosis in patients with CRP after brachytherapy (BT). *Methods*. One hundred four patients with prostate cancer were treated with BT or BT followed by external-beam radiotherapy (BT + EBRT). We retrospectively investigated the 5-year incidence of rectal bleeding and endoscopic findings of CRP using the Vienna Rectoscopy Score (VRS). Twenty patients with VRS ≥ 1 were divided into the improved VRS group without treatment, unchanged VRS group, and treated group. The parameters associated with alteration of VRS were analyzed. *Results*. The incidence of rectal bleeding was 24%. The risk of rectal bleeding was higher in patients treated with BT + EBRT compared to those treated with BT ($p < 0.0001$). The incidence of superficial microulceration was higher in the improved VRS group than in the unchanged VRS group ($p < 0.05$). The incidence of multiple confluent telangiectasia or superficial ulcers $> 1\,\text{cm}^2$ was higher in the treated group than in both the improved and unchanged VRS groups ($p < 0.05$). *Conclusions*. Patients treated with BT + EBRT have a high risk of CRP. Endoscopic findings were useful for prognostic prediction of CRP.

1. Introduction

Prostate cancer is the most commonly diagnosed cancer and the second-leading cause of cancer-related mortality in men over the age of 40 years in the United States [1], with the incidence of prostate cancer in Japan increasing in recent years [2]. For localized prostate cancer, radiation therapy is an effective treatment modality. Since the approval of ^{125}I seed source in 2003, ^{125}I brachytherapy (BT) has become one of the standard treatment modalities for low- to intermediate-risk prostate cancer in Japan. In addition, a combination of BT and external-beam radiation therapy (EBRT) is used for intermediate- to high-risk prostate cancer.

Chronic radiation proctopathy (CRP) is a late gastrointestinal (GI) toxicity and one of the common adverse effects after radiation therapy. Histopathological features of CRP are ischemic endarteritis and fibrosis in the submucosa [3]. The symptoms of CRP include hematochezia, tenesmus, diarrhea, fecal incontinence, and defecatory urgency. The most common complaint is rectal bleeding. CRP is temporary and self-limiting in approximately 95% of all patients; however, patients with severe recurrent hemorrhage may require hospitalization and blood transfusions [3]. Furthermore, various treatment modalities have been reported for the management of CRP, including endoscopic argon plasma coagulation (APC) [4], dilute formalin topical treatment [5], hyperbaric oxygen (HBO) therapy [6], and sucralfate enema [7]. For the evaluation of CRP, endoscopic examination is the most important modality. On endoscopy, the rectal mucosa may show varying appearances, from telangiectasia (TE) to ulceration (UL). Although the relationship between the symptoms and endoscopic findings of CRP has been investigated, literature about long-term follow-up with endoscopic examination is limited [8]. A study has reported the endoscopic findings at 12 and 65 months after EBRT, showing improvement in TE [8]. However, the long-term endoscopic evaluation of CRP after BT has not been reported. Furthermore, the indicators of medical treatment including APC or HBO therapy for rectal bleeding caused by CRP are unclear. Therefore, the purpose of this study was to evaluate the risk and prognostic factors of rectal bleeding after BT for prostate cancer.

2. Patients and Methods

2.1. Patients. A retrospective medical chart review was performed on consecutive patients with prostate cancer underwent brachytherapy between May 2006 and September 2009 at University of Fukui Hospital. This study was approved by institutional review board of University of Fukui, with the IRB number of 20150119. The inclusion criteria consist of histological diagnosis of prostate cancer and treatment with BT alone or BT followed by EBRT boost. The exclusion criteria were subjects with incompletion of follow-up after BT and coexistence of prostate and rectal cancer. Patients were implanted with ^{125}I seeds (OncoSeed; Nihon Medi-physics Co., Japan) by using modified peripheral loading techniques and a Mick applicator (Mick Radionuclear Instruments, Bronx, NY, USA). The prescribed dose was 144 Gy in patients undergoing BT only and 105 Gy in those undergoing BT + EBRT [9]. For combined therapy, BT was performed first, followed by EBRT 4–8 weeks after BT. EBRT was delivered using 10-MV X-rays in two or four fields, with a daily fraction dose of 1.8 Gy, for 5 days per week, up to total dose of 45–55 Gy.

2.2. Evaluation of Late Rectal Toxicity. After radiation therapy, patients were routinely followed up every 3 months to record GI toxicity due to radiotherapy. Rectal bleeding was graded according to the National Cancer Institute Common Terminology Criteria for Adverse Event (CTCAE) version 4.0 [10]. Rectal bleeding was defined as four instances of hematochezia in 4 weeks [11]. No rectal bleeding was defined as CTCAE grade 0 for evaluating the relationship between toxicity grade and endoscopic scoring. We evaluated the incidence of rectal bleeding after BT for 5 years and the factors associated with rectal bleeding, including age, extent of the primary tumor in TMN classification, use of antithrombotic therapy, presence or absence of diabetes mellitus, volume of the prostate gland, presence or absence of EBRT boost, number of seeds, and the use of neoadjuvant androgen depletion therapy (ADT). Tumor staging was performed according to the International Union Against Cancer TMN Classification of Malignant tumors 6th edition [12].

2.3. Evaluation of Endoscopic Findings of CRP. Several endoscopists performed colonoscopy or rectosigmoidoscopy by using the PCF-Q260AI (Olympus, Japan) for symptoms of CRP, as part of a health check-up or as an examination for fecal occult blood. The endoscopic findings of rectal mucosa were graded using the Vienna Rectoscopy Score (VRS), as reported by Wachter et al. [13]. In brief, endoscopic findings including TE, congested mucosa, UL, stricture, and necrosis were graded according to the following graduation system:

TE: grade 0, none; grade 1, single TE; grade 2, multiple nonconfluent TE; and grade 3, multiple confluent TE.

Congested mucosa: grade 0, none; grade 1, focal reddening of the mucosa combined with an edematous mucosa; grade 2, diffuse but nonconfluent reddening of the mucosa combined with an edematous mucosa; and grade 3, diffuse confluent reddening of the mucosa combined with an edematous mucosa.

UL: grade 0, none; grade 1, superficial microulceration $< 1\,cm^2$; grade 2, superficial UL $> 1\,cm^2$; grade 3, deep UL; and grade 4, fistula and perforation.

Stricture: grade 0, none; grade 1, more than two-thirds of the regular diameter; grade 2, one-third to two-thirds of the regular diameter; grade 3, less than one-third of the regular diameter; and grade 4, complete obstruction.

Necrosis: grade 0, none, and grade 1, necrosis.

Each of the five endoscopic parameters were summarized as VRS, from 0 to 5.

The relationship between the VRS and CTCAE grade was analyzed. Furthermore, the 5-year follow-up period was divided into the early period (up to the first 150 weeks after BT) and the late period of posttreatment (more than 150 weeks after BT and thereafter). Patients who had undergone endoscopy in both early and late period were classified into three groups based on their findings, the improved VRS group, the unchanged VRS group, or the treated group (treated with APC or HBO therapy), to evaluate changes of endoscopic findings and to determine their clinical characteristics.

2.4. Statistical Analysis. The distribution of clinical parameters for rectal bleeding and endoscopic parameters associated with rectal mucosal alteration was analyzed using the Student t-test and Fisher's exact test. The cumulative incidence of rectal bleeding was evaluated with the Kaplan-Meier method, and significant differences between treatment modalities were calculated by the log-rank test. The relationship between VRS and the CTCAE grade, obtained at the time of endoscopic examination, was analyzed by using Spearman's correlation test. All statistical analyses were performed using GraphPad Prism 6 (GraphPad Software, Inc., La Jolla, CA). Statistical significance was defined as $p < 0.05$.

3. Results

3.1. Patient Characteristics. A total of 104 patients with localized prostate cancer underwent transperineal ^{125}I prostate

TABLE 1: Patient characteristics.

Characteristic	
Number of patients	104
Age, mean ± SD	68.1 ± 6.6
Clinical stage, n (%)	
T1c	81 (77.8)
T2a	16 (15.4)
T2b	4 (3.8)
T2c	3 (2.9)
Use of antithrombotic drugs (%)	21 (20.2)
Presence of DM (%)	12 (11.5)
Volume of prostate, (cc) mean ± SD	25.6 ± 8.3
Treatment	
EBRT boost (%)	53 (51.0)
Median dose of EBRT (range)	45 (43–55.6)
Median number of seeds (range)	70 (40–100)
ADT (%)	39 (37.5)

DM, diabetes mellitus; EBRT, external-beam radiotherapy; ADT, androgen deprivation therapy.

TABLE 2: Incidence of rectal bleeding, endoscopic examination, and treatment.

	n (%)
CTCAE rectal bleeding scale	
Grade 1	13 (12.5%)
Grade 2	5 (4.8%)
Grade 3	7 (6.7%)
Total	25 (24.0%)
Endoscopic examination	
Number of patients who underwent endoscopy	56 (53.8%)
Total number of endoscopy	101
Number of patients who underwent endoscopy in group of grade ≥ 1 rectal bleeding	24
Treatment	
Iron supplementation	9
Endoscopic argon plasma coagulation	5
Hyperbaric oxygen therapy	2

BT between May 2006 and September 2009 at our institute. The characteristics of these patients are shown in Table 1. The mean age was 68.1 years (range: 54–82 years). According to TMN classification, 81 and 23 patients were classified as having T1 and T2 disease, respectively. Twenty-one patients (20.2%) received antithrombotic drugs for coronary artery diseases or cerebral infarction. A total of 12 patients (11.5%) were treated for diabetes mellitus. The mean prostate volume before RT estimated on ultrasonography was 25.6 mL. Combined therapy with EBRT was performed in 53 (51.0%) patients. The median dose of EBRT was 45 Gy (range: 43–55.6 Gy) and median number of ^{125}I seeds was 70 (range: 40–100). Thirty-nine patients were treated with neoadjuvant ADT consisting of luteinizing hormone-releasing hormone agonists and antiandrogen.

3.2. Risk Factors of Rectal Bleeding after Radiotherapy for Patients with Prostate Cancer. Rectal bleeding was observed in 25 patients (24%), with grade 1 (12.5%) being the most common, followed by grade 2 (4.8%) and grade 3 (6.7%) (Table 2). Endoscopy was performed in 56 (53.8%) patients totally and in 24 of 25 patients who experienced rectal bleeding symptoms of CTCAE grade ≥ 1. Iron supplementation was prescribed for 9 patients with anemia due to rectal bleeding. Endoscopic APC and HBO therapy were administered to 5 and 2 patients, respectively (Table 2). All patients who received endoscopic APC or HBO therapy showed improvement in their rectal bleeding symptoms. The occurrence of rectal bleeding was 41.5% in the BT + EBRT group while it was 5.9% in the BT group, indicating a significant association of the presence or absence of EBRT with rectal bleeding of CTCAE grade ≥ 1 ($p < 0.0001$) (Table 3). No significant differences were observed in other factors. In a log-rank test based on the presence or absence of EBRT, a significantly higher occurrence of rectal bleeding was found in the BT + EBRT group compared to the BT group ($p < 0.0001$) (Figure 1), and the Kaplan-Meier curve showed that the first rectal bleeding occurred before the 150th week after BT in the BT group. Conversely, in the BT + EBRT group, rectal bleeding occurred more frequently in the earlier period after BT (50th to 100th week) compared to the BT group. These results suggest that EBRT boost after BT increased the risk of rectal bleeding.

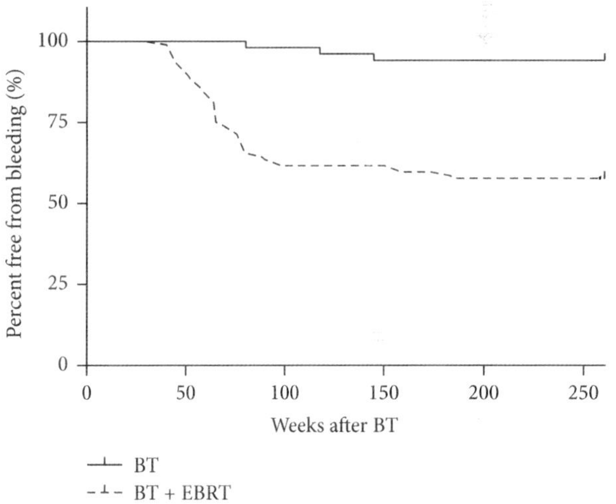

FIGURE 1: Kaplan-Meier curve for grade ≥ 1 rectal bleeding over 5 years ($p < 0.0001$). BT: brachytherapy; EBRT: external-beam radiotherapy.

3.3. Relationship between Endoscopic Findings and Rectal Bleeding Symptoms and Changes in Endoscopic Findings over Time. A total of 101 endoscopies were performed in the investigated patients during 5 years (Table 2). The VRS and CTCAE grade in patients who underwent endoscopies were significantly correlated ($p < 0.01$); CTCAE grade ≥ 1 rectal bleeding was observed in 20.7%, 43.7%, and 84.6% when

Table 3: Clinical parameters associated with rectal bleeding.

Parameter	Grade ≥ 1 rectal bleeding (%)	p value
Age, years		
≥70	14/43 (32.5)	0.11
<70	11/61 (18.0)	
Stage		
T1	19/81 (23.4)	0.79
T2	6/23 (26.1)	
Use of antithrombotic drugs		
Yes	7/21 (33.3)	0.27
No	18/83 (21.6)	
Presence of DM		
Yes	2/12 (16.6)	0.73
No	23/92 (25.0)	
Prostate volume, cc		
≥25	11/49 (22.4)	0.82
<25	14/55 (25.4)	
EBRT boost		
Yes	22/53 (41.5)	<0.0001
No	3/51 (5.9)	
Number of seeds		
≥70	10/52 (19.2)	0.35
<70	15/52 (28.8)	
Use of ADT		
Yes	8/39 (21.0)	0.64
No	17/65 (10.8)	

DM, diabetes mellitus; EBRT, external-beam radiotherapy; ADT, androgen deprivation therapy.

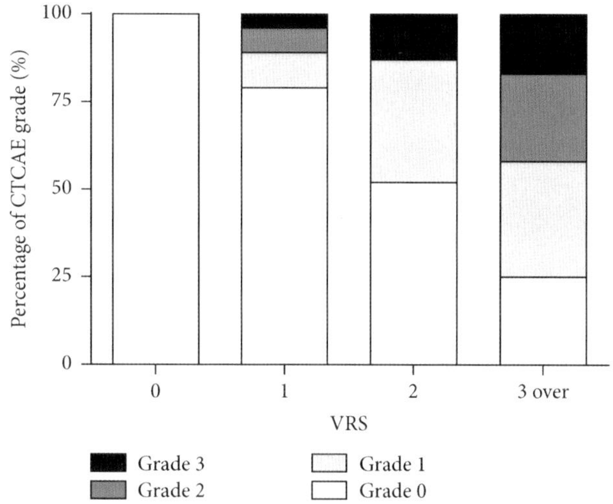

Figure 2: Correlation between VRS and CTCAE grade of rectal bleeding. The statistical significance was analyzed by Spearman's correlation test ($p < 0.01$). VRS: Vienna Rectoscopy Score.

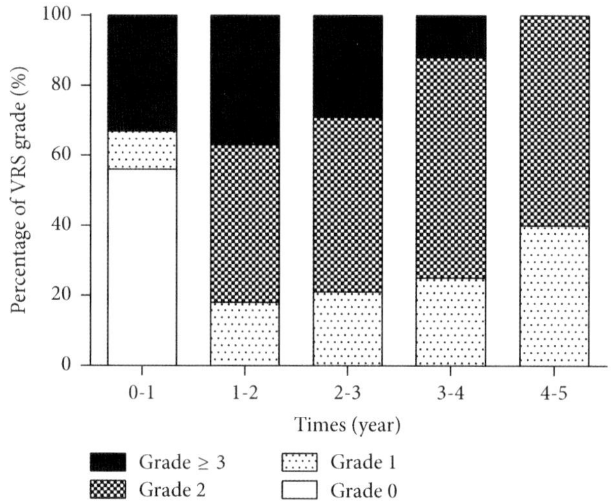

Figure 3: Change in VRS over time, in patients with CTCAE grade ≥ 1. VRS: Vienna Rectoscopy Score.

VRS grade was 1, 2, and 3, respectively (Figure 2). A total of 52 endoscopies were performed in patients with CTCAE grade ≥ 1. VRS 0 (normal) was found in 55.6% of the patients who underwent endoscopy within the first year after BT (0 to 1 year) (Figure 3). VRS 1 or higher was found in all patients who underwent endoscopy between 1 and 2 years after BT. Even though 7 patients who received APC or HBO therapy were included, the percentage of patients with VRS 1 increased with time (5 years) while the percentage of patients with VRS ≥ 3 decreased (Figure 3). In patients with CTCAE grade 0, 49 endoscopies were performed. The evaluation of VRS over time in patients without rectal bleeding revealed that VRS 0 was found in 88.9% of patients who underwent endoscopy between 0 years and 1 year after BT (Figure 4). In contrast, VRS ≥ 1 was found in 80% of patients who underwent endoscopy between 0 years and 1 year after BT (Figure 4). With time, the percentage of patients with VRS 0 increased while the percentage of patients with VRS ≥ 2 decreased in patients with CTCAE grade 0. These results indicated that endoscopic findings were correlated with rectal bleeding symptoms, and abnormal findings that were frequently observed 1 year or longer after BT improved over time.

3.4. Prognostic Factors of CRP Based on Endoscopic Findings after Treatment. The changes in endoscopic findings in the early and late periods were evaluated in 26 patients. Six patients who underwent endoscopy in the early period after BT had VRS 0, and these patients did not show any change in the endoscopic findings and bleeding symptoms in the late period.

Of 20 patients with VRS ≥ 1 in the early period, 4, 5, and 11 patients were from the treated group with APC or HBO therapy, the improved VRS group without treatment, and the unchanged VRS group, respectively (Table 4). All patients with VRS 1 in the early period also did not show any change of VRS. However, improvement of VRS was observed in 2 of 10 patients with VRS 2 and 3 of 6 patients with VRS ≥ 3. Rectal bleeding symptoms improved over the 5-year course in all patients of both the improved VRS and unchanged VRS groups. The percentage of patients with UL grade 1 was significantly higher in the improved VRS group (60%) than

TABLE 4: Endoscopic and clinical factors for improvement of VRS in patients with VRS ≥ 1 who underwent follow-up endoscopic examination.

	Treated group (HBO or APC)	Improved group	Unchanged group	p value
N	4	5	11	
VRS				
1	0	0	4	
2	1	2	7	
≥3	3	3	0	
TE score				
0	0	0	0	
1	0	0	4	
2	1	5	7	
3	3	0	0	
UL score				
0	0	2	11	
1	1	3	0	
2	0	0	0	
3	1	0	0	
UL 1 (+)	1/4	3/5[a]	0/7[a]	<0.05[a]
TE 3 or UL ≥ 2	3/4[b]	0/5[b]	0/5[b]	<0.05[b]
Age, years	71.8 ± 8.3	67.2 ± 3.1	69.7 ± 4.2	NS
Stage T1/T2	2/2	3/2	6/1	NS
Use of ADT	2	2	5	NS
Use of antithrombotic drugs	2	1	1	NS
p volume, mL	22.5 ± 5.5	25.1 ± 7.0	24.6 ± 9.4	NS
Use of EBRT boost	4	5	7	NS
Number of seeds	71.3 ± 6.3	61.0 ± 13.8	62.9 ± 13.3	NS

VRS, Vienna Rectoscopy Score; HBO, hyperbaric oxygen therapy; APC, argon plasma coagulation; TE, telangiectasia; UL, ulceration; ADT, androgen deprivation therapy; EBRT, external-beam radiotherapy; NS, not significant.
[a]The improved group versus the unchanged group, $p < 0.05$.
[b]The treated group versus the improved group; the treated group versus the unchanged group, $p < 0.05$.

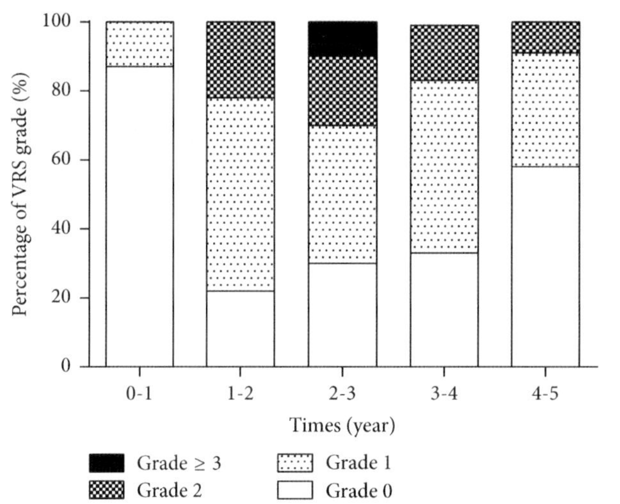

FIGURE 4: Change in VRS over time, in patients with CTCAE grade 0. VRS: Vienna Rectoscopy Score.

in the unchanged VRS group (0%) ($p < 0.05$) (Table 4). When patients had TE grade 3 and UL grade ≥ 2 along with higher endoscopic severity, 75% of patients in the treated group met the criteria while none satisfied the criteria in the improved VRS group and the unchanged VRS group ($p < 0.05$) (Table 4). No differences were observed among the three groups considering the age; extent of the primary tumor (T); use of neoadjuvant ADT, antithrombotic therapy; volume of the prostate gland; and the presence or absence of EBRT. These results indicated that natural recovery of superficial ulceration (UL grade 1) could be expected in patients with VRS ≥ 2.

4. Discussion

In this study, we examined risk factors of rectal bleeding and the prognosis of CRP after BT for prostate cancer. The risk of rectal bleeding significantly increased in the patients treated with BT + EBRT compared to those treated with BT alone. Most episodes of rectal bleeding were observed 1 year or more after BT, and endoscopic findings were correlated with the rectal bleeding score. Overtime evaluation of endoscopic findings after radiotherapy for 5 years revealed that spontaneous recovery was promising if UL grade was 1 or less in the first 150 weeks after BT.

Although the efficacy of radiotherapy for prostate cancer has been recognized, various late toxicities, including rectal bleeding, hematuria, and erectile dysfunction, have been reported, because of the rectum or the urethra adjacent to the prostate gland [14]. The occurrence of rectal bleeding after BT and BT + EBRT is 9.1–27.0% and 18.3–47%, respectively [15–18]. Although BT + EBRT was reported to increase rectal bleeding risk compared to BT [14, 15], no difference in the incidence of toxicity between BT and BT + EBRT has been indicated [11, 18]. Therefore, the rectal bleeding risk and toxicity of these modalities are still controversial. Rectal bleeding risk increased in patients with coronary artery disease while ADT decreased the risk [11]. However, in the present study, no difference was observed in the use of antithrombotic therapy. The use of antithrombotic therapy also results in a rectal bleeding risk after BT or EBRT monotherapy [16, 19]; hence, the limited number of patients in the present study was a possible reason for this difference in results compared to previous studies. In addition, ADT was performed as neoadjuvant therapy and it did not affect rectal bleeding.

As VRS proposed by Wachter et al. varies in grade by TE, congested mucosa, UL, stricture, and necrosis, it is useful for the comprehensive evaluation of endoscopic findings of CRP [13]. VRS has been correlated with rectal GI toxicity caused by pelvic radiotherapy [20, 21]. However, VRS is more sensitive compared to rectal bleeding score systems evaluated by clinical symptoms [13, 21]. A similar result was obtained in our study; no bleeding symptom was observed in 56.3% and 23.1% of patients with VRS 2 and VRS $\geq$ 3, respectively.

In the present study, severity of endoscopic findings increased during 1 to 2 year(s) after treatment and improved over the 5 years of observation. There are only a limited number of reports about the long-term endoscopic evaluation of CRP. Goldner et al. performed proctosigmoidoscopy at 12 and 24 months in patients with prostate cancer who underwent EBRT (range 70 to 75 Gy) and reported that VRS $\geq$ 1 was found in 64% and 62% of the patients at 12 and 24 months, respectively [21]. On the other hand, O'Brien et al. performed proctosigmoidoscopy in prostate cancer patients who underwent EBRT with 65 Gy and showed that the incidence of multiple TE in the rectum at 24 months was higher than that at 12 months and that it was lower at 36 months [22]. Furthermore, Goldner et al. performed a long-term follow-up with endoscopy at 12, 24, and 65 months and showed that the percentage of patients with VRS 1 increased and the percentage of patients with VRS 2 decreased with time [8]. The improving tendency of VRS over the course of a long-term follow-up was similar to the results of our study. In this study, no abnormal endoscopic finding was observed in 50% of the patients who presented with rectal bleeding of grade $\geq$ 1 until the first year after BT. Increased severity of endoscopic findings was observed more often between 1 year and 2 years after BT. Delayed development of rectal mucosal change was observed compared to previous report [21]. This difference can be explained by the fact that EBRT + BT and BT were compared in our study, whereas previous studies evaluated the effects of EBRT alone; moreover, in our study, EBRT boost was initiated at the 4–8th week after BT.

Ippolito et al. performed endoscopy in prostate cancer patients treated with intensity-modulated radiation therapy or three-dimensional conformal radiation therapy, 1 year after treatment, and reported that the occurrence of grade $\geq$ 2 rectal bleeding was 32% and 47% in patients with VRS $\geq$ 2 and VRS $\geq$ 3, respectively, indicating the effectiveness of VRS in predicting rectal bleeding [23]. In the present study, as shown in the Kaplan-Meier curve, most rectal bleeding symptoms occurred between the 50th and 150th week. Hence, we examined whether it would be possible to determine the prognosis of CRP based on the endoscopic findings observed during this period. Our results showed the natural decrease of VRS over time in 31% (5/16) of patients with VRS $\geq$ 2, as well as possible UL 1 improvement, while mild endoscopic findings (VRS 0-1) remained unchanged. No study report has examined factors affecting the recovery of endoscopic findings. Nevertheless, because the number of patients was limited in this study, more patients will be necessary for further investigation in the future. Although the effectiveness and safety of APC therapy have been demonstrated for rectal bleeding due to CRP [4, 24], patients using nonsteroidal anti-inflammatory drugs have shown the development of stenosis after treatment [25] as well as the occurrence of ulcer [26]. Therefore, the endoscopic findings at the occurrence of symptoms are deemed useful for considering treatment indications such as APC or HBO therapy.

5. Conclusion

While the incidence of rectal bleeding is low after BT for prostate cancer, EBRT boost increases its risk. Endoscopy was correlated with bleeding symptoms such as GI toxicity, and it allows an accurate evaluation of rectal mucosal damage. Endoscopy in the first 150 weeks after BT is useful for estimating the long-term prognosis of CRP.

Competing Interests

The authors declare that there are no competing interests regarding the publication of this paper.

Acknowledgments

We would like to thank Editage (http://www.editage.jp/) for English language editing.

References

[1] R. Siegel, D. Naishadham, and A. Jemal, "Cancer statistics for Hispanics/Latinos, 2012," *CA: A Cancer Journal for Clinicians*, vol. 62, no. 5, pp. 283–298, 2012.

[2] T. Matsuda, T. Marugame, K.-I. Kamo, K. Katanoda, W. Ajiki, and T. Sobue, "Cancer incidence and incidence rates in Japan in 2006: based on data from 15 population-based cancer registries in the Monitoring of Cancer Incidence in Japan (MCIJ) project," *Japanese Journal of Clinical Oncology*, vol. 42, no. 2, Article ID hyr184, pp. 139–147, 2012.

[3] V. Appalaneni, R. D. Fanelli, R. N. Sharaf et al., "The role of endoscopy in patients with anorectal disorders," *Gastrointestinal Endoscopy*, vol. 72, no. 6, pp. 1117–1123, 2010.

[4] W. Tam, J. Moore, and M. Schoeman, "Treatment of radiation proctitis with argon plasma coagulation," *Endoscopy*, vol. 32, no. 9, pp. 667–672, 2000.

[5] T. J. Saclarides, D. G. King, J. L. Franklin, and A. Doolas, "Formalin instillation for refractory radiation-induced hemorrhagic proctitis.Report of 16 patients," *Diseases of the Colon and Rectum*, vol. 39, no. 2, pp. 196–199, 1996.

[6] M. A. Dall'Era, N. B. Hampson, R. A. Hsi, B. Madsen, and J. M. Corman, "Hyperbaric oxygen therapy for radiation induced proctopathy in men treated for prostate cancer," *The Journal of Urology*, vol. 176, no. 1, pp. 87–90, 2006.

[7] R. Kochhar, P. V. J. Sriram, S. C. Sharma, R. C. Goel, and F. Patel, "Natural history of late radiation proctosigmoiditis treated with topical sucralfate suspension," *Digestive Diseases and Sciences*, vol. 44, no. 5, pp. 973–978, 1999.

[8] G. Goldner, R. Pötter, A. Kranz, A. Bluhm, and W. Dörr, "Healing of late endoscopic changes in the rectum between 12 and 65 months after external beam radiotherapy," *Strahlentherapie und Onkologie*, vol. 187, no. 3, pp. 202–205, 2011.

[9] N. Oyama, Y. Aoki, H. Ito et al., "Alpha 1-adrenoceptor blocker may improve not only voiding but also storage lower urinary tract symptoms caused by ^{125}I brachytherapy for prostate cancer," *ISRN Urology*, vol. 2014, Article ID 140654, 8 pages, 2014.

[10] National Cancer Institute, National Cancer Institute Common Terminology Criteria for Adverse Events (CTCAE) v.4.0., http://evs.nci.nih.gov/ftp1/CTCAE/About.html.

[11] J. G. Price, N. N. Stone, and R. G. Stock, "Predictive factors and management of rectal bleeding side effects following prostate cancer brachytherapy," *International Journal of Radiation Oncology, Biology, Physics*, vol. 86, no. 5, pp. 842–847, 2013.

[12] L. H. Sobin and Ch. Wittekind, *International Union Against Cancer. Prostate in Classification of Malignant Tumor*, Wiley-Liss, New York, NY, USA, 2002.

[13] S. Wachter, N. Gerstner, G. Goldner, R. Pötzi, A. Wambersie, and R. Pötter, "Endoscopic scoring of late rectal mucosal damage after conformal radiotherapy for prostatic carcinoma," *Radiotherapy and Oncology*, vol. 54, no. 1, pp. 11–19, 2000.

[14] M. Buckstein, S. Kerns, K. Forysthe, N. N. Stone, and R. G. Stock, "Temporal patterns of selected late toxicities in patients treated with brachytherapy or brachytherapy plus external beam radiation for prostate adenocarcinoma," *BJU International*, vol. 111, no. 3, pp. E43–E47, 2013.

[15] M. Aoki, K. Miki, H. Sasaki et al., "Evaluation of rectal bleeding factors associated with prostate brachytherapy," *Japanese Journal of Radiology*, vol. 27, no. 10, pp. 444–449, 2009.

[16] K. Harada, H. Ishikawa, Y. Saito et al., "Risk factors for rectal bleeding associated with I-125 brachytherapy for prostate cancer," *Journal of Radiation Research*, vol. 53, no. 6, pp. 923–929, 2012.

[17] S. K. Kang, R. H. Chou, R. K. Dodge et al., "Gastrointestinal toxicity of transperineal interstitial prostate brachytherapy," *International Journal of Radiation Oncology, Biology, Physics*, vol. 53, no. 1, pp. 99–103, 2002.

[18] D. Y. Gelblum and L. Potters, "Rectal complications associated with transperineal interstitial brachytherapy for prostate cancer," *International Journal of Radiation Oncology, Biology, Physics*, vol. 48, no. 1, pp. 119–124, 2000.

[19] K. Takeda, Y. Ogawa, H. Ariga et al., "Clinical correlations between treatment with anticoagulants/antiaggregants and late rectal toxicity after radiotherapy for prostate cancer," *Anticancer Research*, vol. 29, no. 5, pp. 1831–1834, 2009.

[20] T. G. Kim, S. J. Huh, and W. Park, "Endoscopic findings of rectal mucosal damage after pelvic radiotherapy for cervical carcinoma: correlation of rectal mucosal damage with radiation dose and clinical symptoms," *Radiation Oncology Journal*, vol. 31, no. 2, pp. 81–87, 2013.

[21] G. Goldner, B. Tomicek, G. Becker et al., "Proctitis after external-beam radiotherapy for prostate cancer classified by Vienna Rectoscopy Score and correlated with EORTC/RTOG score for late rectal toxicity: results of a prospective multicenter study of 166 patients," *International Journal of Radiation Oncology, Biology, Physics*, vol. 67, no. 1, pp. 78–83, 2007.

[22] P. C. O'Brien, C. S. Hamilton, J. W. Denham, R. Gourlay, and C. I. V. Franklin, "Spontaneous improvement in late rectal mucosal changes after radiotherapy for prostate cancer," *International Journal of Radiation Oncology Biology Physics*, vol. 58, no. 1, pp. 75–80, 2004.

[23] E. Ippolito, M. Massaccesi, C. Digesù et al., "Early proctoscopy is a surrogate endpoint of late rectal toxicity in prostate cancer treated with radiotherapy," *International Journal of Radiation Oncology, Biology, Physics*, vol. 83, no. 2, pp. e191–e195, 2012.

[24] J. J. Tjandra and S. Sengupta, "Argon plasma coagulation is an effective treatment for refractory hemorrhagic radiation proctitis," *Diseases of the Colon and Rectum*, vol. 44, no. 12, pp. 1759–1765, 2001.

[25] S. Taïeb, A. Rolachon, J.-C. Cenni et al., "Effective use of argon plasma coagulation in the treatment of severe radiation proctitis," *Diseases of the Colon and Rectum*, vol. 44, no. 12, pp. 1766–1771, 2001.

[26] T. Koessler, V. Servois, P. Mariani, E. Aubert, and W. Cacheux, "Rectal ulcer: due to ketoprofen, argon plasma coagulation and prostatic brachytherapy," *World Journal of Gastroenterology*, vol. 20, no. 45, pp. 17244–17246, 2014.

23

Improved Bowel Preparation with Multimedia Education in a Predominantly African-American Population

Shashank Garg,[1] Mohit Girotra,[1] Lakshya Chandra,[1] Vipin Verma,[1] Sumanjit Kaur,[1] Allawy Allawy,[1] Alessandra Sccco,[1] Rohit Anand,[2] and Sudhir K. Dutta[1,3]

[1]*Division of Gastroenterology, Department of Medicine, Sinai Hospital of Baltimore, Baltimore, MD 21215, USA*
[2]*Johns Hopkins University-Sinai Program in Internal Medicine, Baltimore, MD 21215, USA*
[3]*Department of Medicine, University of Maryland School of Medicine, Baltimore, MD 21215, USA*

Correspondence should be addressed to Shashank Garg; shashank.garg@uky.edu

Academic Editor: Patrick J. O'Dwyer

Background and Aim. Inadequate bowel preparation is a major impediment in colonoscopy quality outcomes. Aim of this study was to evaluate the role of multimedia education (MME) in improving bowel preparation quality and adenoma detection rate. *Methods.* This was an IRB-approved prospective randomized study that enrolled 111 adult patients undergoing outpatient screening or surveillance colonoscopy. After receiving standard colonoscopy instructions, the patients were randomized into MME group ($n = 48$) and control group ($n = 46$). The MME group received comprehensive multimedia education including an audio-visual program, a visual aid, and a brochure. Demographics, quality of bowel preparation, and colonoscopy findings were recorded. *Results.* MME group had a significantly better bowel preparation in the entire colon (OR 2.65, 95% CI 1.16–6.09) and on the right side of the colon (OR 2.74, 95% CI 1.12–6.71) as compared to control group ($p < 0.05$). Large polyps (>1 cm) were found more frequently in the MME group (11/31, 35.5% versus 0/13; $p < 0.05$). More polyps and adenomas were detected in MME group (57 versus 39 and 31 versus 13, resp.) but the difference failed to reach statistical significance. *Conclusion.* MME can lead to significant improvement in the quality of bowel preparation and large adenoma detection in a predominantly African-American population.

1. Introduction

Colon cancer is the second most common cancer and also the second leading cause of cancer-related mortality in the United States (http://www.cancer.org/acs/groups/content/@editorial/documents/document/acspc-044552.pdf). Colonoscopy has become the investigation of choice for colorectal cancer (CRC) screening [1]. Several studies have shown that CRC screening with colonoscopy reduced the colon cancer incidence and mortality [2–8]. Quality of bowel preparation is one of the major factors that determine the detection of adenomas during the screening colonoscopy and also the interval to the next colonoscopic examination [1, 9, 10]. However, there are limited data on the effect of patient education in improving the quality of bowel preparation prior to screening colonoscopy [11, 12]. The aim of this study was to evaluate the effect of comprehensive multimedia education (MME) in improving quality of bowel preparation and adenoma detection rate in a predominantly African-American population presenting to an inner city hospital for screening or surveillance colonoscopy.

2. Materials and Methods

2.1. Study Design. This was an IRB-approved prospective, randomized single blind study conducted in the Division of Gastroenterology at Sinai Hospital of Baltimore between September 2012 and December 2013. All authors had access to the study data and had reviewed and approved the final paper.

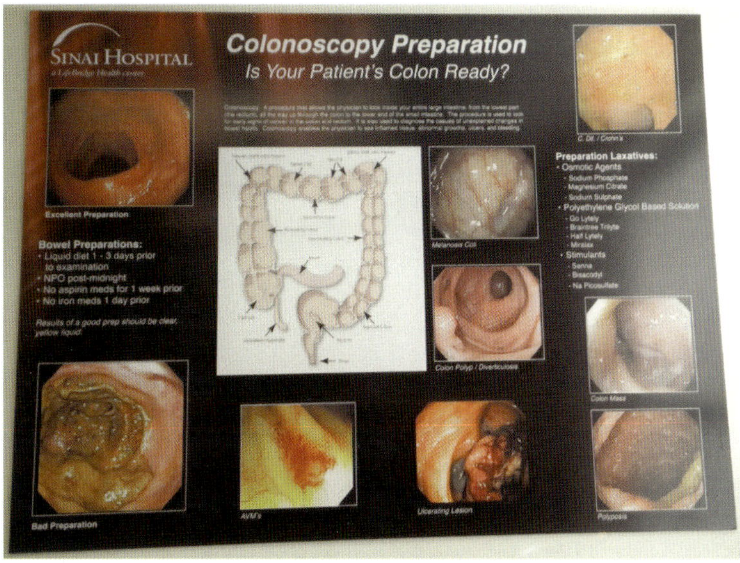

FIGURE 1: Visual aid.

2.2. *Inclusion Criteria.* All adult patients (>18 years of age) undergoing screening or surveillance colonoscopy performed by a single gastroenterologist at Sinai Hospital of Baltimore during the study period were included.

2.3. *Exclusion Criteria.* Patients unable to provide informed consent, patients admitted to the hospital, patients with a known colorectal cancer, or patients undergoing colonoscopy for a reason other than screening or surveillance for colon polyps were excluded.

2.4. *Randomization.* After obtaining informed consent, all of the study patients received standard colonoscopy preparation instructions by the participating gastroenterologist as follows:

Standard Instructions

(1) Take only clear liquid diet on the day before the colonoscopy. Avoid any red or purple color fluids to prevent confusion with blood in the colon.

(2) On the evening prior to colonoscopy, start taking the Golytely© bowel preparation at 6 p.m. Take 8 ounces every 20 minutes and finish by midnight.

A research associate then randomized the patients using simple randomization into study or the multimedia education (MME) group and control group. The gastroenterologist was blinded to the patient group assignment.

2.5. *Multimedia Education.* MME group patients received multimedia education by 3 methods from the research assistant in an education room in the gastroenterology clinic as follows:

Multimedia Education

(1) Visual aid: Figure 1.

(2) Audio-visual education: Supplemental file 1 in Supplementary Material available online at http://dx.doi.org/10.1155/2016/2072401.

(3) American College of Gastroenterology (ACG) questions and answers about quality in colonoscopy: Appendix *Link*: http://patients.gi.org/gi-health-and-disease/questions-and-answers-about-quality-in-colonoscopy/.

First, they were shown a visual aid by the research assistant. It included pictures of good and poor bowel preparation and types of polyps and cancers seen in the colon (Figure 1). Second, patients were given audio-visual education with 3 videos with a total time of 13 minutes and 52 seconds (supplemental file 1). Issues addressed with audio-visual program included importance of CRC prevention by screening or surveillance colonoscopy, importance of good bowel preparation towards doing a good colonoscopic examination, and patient expectations from the bowel preparation. Third, they were given a brochure by American College of Gastroenterology addressing the importance of bowel preparation (see Appendix). After the MME session, the patients were encouraged to seek clarification about bowel preparation instructions from the research assistant.

2.6. *Data Collection.* Patient demographics, past medical history, results of prior colonoscopy(s), and family history of colon cancer were recorded. After the procedure, cecal intubation and scope withdrawal times, quality of bowel preparation, number of polyps, size, location, morphology (sessile or pedunculated), and pathology of the polyps were recorded.

2.7. *Assessing the Quality of Bowel Preparation.* After each procedure, the participating gastroenterologist assessed the quality of bowel preparation based on modified Aronchick scale (Table 1). Aronchick scale is a validated scale used to assess the quality of bowel preparation based on percentage of colon wall visualized [13]. The scale was modified to separately assess the preparation of the right and the left colon. Right side of the colon was defined as the portion of colon extending from cecum to distal transverse colon. Left side of the colon was defined portion of colon extending from splenic flexure to rectum. The category of <90% bowel wall visualized in Aronchick scale was further subcategorized into 2 categories (75–89% and <75%) for a more objective measurement of the bowel preparation quality (Table 1).

2.8. End Points. Primary end points of the study were difference in the quality of bowel preparation and and polyp and adenoma detection rate between the MME group and the control group. Secondary end points included difference in the quality of bowel preparation and polyp and adenoma detection rate separately in the right and left side of the colon between the 2 groups. Post hoc analysis was done for adenoma size and morphology in the 2 groups.

2.9. Data Analysis. Categorical variables were analyzed using chi-square ($n > 5$) or Fischer's exact test ($n \leq 5$). Continuous variables were analyzed using t-test or Wilcoxon rank-sum test depending on distribution. Ordinal data were analyzed using ordinal regression. The data obtained from the patients were analyzed according to their initial assigned group. A two-sided p value < 0.05 was considered as significant. The data was analyzed using STATA (Version 13.1, ©StataCorp, TX, USA).

3. Results

A total of 115 patients underwent screening or surveillance colonoscopy by the participating gastroenterologist during the study period. Four patients declined to participate in the study. Eight patients were excluded after initial enrolment as per exclusion criteria defined above (colon cancer $n = 3$, right hemicolectomy for tubulovillous adenoma with high grade dysplasia $n = 1$, rectal bleeding $n = 3$, and chronic diarrhea $n = 1$). A total of 107 patients were randomized into 2 groups, 55 cases and 48 controls. Seven patients from the study group and 2 patients from control group missed the appointment and did not undergo the procedure. A total of 94 patients (48 cases and 46 controls) were included in the final analysis (Figure 2).

Mean age was 59.27 ± 18.08 years for study group and 57.28 ± 19.40 years for control group ($p > 0.05$). Gender and race distribution in study and control group were similar ($p > 0.05$, Table 2). The two groups were also similar in terms of number of patients with prior colonoscopy, history of colon polyps, and family history of colon cancer.

Cecal intubation times were similar in MME and control group (median time of 6 minutes and range of 2–27 minutes versus median time of 6 minutes and range of 2–15 minutes; p = NS). Similarly scope withdrawal times were similar in both groups (median time of 12 minutes and range of 6–45 minutes versus median time of 13 minutes and range of 6–41 minutes; p = NS). The quality of bowel preparation in the entire colon was significantly better in the MME group as compared to control group (OR 2.65, 95% CI 1.16–6.09, $p < 0.05$, Table 3). Similarly, quality of bowel preparation on the right side of the colon was significantly better in the MME group (OR 2.74, 95% CI 1.12–6.71, $p < 0.05$, Table 4). This difference in the quality of bowel preparation in the entire colon and on the right side of the colon between the two groups remained significant when controlled for age, gender, race, and previous colonoscopy. Quality of bowel preparation in the left side of colon was comparable in the 2 groups ($p > 0.05$).

A higher number of polyps and adenomas were detected in the MME group (57 and 31, resp.) as compared to control group (39 and 13, resp.). Similarly, number of adenomas detected on the right side of the colon was higher in the MME group (19 versus 8). However, these differences failed to reach statistical significance ($p > 0.05$). Similarly, polyp and adenoma detection rate were similar between the MME group (47.91% and 33.33%, resp.) and the control group (34.78% and 19.56, resp.; $p > 0.05$). When classified by size, large polyps were found more commonly in the MME group (11/31, 35.48%) compared to control group (0/13; $p < 0.05$; Table 4).

4. Discussion

This study successfully demonstrates a significant improvement in the quality of bowel preparation in the entire colon and particularly in the right side of the colon with the use of comprehensive multimedia education in a predominantly African-American population. Our results are consistent with

Table 1: Representation of bowel preparation assessment with modified Aronchick scale.

Score	% bowel wall visualized	Right colon	Left colon	Entire colon
1	≥90			
2	75–89			
3	<75			

Table 2: Demographics and clinical characteristics of the study population.

	Study group (n = 48)	Control group (=46)	p value
Mean age in years (±2SD)	59.27 ± 18.08	57.28 ± 19.40	0.31
Gender (F : M)	27 : 21	25 : 21	0.85
Race (AA : other)	43 : 5	41 : 5	0.94
Prior colonoscopy	17	16	0.95
History of colon polyps	4	2	0.68
Family history of colon cancer	8	4	0.36

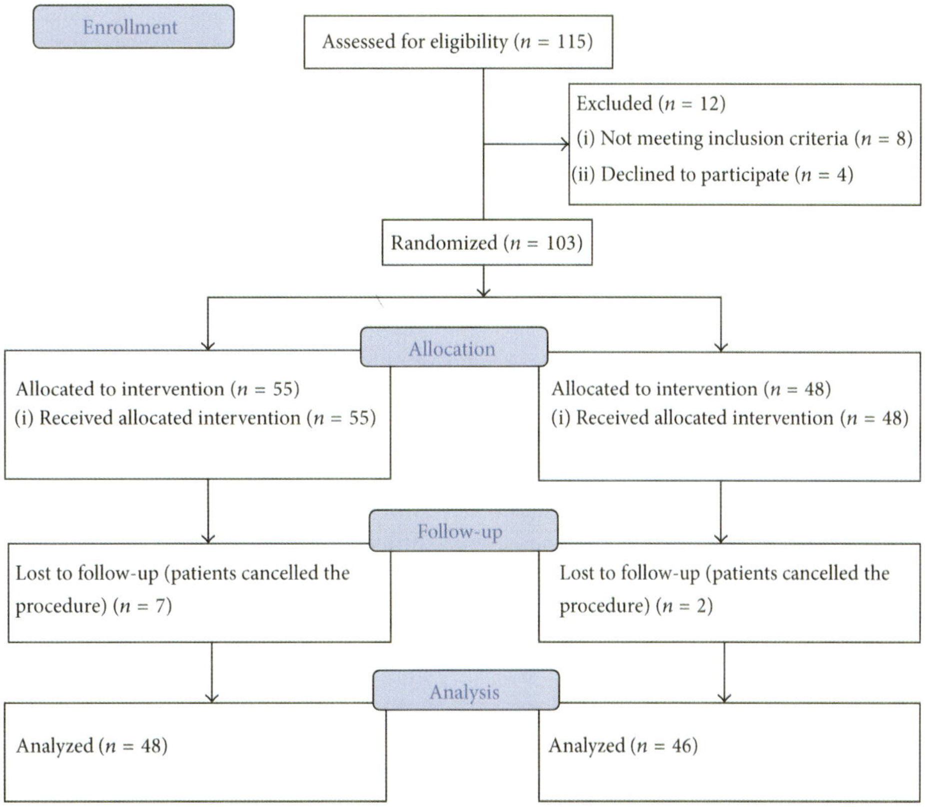

FIGURE 2

TABLE 3: Colonoscopy parameters and quality of bowel preparation in the study population.

	Study group ($n = 48$)	Control group (=46)	p value
Median cecal intubation time in minutes (range)	6 (2–27)	6 (2–15)	0.85
Median scope withdrawal time in minutes (range)	12 (6–45)	13 (6–41)	0.13
Quality of bowel preparation in the entire colon			
(1) >90%	34	22	
(2) 75–90%	11	17	0.02
(3) <75%	3	7	
Quality of bowel preparation in the right colon			
(1) >90%	38	26	
(2) 75–90%	7	16	0.03
(3) <75%	3	4	
Quality of bowel preparation in the left colon			
(1) >90%	37	28	
(2) 75–90%	9	14	0.09
(3) <75%	2	4	

previously reported studies on patient education in improving quality of bowel preparation in the general population in US [12, 14–16] and other countries [11, 17, 18].

Our study employed 3 different methods of patient education. First, the patients were educated, using the visual aide, about the difference between a good and poor bowel preparation and how a good bowel preparation can help in detecting polyps and masses in the colon. Second, audio-visual program was conducted under direct supervision. Third, the patients were provided with a brochure approved by a professional society to read. In contrast, previous studies have utilized only 1 method of patient education, that is, phone based [15], online video based [14], visual aid [17], or reading material based [12] education. Moreover, the patient education was not directly supervised directly in the GI clinic in most of these studies. Instead, the patients were provided with the educational material to read or view at home. This is the first study that was able to show the efficacy of MME

Table 4: Clinical and histological features of colonic polyps detected in the study population.

	Study group (n = 48)	Control group (n = 46)	p value
Total number of adenomas/carcinomas detected	31	13	0.1
(1) Right sided	19	8	
(2) Left sided	12	5	
Total number of small adenomas	20	13	0.38
Total number of large adenomas/carcinomas	11	0	0.03
Total number of sessile adenomas	27	13	0.11
Total number of pedunculated adenomas	2	0	0.33
Adenoma detection rate (%)	16/48 (33.33%)	9/46 (19.56%)	0.13
(1) Right sided	12	7	
(2) Left sided	7	3	
Number of polyps detected	57	39	0.21
(1) Right sided	20	11	
(2) Left sided	37	28	
Polyp detection rate (%)	23/48 (47.91%)	16/46 (34.78%)	0.2

in increasing the detection of large polyps in the study group. This finding could be related to the provision of supervised education to the patients by trained health care providers.

Quality of bowel preparation is vital to performing effective screening or surveillance examination of the colon. It has been shown that adenoma miss rates range within 20–41% from index colonoscopy at 1–3 years when quality of bowel preparation is suboptimal [9, 19]. Poor understanding of the process of bowel preparation by patients remains a major barrier in achieving high rates of good quality bowel preparation at a population level [20–22]. This factor seems to be particularly relevant to African-American population as supported by the fact that African-Americans have a high rate of interval cancer and significantly higher mortality from colorectal cancer compared to other races and ethnic groups (http://www.cdc.gov/cancer/colorectal/statistics/race.htm). Appannagari et al. reported that African-Americans had the highest rate of suboptimal bowel preparation quality (43% versus 25.5% in Caucasians, $p < 0.001$) in large retrospective study involving 3741 subjects [23]. Moreover, poor understanding of the process of bowel preparation has been shown to contribute to inadequate bowel preparation in this population [24].

MME can address the issues related to importance of bowel preparation and CRC screening at individual and population level especially in African-Americans. The audiovisual component of such education supplements the information given to the patient during physician-patient interaction. It provides an opportunity for patients to understand the appearance of different types of polyps and the importance of a good bowel preparation in detecting these polyps. It can also address difficulties of doing a bowel preparation and may help patients deal with these issues with a scientific approach. MME sessions can be performed for a group of patients by trained health care providers utilizing such educational aides.

The strengths of this study include the prospective randomized, single blind design and performance of all the procedures by a single gastroenterologist that avoids interobserver bias. The limitation of the study includes small sample size.

In conclusion, this study showed a significant improvement in the quality of bowel preparation in African-American population undergoing screening and surveillance colonoscopies. These observations need to be further examined in a large multicenter prospective randomized study.

Appendix

American College of Gastroenterology (ACG) Questions and Answers about Quality in Colonoscopy

(1) Why Is Quality Important in Colonoscopy? Although colonoscopy has been available in clinical practice for more than 40 years, only in the past 15 years has awareness developed that the success of colonoscopy in preventing colorectal cancer and minimizing complications is very dependent on the skill and competence of the colonoscopist. Colonoscopists differ substantially in the number of precancerous polyps they detect during colonoscopy and in how often they perform colonoscopy in response to both normal and abnormal findings. Awareness of these differences led the U.S. Multisociety Task Force on Colorectal Cancer in 2002, as well as a joint task force of experts from the American College of Gastroenterology and American Society of Gastrointestinal Endoscopy in 2006, to propose quality indicators that colonoscopists can use to measure how effectively and safely they perform colonoscopy. Obviously, patients have an interest in undergoing the most effective and safe colonoscopy possible, and achieving these goals requires a colonoscopist who is committed to high quality.

(2) Does the Quality of Examination Differ among Colonoscopists from Different Specialties? Studies have shown average performance of colonoscopy by gastroenterologists to be superior to that of primary care physicians in three different

areas of colonoscopy performance. First, three population-based studies have found that gastroenterologists performing colonoscopy are less likely to miss colorectal cancer than primary care physicians who perform colonoscopy. This may reflect the more extensive training that gastroenterologists receive in this procedure and their higher volumes of colonoscopy in practice. Second, gastroenterologists' patients are less likely to incur serious complications during colonoscopy, such as perforation or making a hole in the colon, compared to primary care physicians. Third, gastroenterologists are less likely than both primary care physicians and general surgeons to perform colonoscopy at intervals that are considered too short according to current guidelines. Whether this difference reflects a lack of confidence among primary care physicians and general surgeons in the quality of their colonoscopy or lack of awareness of current guidelines is unknown.

(3) Is There Variation in Quality of Performance among Members of the Same Specialty? Even though gastroenterologists have on average the highest level of training and their examinations have been shown on average to be superior to primary care physicians, there is considerable variation among gastroenterologists in their detection rates of precancerous polyps. Therefore, it is essential that every colonoscopist, regardless of specialty, makes measurements to establish that their examinations are effective. It is very reasonable and appropriate for patients to ask questions of their colonoscopist about whether quality measurements are being made and their results.

(4) How Can I Be Sure That I Will Receive a Careful Examination of My Colon? The measurement that best reflects how carefully colonoscopy is performed is a doctor's "adenoma detection rate." This rate is defined as the percentage of patients aged 50 and older undergoing screening colonoscopy, who have one or more precancerous polyps detected. This rate should be at least 25% in men and 15% in women. A secondary measure of careful examination is that doctors should have an average withdrawal time of at least six minutes. The withdrawal time is the time it takes to remove the scope from the colon. This interval is important because this is the phase of colonoscopy when most doctors actually examine the colon systematically for polyps. It is perfectly reasonable to expect doctors to have measured their adenoma detection rate and to record their withdrawal time. It is also reasonable to ask for a copy of the colonoscopy report that documents that the colonoscope was advanced to the very beginning of the colon and that the landmarks of that portion of the colon (called the "cecum") have been documented by notation in the report and by photography.

(5) Why Is Bowel Preparation for Colonoscopy Important, and What Can I Do to Make Sure My Colon Is Thoroughly Cleansed for the Procedure? Colonoscopy is a video examination of the colon. The video camera and the colonoscope, like any other video camera, cannot see through solids. Therefore, the colon must be thoroughly cleansed to provide the doctor the best opportunity possible for a thorough and detailed examination.

Be sure to pick up and read your written bowel preparation instructions at least several days before your colonoscopy. Go over the instructions and make sure you have all of the materials needed to complete the preparation.

The most effective bowel preparations involve "split" dosing of the laxatives, in which half of the preparation is taken on the morning of the examination, usually 4 to 5 hours before the time of the scheduled colonoscopy, and completed at least 2 to 3 hours before that time. If you are scheduled at 7 or 8 in the morning, this will mean getting up very early to take the second half of the preparation. If the instructions call for split dosing, do not alter the timing of the doses. It is worth the inconvenience of getting up in the middle of the night to make sure that you have a very effective preparation. The timing of the second dose in relationship to the colonoscopy is critical. If too long an interval is allowed between the end of the second half of the preparation and the timing of the colonoscopy, mucus and secretions will come out of the small intestine and stick to the cecum and right colon.

Summary. To ensure an effective and safe colonoscopic examination, find a well-trained colonoscopist who is committed to making quality measurements. It is fair to ask the colonoscopist to be sure to do a slow and careful examination and to provide a copy of the report that documents and photographs the complete extent of examination. Take the bowel preparation instructions seriously. Pick up the written instructions early, read them early, and follow them carefully. When colonoscopy is done carefully and with an effective preparation, it is a very powerful cancer prevention technique.

Disclosure

Shashank Garg and Mohit Girotra are co-first authors for the study.

Acknowledgments

The authors acknowledge Jennifer R. Havens, Ph.D., MPH, Associate Professor, Department of Behavioral Science, University of Kentucky College of Medicine for helping with data analysis, Dayna Sherba, HCA in the Division of Gastroenterology, Sinai Hospital of Baltimore, for helping the study team with procedure scheduling, Laura Thompson, RN, Nancy Scher, RN, and nursing staff at the Gastrointestinal Diagnostic Center at Sinai Hospital for their excellent patient care and collection of patient data. Carolyn and James Frenkil Foundation provided funding to set up the education room in the GI clinic. Eric Cowan Fund provided funding to support the research staff during the study period.

References

[1] D. A. Lieberman, D. K. Rex, S. J. Winawer, F. M. Giardiello, D. A. Johnson, and T. R. Levin, "Guidelines for colonoscopy surveillance after screening and polypectomy: a consensus update by the us multi-society task force on colorectal cancer," *Gastroenterology*, vol. 143, no. 3, pp. 844–857, 2012.

[2] S. J. Winawer, A. G. Zauber, M. N. Ho et al., "Prevention of colorectal cancer by colonoscopic polypectomy. The National Polyp Study Workgroup," *The New England Journal of Medicine*, vol. 329, pp. 1977–1981, 1993.

[3] A. G. Zauber, S. J. Winawer, M. J. O'Brien et al., "Colonoscopic polypectomy and long-term prevention of colorectal-cancer deaths," *The New England Journal of Medicine*, vol. 366, no. 8, pp. 687–696, 2012.

[4] H. Brenner, J. Chang-Claude, L. Jansen, P. Knebel, C. Stock, and M. Hoffmeister, "Reduced risk of colorectal cancer up to 10 years after screening, surveillance, or diagnostic colonoscopy," *Gastroenterology*, vol. 146, no. 3, pp. 709–717, 2014.

[5] D. A. Lieberman, D. G. Weiss, J. H. Bond, D. J. Ahnen, H. Garewal, and G. Chejfec, "Use of colonoscopy to screen asymptomatic adults for colorectal cancer. Veterans Affairs Cooperative Study Group 380," *The New England Journal of Medicine*, vol. 343, no. 3, pp. 162–168, 2000.

[6] P. Schoenfeld, B. Cash, A. Flood et al., "Colonoscopic screening of average-risk women for colorectal neoplasia," *The New England Journal of Medicine*, vol. 352, no. 20, pp. 2061–2068, 2005.

[7] H. Brenner, J. Chang-Claude, C. M. Seiler, A. Rickert, and M. Hoffmeister, "Protection from colorectal cancer after colonoscopy: a population-based, case-control study," *Annals of Internal Medicine*, vol. 154, no. 1, pp. 22–30, 2011.

[8] R. L. Siegel, E. M. Ward, and A. Jemal, "Trends in colorectal cancer incidence rates in the United States by tumor location and stage, 1992–2008," *Cancer Epidemiology Biomarkers and Prevention*, vol. 21, no. 3, pp. 411–416, 2012.

[9] B. Lebwohl, F. Kastrinos, M. Glick, A. J. Rosenbaum, T. Wang, and A. I. Neugut, "The impact of suboptimal bowel preparation on adenoma miss rates and the factors associated with early repeat colonoscopy," *Gastrointestinal Endoscopy*, vol. 73, no. 6, pp. 1207–1214, 2011.

[10] D. K. Rex, J. L. Petrini, T. H. Baron et al., "Quality indicators for colonoscopy," *The American Journal of Gastroenterology*, vol. 101, no. 4, pp. 873–885, 2006.

[11] T. Y. Shieh, M. J. Chen, C. W. Chang et al., "Effect of physician-delivered patient education on the quality of bowel preparation for screening colonoscopy," *Gastroenterology Research and Practice*, vol. 2013, Article ID 570180, 5 pages, 2013.

[12] B. M. R. Spiegel, J. Talley, P. Shekelle et al., "Development and validation of a novel patient educational booklet to enhance colonoscopy preparation," *The American Journal of Gastroenterology*, vol. 106, no. 5, pp. 875–883, 2011.

[13] C. A. Aronchick, W. H. Lipshutz, S. H. Wright, F. Dufrayne, and G. Bergman, "A novel tableted purgative for colonoscopic preparation: efficacy and safety comparisons with Colyte and Fleet Phospho-Soda," *Gastrointestinal Endoscopy*, vol. 52, no. 3, pp. 346–352, 2000.

[14] S. R. Prakash, S. Verma, J. McGowan et al., "Improving the quality of colonoscopy bowel preparation using an educational video," *Canadian Journal of Gastroenterology*, vol. 27, no. 12, pp. 696–700, 2013.

[15] A. R. Sondhi, J. E. Kurlander, A. K. Waljee, and S. D. Saini, "A telephone-based education program improves bowel preparation quality in patients undergoing outpatient colonoscopy," *Gastroenterology*, vol. 148, no. 3, pp. 657–658, 2015.

[16] A. H. Calderwood, E. J. Lai, O. K. Fix, and B. C. Jacobson, "An endoscopist-blinded, randomized, controlled trial of a simple visual aid to improve bowel preparation for screening colonoscopy," *Gastrointestinal Endoscopy*, vol. 73, no. 2, pp. 307–314, 2011.

[17] J. W. Tae, J. C. Lee, S. J. Hong et al., "Impact of patient education with cartoon visual aids on the quality of bowel preparation for colonoscopy," *Gastrointestinal Endoscopy*, vol. 76, no. 4, pp. 804–811, 2012.

[18] F.-C. Hsueh, H.-C. Wang, C.-A. Sun et al., "The effect of different patient education methods on quality of bowel cleanliness in outpatients receiving colonoscopy examination," *Applied Nursing Research*, vol. 27, no. 2, pp. e1–e5, 2014.

[19] S. B. Menees, H. M. Kim, E. E. Elliott, J. L. Mickevicius, B. B. Graustein, and P. S. Schoenfeld, "The impact of fair colonoscopy preparation on colonoscopy use and adenoma miss rates in patients undergoing outpatient colonoscopy," *Gastrointestinal Endoscopy*, vol. 78, no. 3, pp. 510–516, 2013.

[20] M. Martel, A. N. Barkun, C. Menard, S. Restellini, O. Kherad, and A. Vanasse, "Split-dose preparations are superior to day-before bowel cleansing regimens: a meta-analysis," *Gastroenterology*, vol. 149, no. 1, pp. 79–88, 2015.

[21] V. Ghevariya, S. Duddempudi, N. Ghevariya, M. Reddy, and S. Anand, "Barriers to screening colonoscopy in an urban population: a study to help focus further efforts to attain full compliance," *International Journal of Colorectal Disease*, vol. 28, no. 11, pp. 1497–1503, 2013.

[22] C. H. Basch, G. C. Hillyer, C. E. Basch, B. Lebwohl, and A. I. Neugut, "Characteristics associated with suboptimal bowel preparation prior to colonoscopy: results of a national survey," *International Journal of Preventive Medicine*, vol. 5, no. 2, pp. 233–237, 2014.

[23] A. Appannagari, S. Mangla, C. Liao, K. G. Reddy, and S. S. Kupfer, "Risk factors for inadequate colonoscopy bowel preparations in African Americans and whites at an urban medical center," *Southern Medical Journal*, vol. 107, no. 4, pp. 220–224, 2014.

[24] M. Bazargan, C. Ani, S. Bazargan-Hejazi, R. S. Baker, and R. Bastani, "Colorectal cancer screening among underserved minority population: discrepancy between physicians' recommended, scheduled, and completed tests," *Patient Education and Counseling*, vol. 76, no. 2, pp. 240–247, 2009.

24

Factors Significantly Contributing to a Failed Conventional Endoscopic Stone Clearance in Patients with "Difficult" Choledecholithiasis: A Single-Center Experience

Emmanuel Christoforidis,[1] Konstantinos Vasiliadis,[2] Konstantinos Tsalis,[1] Dimitrios Patridas,[1] Konstantinos Blouhos,[3] Manousos-Georgios Pramateftakis,[1] Moysis Moysidis,[1] and Charalampos Lazaridis[1]

[1] *Fourth Surgical Department, Endoscopic Unit, "George Papanikolaou" Hospital, Aristotle University, Exohi, 57010 Thessaloniki, Greece*
[2] *First Department of General Surgery, Section of Hepatopancreatobiliary Surgery, "Papageorgiou" Hospital, Nea Efkarpia, 56 403 Thessaloniki, Greece*
[3] *Department of General Surgery, General Hospital of Drama, End of Hippokratous Street, 66100 Drama, Greece*

Correspondence should be addressed to Konstantinos Vasiliadis; keva@med.auth.gr

Academic Editor: Tony C. K. Tham

The objective of this study is to retrospectively evaluate factors significantly contributing to a failed stone extraction (SE) in patients with difficult to extract bile duct stones (BDS). *Patients and Methods.* During a 10-year period 1390 patients with BDS underwent successfully endoscopic sphincterotomy. Endoscopic SE was graded as easy; relatively easy; difficult; and failed. Difficult SE was encountered in 221 patients while failed SE was encountered in 205. A retrospective analysis of the criteria governing the difficulty of endoscopic SE following the index endoscopic intervention was performed to evaluate their significance in determining failure of complete SE among patients with difficult to extract bile duct stones. *Results.* Age ≥ 85 years, periampullary diverticula, multiple CBD stones (>4), and diameter of CBD stones (≥15 mm) were all significant contributing factors to a failed SE in univariate statistical tests. In the definitive multivariate analysis age, multiple stones and diameter of stones were found to be the significant, independent contributors. *Conclusion.* Failed conventional endoscopic stone clearance in patients with difficult to extract BDS is more likely to occur in overage patients, in patients with multiple CBD stones >4, and in patients with CBD stone(s) diameter ≥15 mm.

1. Introduction

Common bile duct (CBD) lithiasis is present in 7%–12% of patients with cholecystolithiasis and represents a well-established indication for endoscopic retrograde cholangiopancreatography (ERCP) with endoscopic sphincterotomy and basket or balloon stone extraction (SE) techniques [1]. Bile duct stones vary in size ranging from rather small (1-2 mm) to very large (>3 cm) [2]. The vast majority of them (85%–95%) can be removed with the use of conventional endoscopic techniques [3, 4]. Balloon dilatation following endoscopic sphincterotomy is an easy to use alternative for *difficult to extract* BDS with an acceptable safety profile [5]. However, despite the refinements in endoscopic removal of BDS, complete SE can be occasionally difficult posing an endoscopic challenge.

Extraction of BDS can be difficult for anatomic alteration and stone, duct, and patients' factors [6–9]. The size and number of BDS are major determinants of their resistance to extraction. Among other important factors, the acute distal angulation of the CBD and the shorter length of its distal CBD "arm," the altered postsurgical anatomy, and the firmness and diameter of BDS relative to the width of the distal CBD [6–9] are included.

Failure of SE exposes the patients to a substantial risk of complications, thereby increasing morbidity and mortality [10]. In such scenario, further treatment is mandatory to avert life threatening complications [11]. Consequently, if endoscopic SE fails, patients are often referred for surgery even in the presence of substantial comorbidity [12]. The need for a definitive minimally invasive management of difficult to extract BDS forced the medical community to develop several therapeutic fragmentation modalities through shock waves both internally and externally. However, these methods are not widely available; their cost and indications are still under clinical evaluation [13]. Despite the fact that the clinical significance of factors governing the difficulty of endoscopic SE is well known, accurate identification and evaluation of these factors have attracted little investigative attention.

The objective of this study is to retrospectively evaluate factors significantly contributing to a failed SE in patients with difficult to extract BDS and to present the efficacy of conventional endoscopic management of difficult to extract BDS combined with biliary stenting when modern stone fragmentation modalities are not available.

2. Methods

2.1. Patients. During a 10-year period (2004 to 2014) 1390 from a total of 1448 patients with BDS underwent successful endoscopic sphincterotomy. *Among these,* 221 *patients with difficult and* 205 *patients with failed SE were included in this retrospective clinical study.* Patients with acute suppurative cholangitis were excluded. No oral dissolution agent was administered to the patients included in the study. Before the procedure, each patient status was classified according to the physical status classification of the American Society of Anesthesiologists (ASA) [14]. Patients with ASA score greater than 2 were excluded. Preprocedural work-up included complete blood cell count, liver function tests, serum electrolytes, and coagulation studies. All patients underwent ERCP within 24 h of admission. Patients were monitored during the procedure while sedation and analgesia were achieved with intravenous midazolam and fentanyl titrated to suit age and tolerance. General anesthesia was undertaken whenever this was necessary. An informed written consent was obtained from all patients. Diagnosis of BDS was based on radiologic and endoscopic findings.

2.2. Identification of Patients with Difficult Endoscopic SE-Grading of Difficulty of Endoscopic SE. Although multiple factors have been postulated to govern the difficulty of endoscopic SE, it is rather difficult to objectively determine which of them represent significant and independent contributors to the failure of endoscopic clearance. In the present study, selected literature-based criteria [5–9, 15–17], added by criteria drawn from our units experience potentially contributing to the difficulty of endoscopic SE, were used for pre- and periprocedural identification of patients with presumable difficult to extract BDS. The selected criteria are listed in Table 1.

Endoscopic retrograde cholangiopancreatography (ERCP) represents the most difficult and technically demanding endoscopic procedure. Therefore, the need to objectively evaluate the difficulty of ERCP procedures has long been acknowledged. Although several US endoscopic centers have attempted to introduce ERCP technical difficulty grading scales [18, 19], there has been no data concerning a validated, internationally acceptable, easily understandable, reproducible grading scale, which can be applied in everyday practice as a tool to objectively evaluate the difficulty of ERCP procedures and especially the difficulty of endoscopic removal of bile duct stones. Therefore, in this study we devised an easily understood difficulty grading system according to the number of attempts at CBD stone extraction with a basket or balloon catheter taking also into consideration the patient's discomfort and the feeling of difficulty by the endoscopist. Although this grading system has not been validated, it can be easily applied in everyday practice. Besides, a similar grading scale has been used in a relevant study by Kim and coworkers [6].

Following the index endoscopic session the technical difficulty of SE was graded as follows, based on number of attempts of basket grasping or balloon sweeping: easy: completely extracted by 1 to 3 attempts; relatively easy: completely extracted by 4 to 7 attempts; difficult: completely extracted by 8 or more attempts; failed: stones incompletely removed.

2.3. Endoscopic Procedure-Therapeutic Algorithm. All procedures of ERCP, endoscopic sphincterotomy, and SE were done by the same endoscopist with a side-viewing duodenoscope, and a standard type papillotome, using the same technique with a low osmolarity, nonionic contrast media (Iopromide, Ultravist 370: Schering, Berlin, Germany). Identified patients with a presumable difficult to extract BDS followed a specific therapeutic algorithm. The first step was the catheterization of the ampulla and injection of contrast media. In case of inability to perform a cholangiogram a guide-wire was inserted into the bile duct. Provided that the latter step was successful, an endoscopic sphincterotomy was performed, followed by attempts to extract the BDS by basket-mechanical lithotripsy and/or retrieval balloon or combination of both. All sphincterotomies were complete in type, resulting in a gush of bile and the cholangiographic confirmation of air in the biliary tree. After SE, contrast media were injected in the biliary tree and the inflated balloon catheter was withdrawn along the CBD to the duodenum to confirm clearance. *Clearance was then classified as difficult-successful, or failed.* In the latter event, bile duct drainage was *always* obtained by the insertion of a plastic stent (Amsterdam type stent) or a nasobiliary catheter. Stable patients with failed SE were scheduled for a repeated, elective intervention, at which time standard techniques were again implemented. Needle knife fistulotomy (NFK) was applied in cases of inability to catheterize the ampulla and was reserved only for older patients with a dilated CBD. In our unit NFK was performed by using the NK fistulotomy technique [20].

Table 1: Selected criteria potentially contributing to the difficulty of endoscopic SE.

Anatomic variations/alterations	Stone factors	Duct factors	Patients factors
Periampullary diverticula[a]	>15 mm in diameter	Acute distal CBD angulation[b]	Age ≥ 85 years
Postgastrectomy Billroth type II or Roux-en-Y reconstruction	>4 in number (multiple stones)		
Presence of T-tube in situ + proximal lithiasis	Impacted stones		
Iatrogenic injury to the extrahepatic biliary tree + lithiasis	Intrahepatic or cystic duct stones		

[a]Defined endoscopically as a depressed lesion of 5 mm or more with intact mucosa and with the major papilla either within it or close by [17].
[b]Defined as the sharpest angle along the CBD from 1 cm below the bifurcation to 1 cm above the papilla [15].

2.4. Collection and Evaluation of Factors Significantly Determining Failure in Endoscopic BDS Clearance. Selected preprocedural criteria added by periprocedural parameters (including parameters identified on cholangiogram and endoscopy) that contributed to the difficulty of endoscopic SE were retrospectively collected and analyzed for their significance in determining failure in stone clearance in patients with difficult to extract BDS.

2.5. Statistical Analysis. Statistical analysis was conducted using SPSS 20.0 (SPSS Inc., Chicago, IL). The chi-squared test for independence was used in order to study univariate relationships between failure in complete SE and binary categorical variables. Factors found to be nominally significant in exploratory univariate statistical analysis were included in the binary logistic regression model to determine the significant contributors to the failure of SE. Binary logistic regression analysis was used with a stepwise procedure for model selection in order to study covariate effects on failure in endoscopic SE in a multivariable setting. The definitive results arise from the multivariate logistic regression analysis, which estimates the independent effect of each factor after adjustment for the contributions of each of the other parameters. All tests were two-sided and P values less than 0.05 were considered statistically significant.

3. Results

All ERCPs were performed in a hospital setting. Difficult but ultimately successful SE was encountered in 221 patients while failed SE was encountered in 205 patients. The clinical characteristics and contributing factors to the difficulty of endoscopic SE in patients with difficult and failed intervention are shown in Table 2. In *all* patients with failed BDS clearance, endoprosthesis insertion establishing biliary drainage was a definitive measure. Patients with a failed index intervention underwent further endoscopic sessions that accomplished complete SE in either 2 (152/205, 74.1%) or 3 sessions (47/205, 22.9%). All patients with a failed third endoscopic session were treated successfully surgically (6/205, 2.9%).

Postprocedural ERCP-related complications occurred in 34 (7.98%) patients with difficult BDS (difficult and failed): acute cholangitis in 12; post-ERCP pancreatitis in 7; pulmonary complications in 7; acute cholecystitis in 5; and bleeding in 3. These complications were mild and were managed successfully conservatively with no ERCP-related deaths.

Following the index endoscopic intervention the selected contributing parameters were analyzed for the patients with difficult and failed endoscopic SE. Older age ≥ 85 years ($P = 0.028$), periampullary diverticula ($P = 0.016$), multiple stones >4 ($P = 0.046$), and diameter of CBD stones ≥ 15 mm ($P = 0.012$) were nominally significant contributing factors to the failure of endoscopic clearance of CBD stone(s) in exploratory univariate testing (Table 3). Presence of T-tube in situ in addition to proximal lithiasis, iatrogenic injury to the extrahepatic biliary tree in addition to CBD lithiasis, intrahepatic stones, previous gastrojejunostomy, acute distal CBD angulation, and impacted stones were not significant contributors to the failure of SE in exploratory univariate testing (Table 3). In the multivariate analysis it was found that age ≥ 85 years, odds ratio (OR) = 1.779, CI (1.110–2.850), $P = 0.017$; multiple stones >4, OR = 1.647, CI (1.060–2.559), $P = 0.026$; and CBD stone(s) diameter ≥ 15 mm, OR = 1.804, CI (1.210–2.691), $P = 0.004$, were the independent contributors to the failure of CBD stone removal (Table 4).

4. Discussion

Since its inception nearly 40 years ago, ERCP represents the therapeutic cornerstone for the removal of CBD stones. Following endoscopic sphincterotomy with standard extraction techniques, the vast majority of stones can be successfully removed [21]. However, in approximately 10% to 15% of patients, CBD stone removal can be difficult, predisposing to a failed endoscopic clearance [22]. Failure of SE renders the patients susceptible to the risk of cholangitis, pancreatitis, and obstructive jaundice, which add further to the significant burden of morbidity and mortality of choledocholithiasis. Therefore, assessment of contributing factors to the technical difficulty and/or failure of endoscopic SE would be extremely useful to predict a long and difficult endoscopic intervention that will require, on the one hand, special periprocedural measures, such as conscious sedation, and on the other hand, proper planning of alternative, minimally invasive therapeutic modalities, which must be carefully balanced

TABLE 2: Clinical characteristics, preprocedural criteria, and periprocedural factors that contributed to the difficulty of endoscopic SE of patients with (a) difficult ($n = 221$) and (b) failed ($n = 205$) endoscopic BDS clearance.

Clinical characteristics	Failed n (%)	Difficult, n (%)
Median age in years	78,3	77,1
Gender, n (%)		
Men	97 (47.3)	100 (45.25)
Women	108 (52.7)	121 (54.75)
Clinical picture, n (%)		
Jaundice/pain	52 (25.4)	42 (19)
Abnormal blood liver test	49 (23.9)	51 (23.1)
Acute cholangitis	12 (5.8)	24 (10.6)
Acute pancreatitis	9 (4.4)	11 (64.7)
Shock	3 (1.5)	1 (0.45)
Preprocedural criteria and periprocedural factors		
Age ≥ 85	38 (38)	62 (62)
Periampullary diverticula, n (%)	84 (56.4)	65 (43.6)
Multiple stones > 4	136 (44.9)	167 (55,1)
Diameter of CBD stone(s) ≥ 15 mm	92 (42)	127 (58)
Presence of T-tube in situ + proximal lithiasis	25 (56.8)	19 (43.2)
Extrahepatic biliary tree iatrogenic injury + lithiasis	11 (57.9)	8 (42.1)
Intrahepatic stone(s)	8 (38.1)	13 (61.9)
Previous gastrojejunostomy	6 (35.3)	11 (64.7)
Acute distal CBD angulation	7 (46.7)	8 (53.3)
Impacted stone(s)	45 (44.6)	56 (55.4)

against each other and finally with surgery, in the unfortunate event of a failed conventional endoscopic intervention. Notwithstanding, accurate determination and evaluation of factors significantly contributing to the failure of endoscopic SE have attracted little investigative attention.

Various factors have been postulated to be inversely associated with endoscopic SE, including sigmoid shaped CBD, postgastrectomy anatomy, large number of stones, intrahepatic and cystic duct stones, and stones proximal to bile duct strictures [23]. Endoscopic retrieval of bile duct stones becomes also formidable in Mirizzi syndrome and in the presence of T-tube in situ with CBD stones proximal to the T-tube [23]. However, with the exception of stone size [24], the exact role of various parameters in the success or failure of endoscopic SE remains practically unsettled.

A valuable contribution to the exceedingly sparse literature regarding the evaluation of factors contributing to the difficulty of endoscopic SE is the study by Kim and coworkers [6]. In their prospective study it was established that older age (>65 years), previous gastrojejunostomy, larger stone size (≥15 mm), impaction of stones, shorter length of the distal CBD arm (≤36 mm), and more acute distal CBD angulation (≤135 degrees) were all significant contributors to the technical difficulty for endoscopic SE. In the same study insignificant factors were found to be patients' comorbidity, previous cholecystectomy, CBD diameter ≥ 15 mm, periampullary diverticula, number of CBD stones ≥ 5, stone impaction, and stone CBD ratio > 1. Among the aforementioned significantly contributing factors, only the shorter length of the distal CBD arm and the more acute distal CBD angulation were in the definitive multivariate analysis significant and independent contributors to the difficulty of SE [6]. However, in a similar recent prospective study by García [25], no association was found between the difficulty of endoscopic SE and the shorter length of the distal CBD arm and the more acute distal CBD angulation. Furthermore, in the study by García [25], no association was found between SE and age; previous cholecystectomy and number of stones; and stone impaction and periampullary diverticula on the contrary; stone size ≥ 15 mm, CBD diameter ≥ 15 mm, and mechanical lithotripsy were all found to be significant independent contributors to the difficulty of SE.

In the present study, *which is probably the first evaluating certain factors that can significantly contribute to a failed endoscopic clearance in patients with difficult to extract bile duct stones*, following definitive multivariate analysis, it was found that age ≥ 85 years, multiple CBD stones (>4), and the diameter of CBD stones (≥15 mm) were the significant, independent contributors to a failed endoscopic BDS clearance. In addition, the present study showed that the presence of T-tube in situ and proximal lithiasis, iatrogenic injury to the extrahepatic biliary tree in addition to CBD lithiasis, intrahepatic stones, previous gastrojejunostomy, impacted stones, and acute distal CBD angulation were not significant contributors to the failure of endoscopic clearance of CBD stones.

With regard to acute distal CBD angulation, it is rather logical to hypothesize that the endoscopist will encounter

TABLE 3: Univariate analyses of contributing factors to failed endoscopic stone extraction.

	SE		*P* value
	Failed 205 (%)	Difficult successful 221 (%)	
Age			
<85	167 (51.2)	159 (48.8)	0.028
≥85	38 (38.0)	62 (62.0)	
Periampullary diverticula			
No	121 (43.7)	156 (56.3)	0.016
Yes	84 (56.4)	65 (43.6)	
Multiple stones			
No	69 (56.1)	54 (43.9)	0.046
Yes	136 (44.9)	167 (55.1)	
Diameter of CBD stones			
<15 mm	113 (54.6)	94 (45.4)	0.012
≥15 mm	92 (42.0)	127 (58.0)	
Presence of T-tube in situ + proximal lithiasis			
No	180 (47.1)	202 (52.9)	NS
Yes	25 (56.8)	19 (43.2)	
Iatrogenic injury to the extrahepatic biliary tree + lithiasis			
No	194 (47.7)	213 (52.3)	NS
Yes	11 (57.9)	8 (42.1)	
Intrahepatic stones			
No	197 (48.6)	208 (51.4)	NS
Yes	8 (38.1%)	13 (61.9)	
Previous gastrojejunostomy			
No	199 (48.7)	210 (51.3)	NS
Yes	6 (35.3)	11 (64.7)	
Acute distal CBD (common bile duct) angulation			
No	198 (48.2)	213 (51.8)	NS
Yes	7 (46.7)	8 (53.3)	
Impacted stone			
No	160 (49.2)	165 (50.8)	NS
Yes	45 (44.6)	56 (55.4)	

TABLE 4: Multivariate analysis of contributing factors to successful or unsuccessful stone extraction.

	OR	95% CI	*P* value
Age	1.779	1.110–2.850	0.017
Periampullary diverticula	0.684	0.452–1.034	NS
Multiple stones	1.647	1.060–2.559	0.026
Diameter of CBD stones > 15 mm	1.804	1.210–2.691	0.004

OR: odds ratio, NS: not significant.

technical difficulties when manipulating into an abruptly deviated common duct, just above the hepatopancreatic ampulla. This difficulty owing to the tortuosity of the distal part of CBD can cause improper positioning and inadequate manipulation of stone retrieval devices. In accordance with the study by García [25] and contrary to the study by Kim et al. [6], the present study showed that acute angulation of the distal CBD proved to be an insignificantly contributing factor to a failed endoscopic SE. In our view, acute distal CBD angulation could play a decisive role in the difficulty of endoscopic SE in the case of coexisting dilatation of the distal CBD. In such scenario, the inflated stone extraction balloon cannot sufficiently rest against the wall of the dilated duct, making the retrieval of stones extremely difficult. On the contrary, in the case of an acute angulation of a nondilated distal CBD, we believe that proper manipulations, such as the "loop" handling, following the insertion of a "Jagwire" type hydrophilic guide-wire (0.035 in, Boston Scientific) proximal to the CBD angulation, can succeed in a rather straightforward SE.

These conflicting data may be explained in part by variation in operator expertise and by the fact that ERCP is a highly operator-depended intervention. However, these intrinsic procedure-related drawbacks should not discourage investigators from further clarifying and analyzing factors contributing to a failed endoscopic SE.

The present study also showed that conventional endoscopic management of difficult to extract BDS proved for the vast majority of patients safe and effective, on the condition that bile duct drainage can be obtained and patients are capable of allowing for a repeated intervention. In fact, according to the results of the present study conventional endoscopic management cleared completely the duct in the vast majority of cases with, however, the expense of multiple treatment sessions and endoprosthesis insertion. This outcome underlines the significant role of stenting when managing patients with difficult to extract BDS, which can be lifesaving [11]. Deployment of a biliary endoprosthesis is an easy and effective alternative, especially for frail, elderly, and high risk patients. Stent insertion results in immediate biliary drainage, accomplishing treatment and/or prevention of cholangitis, serves as a "bridge" to a safe, elective, repeated session or as a dissolution therapy, and prevents impaction of stones in the distal CBD thereby maintaining the biliary flow [7, 8].

It is worth mentioning the findings of several studies which documented that after biliary stenting for a time period ranging from three to six months, a significant proportion of large CBD stones disintegrated, decreased in size, or even disappeared [26–28]. These effects of biliary stenting, which we affirm, can serve as an adjuvant measure to finally clear initially deemed "unextractable" CBD stones.

Despite the fact that in the present study conventional endoscopic management of difficult to extract BDS proved in the vast majority of patients safe and effective, this finding should not underestimate the important role of modern stone fragmentation modalities which definitively contribute to a conclusive minimally invasive treatment, especially in cases in which various conventional therapeutic strategies fail. However, one should keep in mind that the choice, if any, of which lithotripsy technique to utilize depends on availability, expertise, and certainly economic resources.

In conclusion, failed conventional endoscopic SE in patients with difficult to extract BDS is more likely to occur in overage patients, in patients with CBD stones >4, and in patients with CBD stone(s) diameter $\geq 15\,\text{mm}$. Endoprosthesis insertion in the event of a failed endoscopic CBD SE providing bile duct drainage offers a safety bridge to a repeated, elective, and ultimately successful minimally invasive intervention.

Disclosure

Emmanuel Christoforidis and Konstantinos Vasiliadis are equal first authors.

Acknowledgment

The authors gratefully thank Mrs. Krystallia Moshota, the former head nurse of their endoscopy unit, for her invaluableness assistance.

References

[1] M. L. Freitas, R. L. Bell, and A. J. Duffy, "Choledocholithiasis: evolving standards for diagnosis and management," *World Journal of Gastroenterology*, vol. 12, no. 20, pp. 3162–3167, 2006.

[2] S. Tazuma, "Epidemiology, pathogenesis, and classification of biliary stones (common bile duct and intrahepatic)," *Best Practice and Research: Clinical Gastroenterology*, vol. 20, no. 6, pp. 1075–1083, 2006.

[3] J. Samardzic, F. Latic, D. Kraljik et al., "Treatment of common bile duct stones—is the role of ERCP changed in era of minimally invasive surgery?" *Medicinski arhiv*, vol. 64, no. 3, pp. 187–188, 2010.

[4] C. Strömberg and M. Nilsson, "Nationwide study of the treatment of common bile duct stones in Sweden between 1965 and 2009," *British Journal of Surgery*, vol. 98, no. 12, pp. 1766–1774, 2011.

[5] G. Trikudanathan, U. Navaneethan, and M. A. Parsi, "Endoscopic management of difficult common bile duct stones," *World Journal of Gastroenterology*, vol. 19, no. 2, pp. 165–173, 2013.

[6] H. J. Kim, H. S. Choi, J. H. Park et al., "Factors influencing the technical difficulty of endoscopic clearance of bile duct stones," *Gastrointestinal Endoscopy*, vol. 66, no. 6, pp. 1154–1160, 2007.

[7] G. D. de Palma and C. Catanzano, "Stenting or surgery for treatment of irretrievable common bile duct calculi in elderly patients?" *American Journal of Surgery*, vol. 178, no. 5, pp. 390–393, 1999.

[8] J. J. G. H. M. Bergman, E. A. J. Rauws, J. G. P. Tijssen, G. N. J. Tytgat, and K. Huibregtse, "Biliary endoprostheses in elderly patients with endoscopically irretrievable common bile duct stones: report on 117 patients," *Gastrointestinal Endoscopy*, vol. 42, no. 3, pp. 195–201, 1995.

[9] S. Amplatz, L. Piazzi, M. Felder et al., "Extracorporeal shock wave lithotripsy for clearance of refractory bile duct stones," *Digestive and Liver Disease*, vol. 39, no. 3, pp. 267–272, 2007.

[10] M. A. Parsi, T. Stevens, J. A. Dumot, and G. Zuccaro, "Endoscopic therapy of recurrent acute pancreatitis," *Cleveland Clinic Journal of Medicine*, vol. 76, no. 4, pp. 225–233, 2009.

[11] T. Tsujinoa, R. Sugitaa, H. Yoshidaa et al., "Risk factors for acute suppurative cholangitis caused by bile duct stones," *European Journal of Gastroenterology & Hepatology*, vol. 19, pp. 585–588, 2007.

[12] D. J. Martin, D. R. Vernon, and J. Toouli, "Surgical versus endoscopic treatment of bile duct stones," *Cochrane Database of Systematic Reviews*, no. 2, Article ID CD003327, 2006.

[13] S. P. Misra and M. Dwivedi, "Large-diameter balloon dilation after endoscopic sphincterotomy for removal of difficult bile duct stones," *Endoscopy*, vol. 40, no. 3, pp. 209–213, 2008.

[14] W. D. Owens, J. A. Felts, and E. L. Spitznagel Jr., "ASA physical status classifications: a study of consistency of ratings," *Anesthesiology*, vol. 49, no. 4, pp. 239–243, 1978.

[15] D. Keizman, M. I. Shalom, and F. M. Konikoff, "Recurrent symptomatic common bile duct stones after endoscopic stone extraction in elderly patients," *Gastrointestinal Endoscopy*, vol. 64, no. 1, pp. 60–65, 2006.

[16] D. Keizman, M. I. Shalom, and F. M. Konikoff, "An angulated common bile duct predisposes to recurrent symptomatic bile duct stones after endoscopic stone extraction," *Surgical Endoscopy and Other Interventional Techniques*, vol. 20, no. 10, pp. 1594–1599, 2006.

[17] D. N. Lobo, T. W. Balfour, S. Y. Iftikhar, and B. J. Rowlands, "Periampullary diverticula and pancreaticobiliary disease," *British Journal of Surgery*, vol. 86, no. 5, pp. 588–597, 1999.

[18] S. M. Schutz and R. M. Abbott, "Grading ERCPs by degree of difficulty: a new concept to produce more meaningful outcome data," *Gastrointestinal Endoscopy*, vol. 51, no. 5, pp. 535–539, 2000.

[19] R. Madhotra, P. B. Cotton, J. Vaughn et al., "Analyzing ERCP practice by a modified degree of difficulty scale: a multicentre database analysis," *The American Journal of Gastroenterology*, vol. 95, pp. 2480–2481, 2000.

[20] C. Mavrogiannis, C. Liatsos, A. Romanos, C. Petoumenos, A. Nakos, and G. Karvountzis, "Needle knife fistulotomy versus needle knife precut papillotomy for the treatment of common bile duct stones," *Gastrointestinal Endoscopy*, vol. 50, no. 3, pp. 334–339, 1999.

[21] K.-S. Yoo and G. A. Lehman, "Endoscopic management of biliary ductal stones," *Gastroenterology Clinics of North America*, vol. 39, no. 2, pp. 209–227, 2010.

[22] L. McHenry and G. Lehman, "Difficult bile duct stones," *Current Treatment Options in Gastroenterology*, vol. 9, no. 2, pp. 123–132, 2006.

[23] K. F. Binmoeller, M. Brückner, F. Thonke, and N. Soehendra, "Treatment of difficult bile duct stones using mechanical, electrohydraulic and extracorporeal shock wave lithotripsy," *Endoscopy*, vol. 25, no. 3, pp. 201–206, 1993.

[24] A. Lauri, R. C. Horton, B. R. Davidson, A. K. Burroughs, and J. S. Dooley, "Endoscopic extraction of bile duct stones: management related to stone size," *Gut*, vol. 34, no. 12, pp. 1718–1721, 1993.

[25] J. R. García, "Factors related to therapeutic failure in the extraction of bile duct stones for endoscopic retrograde colangiopancreatography ERCP," *Revista de Gastroenterología del Perú*, vol. 31, no. 4, pp. 330–334, 2011.

[26] Z. Fan, R. Hawes, C. Lawrence, X. Zhang, X. Zhang, and W. Lv, "Analysis of plastic stents in the treatment of large common bile duct stones in 45 patients," *Digestive Endoscopy*, vol. 23, no. 1, pp. 86–90, 2011.

[27] T. H. Lee, J.-H. Han, H. J. Kim, S. M. Park, S.-H. Park, and S.-J. Kim, "Is the addition of choleretic agents in multiple double-pigtail biliary stents effective for difficult common bile duct stones in elderly patients? A prospective, multicenter study," *Gastrointestinal Endoscopy*, vol. 74, no. 1, pp. 96–102, 2011.

[28] A. Horiuchi, Y. Nakayama, M. Kajiyama et al., "Biliary stenting in the management of large or multiple common bile duct stones," *Gastrointestinal Endoscopy*, vol. 71, no. 7, pp. 1200–1203, 2010.

25

Endoscopic Submucosal Dissection Outcomes for Gastroesophageal Tumors in Low Volume Units: A Multicenter Survey

Ahmad Najib Azmi,[1,2] Christopher J. L. Khor,[3] Khek-Yu Ho,[4] Rapat Pittayanon,[5] Rungsun Rerknimitr,[5] Thawee Ratanachu-ek,[6] Doreen S. C. Koay,[3] Jianyi Calvin Koh,[4] Shiaw-Hooi Ho,[1] Khean-Lee Goh,[1] and Sanjiv Mahadeva[1]

[1]*Division of Gastroenterology, Department of Medicine, University Malaya Medical Center, Kuala Lumpur, Malaysia*
[2]*Faculty of Medicine and Health Sciences, Universiti Sains Islam Malaysia, Malaysia*
[3]*Department of Gastroenterology & Hepatology, Singapore General Hospital, Singapore*
[4]*Department of Gastroenterology, National University Hospital, Singapore*
[5]*Division of Gastroenterology, Department of Medicine, Chulalongkorn University Hospital, Bangkok, Thailand*
[6]*Department of Surgery, Rajavithi Hospital, Bangkok, Thailand*

Correspondence should be addressed to Ahmad Najib Azmi; drahmadnajib@gmail.com

Academic Editor: Patrick J. O'Dwyer

Background and Aims. Endoscopic submucosal dissection (ESD) outcomes have traditionally been reported from high volume centers in East Asia. Data from low volume centers in other parts of Asia remain sparse. *Methods.* A retrospective survey with a structured questionnaire of 5 tertiary centers in 3 countries in South East Asia was conducted. Details of training and clinical outcomes of ESD cases, with follow-up data from these centers, were analyzed. *Results.* Seven endoscopists from the 5 centers performed a total of 35 cases of ESD in the upper gastrointestinal tract (UGIT) over a 6-year duration. Details of the lesions excised were as follows: median size was 20 mm, morphologically 20 (68.6%) were flat/depressed and 6 (17.1%) were submucosal, and histologically 27 (77.1%) were neoplastic. The median duration of ESD procedures was 105 minutes, with an en-bloc resection rate of 91.4%. There was 1 (2.9%) case of delayed bleeding, but no perforation nor mortality in any of the cases. The recurrence rate after ESD was 5.7%. A prolonged ESD duration was influenced by a larger size of lesion (25 mm, $p = 0.02$) but not by factors related to the training experience of endoscopists. *Conclusions.* ESD in the UGIT is feasible and safe in low volume centers in Asia.

1. Introduction

Endoscopic resection is the least invasive and cost-effective way of treating superficial malignant lesions in the digestive tract. Endoscopic submucosal dissection (ESD) has now become the accepted technique of resection of early tumors in the upper gastrointestinal (GI) tract, although it has long been practiced among Japanese endoscopists who pioneered this technique. ESD, however, is technically challenging and is rarely practiced outside of Japan or Korea [1]. A steep learning curve to master ESD, prolonged procedure duration, increased procedure risks, lack of commensurate reimbursement, and need for specialized tools have become challenges in mastering ESD [2]. Endoscopic mucosal resection (EMR) is technically less demanding and seen by many as an alternate method of endoscopic resection for early GI neoplasia. However, EMR is unable to achieve en-bloc resection for lesions >20 mm in size and has been shown to have a higher rate of tumor recurrence compared to ESD.

In Japan, several experts have suggested that competency in ESD can only be achieved following supervised performance of between 30 and 80 ESD cases [3]. Such a volume of ESD cases may be easily achieved in a short space of time in Japan and Korea, where a high incidence of early gastric cancer detection resulting from an active screening programme is present [4, 5], but this is clearly not the case elsewhere in Asia or in the West [6]. This does not necessarily indicate then that ESD should not be practiced outside of East Asia, as there is a growing indication for ESD beyond early gastric malignancy, such as for submucosal GI tumors [7–9]. As such, recent experts from the West have proposed a variation to the Japanese recommendation for training in ESD. In addition to being experienced in general therapeutic GI endoscopy, Draganov et al. have suggested that proficiency in conventional EMR, together with animal model training, may be sufficient for endoscopists in the West to embark on ESD in humans [10].

The incidence of gastric cancer in South East Asia is low at 10.1 per 100,000 populations (age-standardised rates) [11]. Nevertheless, with its moderate/low prevalence of *H. pylori* infection, early gastric cancer is not totally unrecognized in the Southeast Asian region [12]. Recognizing the need to develop ESD within their respective countries, several endoscopic centers in South East Asia, namely, in Thailand, Singapore, and Malaysia, had embarked on ESD for upper GI tumors over the last 6 years. Specific individuals in each center, usually with a background of EMR experience, underwent training on animal models and performed ESD under supervision by experts before embarking on the procedure independently. This report aims to document the collective feasibility and safety of ESD in the main centers performing ESD in South East Asia.

2. Methods

ESD in the upper GI tract had been commenced in the following 5 centers in South East Asia over the past several years: Chulalongkorn University Hospital and Rajavithi Hospital in Bangkok; National University Hospital and Singapore General Hospital in Singapore; and University Malaya Medical Center in Kuala Lumpur. Prospective data on experience of ESD operators, procedure details, and clinical follow-up information were obtained in all cases using a structured clinical record form.

Data on ESD in the upper GI tract alone were collected in this study, as mucosal or submucosal lesions in the esophagus and stomach were the commonest indication for ESD in all centers.

2.1. ESD Technique. Prior to ESD, all gastric lesions were carefully evaluated with chromoendoscopy and endoscopic ultrasound (EUS) where indicated. The endoscopic appearances of mucosal lesions were classified based on the Paris Classification of superficial tumors [13]. Tissue biopsies were taken in cases prior to ESD where indicated. ESD was performed in a standard manner [14]. All patients had sedation, which was administered by an anaesthetist. After chromoendoscopy with 0.2% Indigo carmine dye to delineate the border of the tumor, circumferential marking with a needle knife (KD-1L-1, Olympus, Tokyo, Japan) or ERBE hybrid knife (Erbe Elektromedizin GmbH, Tuebingen, Germany) was made. Submucosal injection was performed using a standard solution (Gelafundin or normal saline with Adrenaline and Indigo carmine in a ratio of 20 : 1 : 1) [15]. After an adequate submucosal lift of the periphery of the tumor was made, an initial mucosal incision was performed (needle knife KD-1L-1, Olympus, Tokyo, Japan, or ERBE hybrid knife). This was followed by a circumferential incision and subsequent submucosal dissection using the IT2 knife, Dual knife (Olympus, Tokyo, Japan) or ERBE hybrid knife (Erbe Elektromedizin GmbH, Tuebingen, Germany), with repeated submucosal injection where necessary. Following en-bloc resection of the tumor, the mucosal defect was carefully inspected and areas of bleeding or prominent vessels were cauterized using hemostatic forceps (Olympus, Tokyo, Japan). After ESD, all patients had a routine follow-up endoscopic examination at 1 month to check for ulcer healing and subsequently at 6 and 12 months. Further assessment was made depending on the findings at repeat endoscopy.

2.2. Clinical Data Parameters. All resected specimens were examined histologically based on the Vienna Classification [16]. Involvement or clearance of the margins was recorded. All patients' vital signs were monitored after procedure. Hemoglobin levels were checked on the day after the procedure routinely and were clinically indicated. Procedure duration was described from the time the endoscope entered the oral cavity until the time it was removed from the patients' mouth. Complications were divided into intraprocedure and postprocedure. These included immediate and delayed bleeding, perforation, and complications associated with sedation.

Patients who had a reduction in hemoglobin by 2 g/dL or requiring blood transfusion after procedure were labeled as delayed bleeding. All patients were followed up for a median period of 24 weeks. The endoscopic findings during follow-up were recorded. "Local recurrence" was defined as the presence of tumor after 2 negative gastroscopy follow-up examinations.

2.3. Main Outcomes. The main outcomes of this study were to examine the feasibility and safety of ESD in low volume centers. Feasibility will be assessed with the following parameters: duration of ESD procedure, completeness of tissue resection (by histological assessment), and recurrence rate at follow-up endoscopy. The safety of ESD will be based on the rates of immediate and delayed complications after ESD. Comparisons with published data on ESD in both European and Eastern (Korean and Japanese) series will be explored.

2.4. Statistical Analysis. All raw data obtained from each center were recorded and analyzed using a standard software package (SPSS version 21, Chicago, IL). Mean and median values of variables were calculated and presented accordingly. Basic analyses on predictors of ESD technical success and complications will be performed. Statistical significance was assumed at a p value of <0.05.

3. Results

3.1. Endoscopists. A total of 7 endoscopists from the 5 centers were involved in this study: Thailand $n = 3$, Singapore

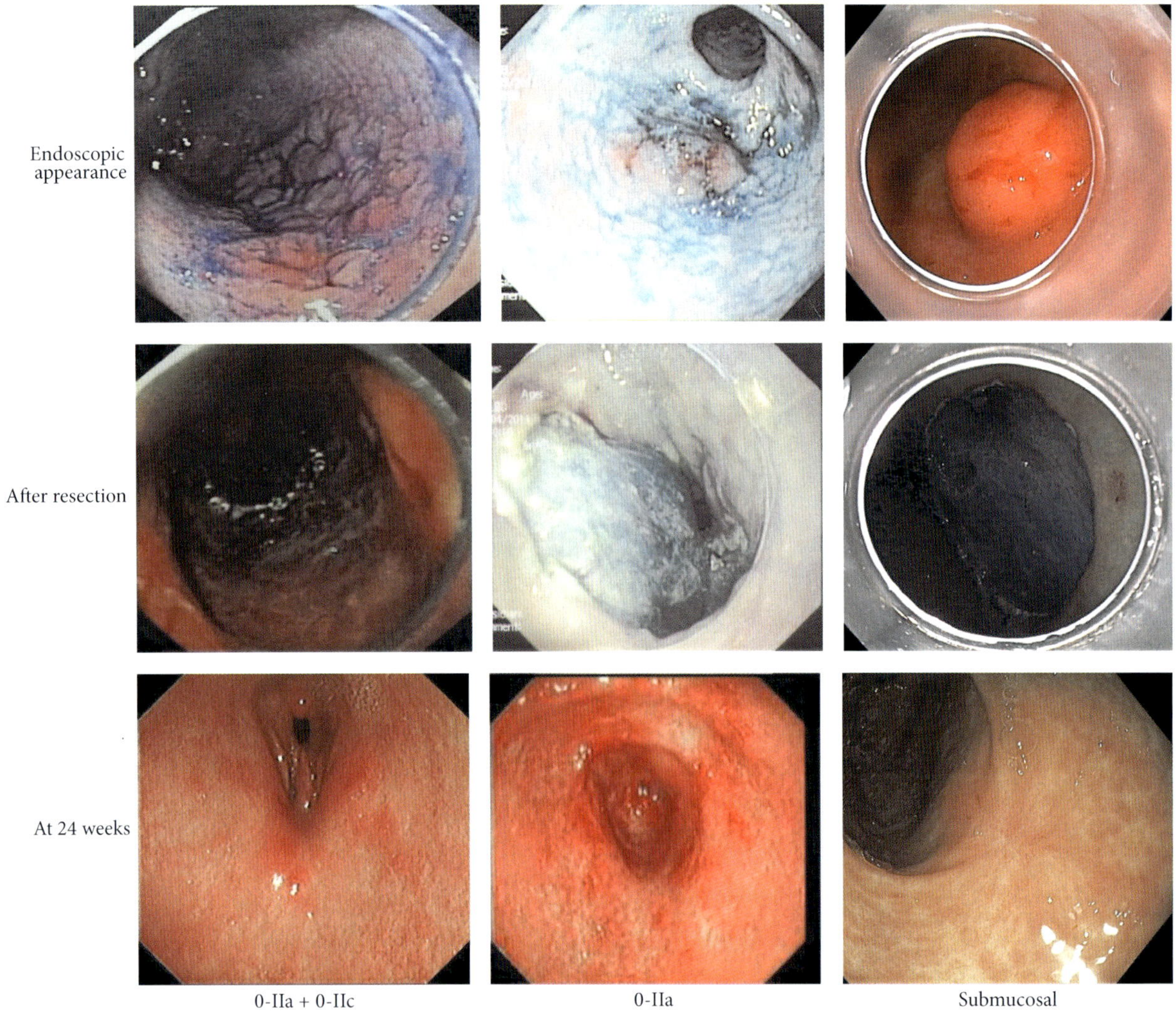

Figure 1: Endoscopic images of various lesions excised by ESD in this series.

$n = 2$, and Malaysia $n = 2$. The median general endoscopy experience was 17 (range 5–22) years and all endoscopists had prior EMR experience before embarking on ESD (median 11 years, range 3–15 years). All 7 endoscopists had undergone animal model training for ESD and 3 of them were trained in Japan. A median of 25 ESD cases (min 15, max 40) had been observed prior to commencing ESD individually in patients.

3.2. Case Description. A total of 35 patients had undergone ESD between 2009 and 2015. 18 (51.4%) cases were female and the median age was 71 (range 21–85) years. Details of the lesions are summarized in Table 1. The majority of lesions identified were in the lower stomach (54.3%). There were a range of lesions morphologically, with Type 0-IIa being the commonest; examples of some of these lesions are shown in Figure 1. ESD was performed for 6 submucosal lesions, as they were suspected neuroendocrine tumors (NET). The median size of lesions was 20 mm (IQR 15–25 mm), with a range from 5 mm to 60 mm. Based on histological evaluation of the resected specimens (Table 1), the lesions were subsequently categorized as neoplastic (mucosal dysplasia, neoplasia, or NET) $n = 27$ (77.1%) and benign mucosal/benign submucosal lesions $n = 8$ (22.9%).

3.3. ESD Feasibility. 23 (65.7%) cases were performed under general anaesthesia, 9 (25.7%) cases with Propofol sedation, and 3 (8.6%) cases with Midazolam sedation alone. The median duration of ESD procedures was 105 IQR (65–184) minutes, with a range from 15 to 480 minutes. Figure 2 illustrates the linear relationship between lesion size and the median duration of ESD procedures.

En-bloc resection was successful in 32/35 lesions (91.4%) and the remaining 3 lesions were resected in a piecemeal manner. From en-bloc resected specimens, histologically, 30/35 (85.7%) specimens showed complete resection (R0) and 2/35 (5.7%) samples had R1 resection (see Table 2). Six patients had histology suggesting incomplete margin clearance (duodenal NET $n = 1$, gastric NET $n = 1$, and gastric adenocarcinoma $n = 4$) and were referred for surgical resection.

TABLE 1: Clinical characteristics of ESD lesions ($n = 35$).

Location	
Esophagus	3 (8.6%)
Upper stomach	4 (11.4%)
Mid stomach	8 (22.9%)
Lower stomach	19 (54.3%)
Duodenum	1 (2.9%)
Morphology	
0-I	4 (11.4%)
0-Is	1 (2.9%)
0-IIa	12 (34.3%)
0-IIc	4 (11.4%)
0-IIa + 0-IIc	8 (22.9%)
Submucosal	6 (17.1%)
Size	Median 20 (range 5–60) mm
Histology	
Adenocarcinoma	17 (45.8%)
Severe dysplasia	6 (17.1%)
Intestinal metaplasia	1 (2.9%)
Neuroendocrine tumor	3 (8.6%)
Leiomyoma	3 (8.6%)
Ectopic pancreatic tissue	2 (5.7%)
Hyperplastic	1 (2.9%)
Lipoma	2 (5.7%)

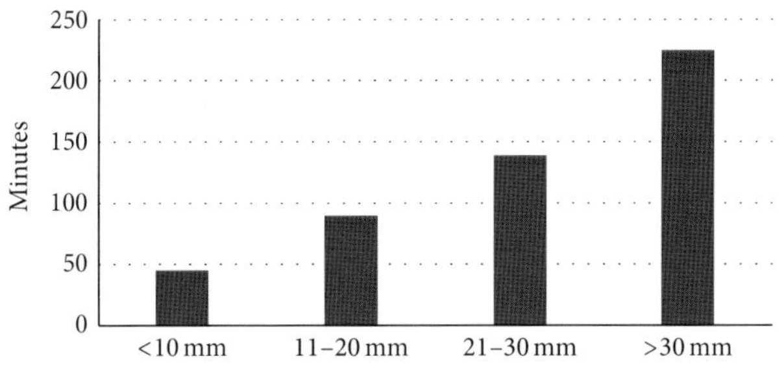

FIGURE 2: Duration of ESD procedure in relation to the size of lesion.

3.4. ESD Safety. Significant profuse bleeding was reported in only 1 (2.9%) case, but this was successfully treated with hemoclips. All minor bleeding during ESD was managed immediately with either hemostatic forceps or hemoclips. No patient required a blood transfusion during or 24 hours after procedure. There were no perforations and no immediate mortality resulting from ESD. No complications relating to sedation/anaesthesia, such as hypoxia or aspiration, were observed in this series.

3.5. Follow-Up. All patients were followed-up for a median duration of 24 weeks (range 4–224 weeks). Recurrence was detected in 2/35 (5.7%) cases—1 with adenocarcinoma (en bloc, R1) and the other with a gastric NET (en bloc, R0). EMR was performed for the adenocarcinoma recurrence with complete marginal clearance. The gastric NET recurrence is being monitored without immediate plans for resection as the original histology was a low-grade NET.

TABLE 2: Outcomes of ESD ($n = 35$ cases).

Median duration (minutes)	105 (15–480)
Complete resection	
En bloc resection	32 (91.4%)
R0 resection (includes en bloc and piecemeal specimens)	29 (82.9%)
En bloc with R0 resection	27 (77.1%)
Complications	
Delayed bleeding	1 (2.9%)
Perforations	0
Recurrence	
Recurrence	2 (9.8%)

3.6. Predictors of ESD Outcomes. Due to the low number of complications and high number of en-bloc resections, predictors of these outcomes could not be analyzed in this study. "Procedure duration" was therefore evaluated as a proxy of ESD outcomes in this study. The median duration of ESD was 105 minutes and procedure duration beyond this was defined as a poorer outcome. Factors which may have influenced procedure duration were explored by univariate analysis (Table 3). Factors related to training (duration of EMR experience, number of ESD cases observed, and prior experience in Japan) did not influence ESD procedure duration. The main predictor for a prolonged ESD procedure was the size of the lesion (25 mm versus 15 mm, $p = 0.02$).

4. Discussion

Most publications of ESD case series have been derived from high volume centers in Japan and Korea [17, 18], but reports from Western countries and smaller Asian nations are gradually emerging. A recent nationwide survey from 14 centers in France performing ESD in the UGIT reported a mean procedure duration of 108.2 ± 62 (range of 37 to 330) minutes, en-bloc resection, and R0 rate 91.7% and 71.2%, respectively [19]. In Taiwan, a multicenter case series reported a median procedure duration of gastric ESD of 92.4 minutes for lesions of a median size of 18 mm, with an en-bloc resection rate of 91% [8]. In this multicenter, multinational case series from South East Asia, the median procedure duration of 105 minutes for lesions with a median size of 20 mm, with an RO resection rate of 85.7%, compares favourably to these published reports from non-Japanese/Korean centers. Table 4 is a brief summary comparing ESD experiences from low volume centers from different regions.

There were no major complications from this case series, probably due to the smaller number of cases. Perforations complicating ESD have been reported to range from 1.2% to 5.2% and delayed bleeding from 0% to 15.6% [20]. However, the <100% en-bloc resection rate, with tumor recurrence, was probable indicator of operator inexperience. In our

Table 3: Predictive factors for a prolonged ESD duration.

	Prolonged ESD duration (>105 mins)		p
	Yes (n = 17)	No (n = 18)	
Cases done by endoscopists with training in Japan (total n = 16)	9 (56.3%)	7 (43.7%)	0.4[#]
Endoscopy training (median years)	18	17	0.62[*]
ESD cases observed (median number)	30	40	0.06[*]
Previous EMR experience (median years)	11	9.5	0.40[*]
Location of lesion			
Lower stomach	4 (21.1%)	15 (78.9%)	0.29[#]
Non-lower stomach	6 (37.5%)	10 (62.5%)	
Lesion morphology			
Flat/depressed (0-IIc)	8 (42.1%)	11 (58.9%)	0.51[#]
Elevated (0-IIa)	9 (56.3%)	7 (44.7%)	
Size of lesion (median mm)	25	15	0.02[*]

[*]Mann–Whitney U test.
[#]Chi-square test.

Table 4: Summary of ESD in upper GI tract outcomes from low-volume centres in the world.

	Taiwan [8]	Italy [23]	Portugal [27]	France [19]	South East Asia (this study)
Year	2004–2007	2005–2011	2005–2008	2010–2013	2009–2015
Centers	8	2	1	14	5
Study method	Retrospective	Retrospective	Retrospective	Prospective	Retrospective
Number of ESD cases	70	20	19	177 (upper GI only)	35
Size (mm)	Mean 32.6 ± 13.9	Median 29 (15–60)	Median 25 (15–30)	Mean 39 ± 23	Median 20 (5–60)
Procedure time (minutes)	Median 92.4 (25–210)	Medial 119.1 (40–240)	Median 90 (40–300)	Mean 108.2 ± 62	Median 105 (15–480)
Knife used	IT knife Needle knife	IT knife Hook knife	IT knife Hook knife	Dual knife Flush knife	IT knife Hybrid knife
Outcomes					
En bloc resection, n (%)	64/70 (91.4%)	—	15/19 (79%)	292/319 (91.5%)	32/35 (91.4%)
R0 en bloc resection, n (%)	NA	18/20 (90%)	13/19 (68%)	277/319 (71.2%)	27/32 (77.1%)
Complications					
Bleeding, n (%)	4/70 (5.7%)	0	1/19 (5.3%)	15 (4.7%)	1 (2.9%)
Perforation, n (%)	3/70 (4.3%)	3/20 (15%)	0	26 (8.1%)	0
Recurrence					
Esophagus, n (%)	—	NA	—	4/60 (6.7%)	0
Stomach, n (%)	2/70 2.8%	NA	0	5/63 (6.1%)	2/35 (9.8%)

ESD: Endoscopic submucosal dissection; R0: complete resection with no margin involvement; NA: not available; and IT: insulated tip.

series, 19 (54.3%) lesions located in the lower portion of the stomach had a successful en-bloc resection, except for a single lesion. Location of a lesion in the upper part of stomach, previous scars, and an undifferentiated pathologic type have been identified as risk factors for not achieving an en-bloc resection [18]. Local recurrence occurred in 2 (5.7%) cases in this series. A previous meta-analysis by Lian et al. has suggested that tumor recurrence is much lower for ESD when compared to EMR [17]. However rates of tumor recurrence post ESD have been shown to vary from 2% to 35% [21]. Piecemeal resection and resection margin involvement by tumor are two main reasons for recurrence after ESD. En-bloc resection is the single most important factor for a curative ESD without recurrence, which can give a disease-specific 5-year overall survival of 97.1%–100% [22]. Six patients who had incomplete histological clearance had subsequent surgery. However, no residual tumor cells were present in surgically resected specimens. It is likely that the ESD had actually been successful, but histology had been inaccurate or cautery effect at the resection margin may have ablated tumor outside the resected specimen.

A prolonged duration of ESD can lead to unwanted complications resulting from sedative or anaesthetic medications. Furthermore, many of the patients requiring an

ESD procedure are elderly (median age 71 years in this case series), with the potential of cardiorespiratory complications with sedation/anaesthesia. Hence, a prolonged duration of procedure has been accepted as an undesirable outcome of ESD [18]. In a large retrospective series of 1000 ESD cases from Korea, Chung et al. defined >60 minutes as a prolonged ESD duration and identified large size of lesion, upper stomach location of tumor, presence of scar, recurrent lesion, and flat macroscopic morphology as predictors [18]. Of these factors, large size of lesion (OR 4.5) and recurrent lesion (OR 3.0) were the most predictive of a prolonged duration of procedure. In our small series, we similarly identified that a larger size of lesion, but no other characteristics, influenced the duration of ESD procedure. It is likely that the small sample size in this series prohibited an accurate assessment of the other factors other than size, that is, Type 2 statistical error.

ESD was initially developed for en-bloc resection of mucosal tumors. Due to its technical success and an improvement in accessories which can be used for closure of transmural perforations, ESD has expanded to include resection of various submucosal tumors in the stomach. An initial study by Li et al. on 29 neuroendocrine tumors showed that 28 lesions (96.6%) in the upper GI tract could be completely resected, with only 1 case of delayed bleeding, 0 perforations, and 1 recurrence [9]. Several other case series have recently reported successful ESD for various gastric submucosal tumors such as ectopic pancreas, ectopic spleen, leiomyoma, and gastrointestinal stromal tumor (GIST) [23, 24]. In another case series from France, the authors reported successful resection of 33 submucosal lesions in the stomach for lesions <20 mm, with the majority of lesions being resected by ESD [25]. In this study, 6 lesions dissected were submucosal in origin. All lesions were resected safely without any complications, indicating that ESD for these deeper lesions was feasible even in low volume centers.

Data from this case series may have been limited by the self-reporting method of individual endoscopists. Nevertheless, the modest records of procedure duration are indicative of ESD being performed in a low volume setting. The recent large series of ESD in multiple centers in France [19] and a prior study in Nagano [26] suggest that center volume may not necessarily be the sole factor affecting outcomes in ESD. Unlike young Japanese endoscopists who embark on ESD, endoscopists here develop a significant amount of experience in therapeutic endoscopy prior to performing ESD. In particular, standard EMR for lesions in the GI tract share many technical aspects with ESD, namely, chromoendoscopy, submucosal elevation prior to resection, and use of electrocautery devices and that of clips for closure of mucosal defects after resection. We concur with a recent review article which suggested that ESD can be taken up by non-Japanese endoscopists who were proficient in conventional EMR and had undergone sufficient training in animal models [10]. Although EGC may not be common in this region, the expanding role of ESD as a minimally invasive therapeutic modality for gastric submucosal tumors and other such lesions indicates that there is still a need for developing this skill among endoscopists in this region.

Competing Interests

The authors declare that there is no conflict of interests regarding the publication of this paper.

References

[1] M.-Y. Kim, J.-H. Cho, P. Jain, and J. Y. Cho, "ESD around the world: Asia," *Gastrointestinal Endoscopy Clinics of North America*, vol. 24, no. 2, pp. 283–293, 2014.

[2] A. Y. Wang, "The international emergence of endoscopic submucosal dissection for early gastric cancer," *Gastrointestinal Endoscopy*, vol. 73, no. 5, pp. 928–931, 2011.

[3] R. M. Coman, T. Gotoda, and P. V. Draganov, "Training in endoscopic submucosal dissection," *World Journal of Gastrointestinal Endoscopy*, vol. 5, no. 8, pp. 369–378, 2013.

[4] K. S. Lee, D. K. Oh, M. A. Han et al., "Gastric cancer screening in Korea: report on the national cancer screening program in 2008," *Cancer Research and Treatment*, vol. 43, no. 2, pp. 83–88, 2011.

[5] C. Hamashima, D. Shibuya, H. Yamazaki et al., "The Japanese guidelines for gastric cancer screening," *Japanese Journal of Clinical Oncology*, vol. 38, no. 4, pp. 259–267, 2008.

[6] S. M. Everett and A. T. R. Axon, "Early gastric cancer in Europe," *Gut*, vol. 41, no. 2, pp. 142–150, 1997.

[7] C.-T. Lee, C.-Y. Chang, C.-M. Tai et al., "Endoscopic submucosal dissection for early esophageal neoplasia: a single center experience in South Taiwan," *Journal of the Formosan Medical Association*, vol. 111, no. 3, pp. 132–139, 2012.

[8] C.-C. Chang, I.-L. Lee, P.-J. Chen et al., "Endoscopic submucosal dissection for gastric epithelial tumors: a multicenter study in Taiwan," *Journal of the Formosan Medical Association*, vol. 108, no. 1, pp. 38–44, 2009.

[9] Q.-L. Li, Y.-Q. Zhang, W.-F. Chen et al., "Endoscopic submucosal dissection for foregut neuroendocrine tumors: An Initial Study," *World Journal of Gastroenterology*, vol. 18, no. 40, pp. 5799–5806, 2012.

[10] P. V. Draganov, T. Gotoda, D. Chavalitdhamrong, and M. B. Wallace, "Techniques of endoscopic submucosal dissection: application for the Western endoscopist?" *Gastrointestinal Endoscopy*, vol. 78, no. 5, pp. 677–688, 2013.

[11] J. Ferlay, H.-R. Shin, F. Bray, D. Forman, C. Mathers, and D. M. Parkin, "Estimates of worldwide burden of cancer in 2008: GLOBOCAN 2008," *International Journal of Cancer*, vol. 127, no. 12, pp. 2893–2917, 2010.

[12] K. M. Fock and T. L. Ang, "Epidemiology of *Helicobacter pylori* infection and gastric cancer in Asia," *Journal of Gastroenterology and Hepatology*, vol. 25, no. 3, pp. 479–486, 2010.

[13] "The Paris endoscopic classification of superficial neoplastic lesions: esophagus, stomach, and colon: November 30 to December 1, 2002," *Gastrointestinal Endoscopy*, vol. 58, no. 6, pp. S3–S43, 2003.

[14] M. Fujishiro, "Endoscopic submucosal dissection for stomach neoplasms," *World Journal of Gastroenterology*, vol. 12, no. 32, pp. 5108–5112, 2006.

[15] S. Mahadeva and B. J. Rembacken, "Standard 'inject and cut' endoscopic mucosal resection technique is practical and effective in the management of superficial colorectal neoplasms," *Surgical Endoscopy*, vol. 23, no. 2, pp. 417–422, 2009.

[16] R. J. Schlemper, R. H. Riddell, Y. Kato et al., "The vienna classification of gastrointestinal epithelial neoplasia," *Gut*, vol. 47, no. 2, pp. 251–255, 2000.

[17] J. Lian, S. Chen, Y. Zhang, and F. Qiu, "A meta-analysis of endoscopic submucosal dissection and EMR for early gastric cancer," *Gastrointestinal Endoscopy*, vol. 76, no. 4, pp. 763–770, 2012.

[18] I.-K. Chung, J. H. Lee, S.-H. Lee et al., "Therapeutic outcomes in 1000 cases of endoscopic submucosal dissection for early gastric neoplasms: Korean ESD Study Group multicenter study," *Gastrointestinal Endoscopy*, vol. 69, no. 7, pp. 1228–1235, 2009.

[19] M. Barret, V. Lepilliez, D. Coumaros et al., "The expansion of endoscopic submucosal dissection in France: a prospective nationwide survey," *United European Gastroenterology Journal*, 2016.

[20] I. Oda, H. Suzuki, S. Nonaka, and S. Yoshinaga, "Complications of gastric endoscopic submucosal dissection," *Digestive Endoscopy*, vol. 25, no. 1, pp. 71–78, 2013.

[21] T. Kojima, A. Parra-Blanco, H. Takahashi, R. Fujita, and C. J. Lightdale, "Outcome of endoscopic mucosal resection for early gastric cancer: review of the Japanese literature," *Gastrointestinal Endoscopy*, vol. 48, no. 5, pp. 550–555, 1998.

[22] H. Isomoto, S. Shikuwa, N. Yamaguchi et al., "Endoscopic submucosal dissection for early gastric cancer: a large-scale feasibility study," *Gut*, vol. 58, no. 3, pp. 331–336, 2009.

[23] F. Catalano, L. Rodella, F. Lombardo et al., "Endoscopic submucosal dissection in the treatment of gastric submucosal tumors: results from a retrospective cohort study," *Gastric Cancer*, vol. 16, no. 4, pp. 563–570, 2013.

[24] S. Zhang, G.-Q. Chao, M. Li, G.-B. Ni, and B. Lv, "Endoscopic submucosal dissection for treatment of gastric submucosal tumors originating from the muscularis propria layer," *Digestive Diseases and Sciences*, vol. 58, no. 6, pp. 1710–1716, 2013.

[25] S. Godat, M. Robert, F. Caillol et al., "Efficiency and safety of endoscopic resection in the management of subepithelial lesions of the stomach," *United European Gastroenterology Journal*, vol. 4, no. 2, pp. 250–256, 2016.

[26] K. Hotta, T. Oyama, T. Akamatsu et al., "A comparison of outcomes of endoscopic submucosal dissection (ESD) For early gastric neoplasms between high-volume and low-volume centers: multi-center retrospective questionnaire study conducted by the Nagano ESD Study Group," *Internal Medicine*, vol. 49, no. 4, pp. 253–259, 2010.

[27] M. Dinis-Ribeiro, P. Pimentel-Nunes, M. Afonso, N. Costa, C. Lopes, and L. Moreira-Dias, "A European case series of endoscopic submucosal dissection for gastric superficial lesions," *Gastrointestinal Endoscopy*, vol. 69, no. 2, pp. 350–355, 2009.

Endoscopic Ultrasound Guided Rendezvous Drainage of Biliary Obstruction Using a New Flexible 19-Gauge Fine Needle Aspiration Needle

Zhouwen Tang,[1] Efehi Igbinomwanhia,[2] Sherif Elhanafi,[3] and Mohamed O. Othman[1]

[1] *Section of Gastroenterology and Hepatology, Department of Medicine, Baylor College of Medicine, Houston, TX, USA*
[2] *School of Public Health, University of Texas Science Health Center at Houston, Houston, TX, USA*
[3] *Division of Gastroenterology, Department of Medicine, University of Pennsylvania, Perelman School of Medicine, Philadelphia, PA, USA*

Correspondence should be addressed to Mohamed O. Othman; mohamed.othman@bcm.edu

Academic Editor: Lars Aabakken

Background and Aim. A successful endoscopic ultrasound guided rendezvous (EUS-RV) biliary drainage is dependent on accurate puncture of the bile duct and precise guide wire manipulation across the ampulla of Vater. We aim to study the feasibility of using a flexible 19-gauge fine aspiration needle in the performance of EUS-RV biliary drainage. *Method.* This is a retrospective case series of EUS-RV biliary drainage procedures at a single center. Patients who failed ERCP during the same session for benign or malignant biliary obstruction underwent EUS-RV using a flexible, nitinol covered, 19-gauge needle for biliary access and guide wire manipulation. *Result.* 24 patients underwent EUS-RV biliary drainage via extrahepatic access while 1 attempt was via intrahepatic access. The technical success rate was 80%, including 83.3% of cases via extrahepatic access. There was no significant difference in success rate of inpatient and outpatient procedures, benign or malignant indications, or type of guide wire used. Adverse events included mild pancreatitis (3 patients) and cholangitis (1 patient). *Conclusion.* A flexible 19-gauge needle for biliary access can be safe and effective when used to perform EUS-RV biliary drainage. Direct comparison between the nitinol needle and conventional metal needles in the performance of EUS guided biliary drainage is needed.

1. Introduction

Endoscopic retrograde cholangiopancreatography (ERCP) is a standard method for diagnostic and therapeutic intervention in many benign or malignant pancreaticobiliary conditions [1]. But every ERCP based intervention must start with successful initial cannulation of the major duodenal papilla, which is achieved approximately 90% of the time [2].

Various strategies have been developed to assist in cannulation of the common bile duct (CBD). In addition to cannulation with the standard biliary catheter or sphincterotome, biliary guide wire assisted cannulation [3], pancreatic duct guide wire assisted cannulation [4], pancreatic duct stent assisted cannulation [5], needle-knife papillotomy [6], and suprapapillary fistulotomy [7] have been described and are in clinical use [8]. Yet when access sphincterotomy fails to result in deep biliary cannulation or when the papilla is inaccessible such as in the setting of surgically altered anatomy, gastrointestinal tract obstruction, or high grade biliary obstruction, alternative methods of biliary access and drainage are required.

Radiological methods such as percutaneous transhepatic cholangiography (PTC) and surgical intervention are well described as alternative methods but suffer from high complication rates and significant morbidity [9, 10]. PTC is further limited by the cosmetic and nonphysiological sequelae of external biliary drainage [11].

Linear array endoscopic ultrasound (EUS) was developed as a diagnostic modality for biliary and pancreatic neoplasms but its use has since been extended, with the aid of Doppler capabilities, to a broad collection of interventional procedures, including EUS guided biliary drainage (EUS-BD) [12].

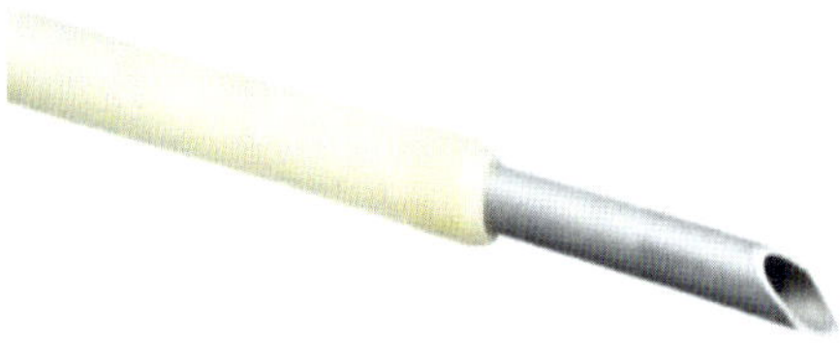

Figure 1: Flexible 19-gauge fine needle aspiration needle.

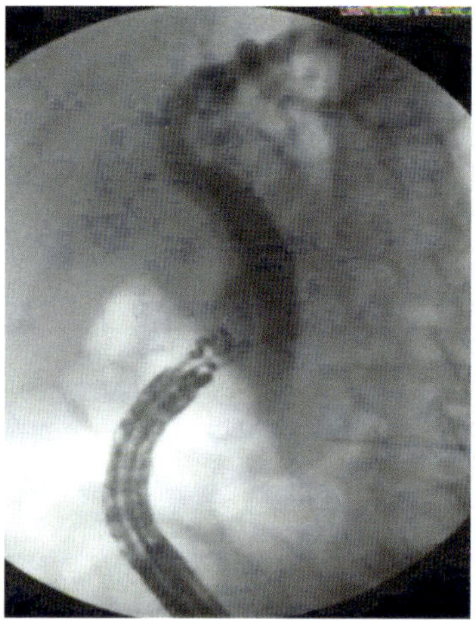

Figure 2: EUS guided cholangiogram.

EUS-BD may be categorized according to access method and drainage route. The bile duct may be accessed by either the intrahepatic or extrahepatic portions, typically with a 19- or 22-gauge fine needle aspiration (FNA) needle. Intrahepatic access may be transgastric, transesophageal, or transjejunal (in surgically altered anatomy) with typical initial puncture into the left hepatic lobe. Extrahepatic access is usually transduodenal and progresses into the CBD. Once accessed, biliary drainage methods include direct transmural or transluminal drainage, antegrade transpapillary placement of a biliary stent, or guide wire rendezvous with a duodenoscope allowing subsequent conventional ERCP management. This last method, termed EUS guided rendezvous (EUS-RV), is preferred as the initial option for EUS-BD by many practitioners because it avoids the creation of a permanent biliary-enteric fistula and complications of fistula creation including bile leak and perforation [13, 14].

Extrahepatic EUS-RV may be performed with the echoendoscope in either long or short positions. In the short position, the point of puncture is in the second portion of the duodenum with the needle pointed toward the papilla. However, this position suffers from relative echoendoscope instability. In the long position, the echoendoscope is stabilized in the duodenal bulb but the needle typically points toward the hepatic hilum due to the stiffness of conventional stainless steel FNA needles therefore hindering passage of the guide wire across the papilla [15].

Recently, Varadarajulu et al. [16] described the successful technical performance of a flexible nitinol covered FNA needle (Expect™ 19-gauge flex, Boston Scientific, Marlborough, MA, USA) for transduodenal sampling of the pancreatic head/uncinate, a process that had also suffered from technical limitations with conventional stiff stainless steel FNA needles [17, 18].

Experience with this flexible needle in EUS-RV has not been specifically described in the literature. Since guide wire manipulation may be a leading factor in failed EUS-BD [19], we hypothesized that using a nitinol covered flexible 19-gauge FNA needle (Figure 1) will improve the ease of performance of EUS-RV and hence serve as a viable access device. Therefore, we aim to assess the technical and clinical performance of the flexible 19-gauge FNA needle in EUS-RV.

2. Methods

This is a single center retrospective study of EUS guided rendezvous biliary drainage procedures. We reviewed the electronic medical and endoscopic records at University Medical Center (El Paso, TX, USA) to identify all consecutive EUS-BD procedures using the Expect 19-gauge flexible needle for biliary access from January 2012 until March 2014. Patients needing EUS-BD following failed ERCP for biliary obstruction within the same session were included. The study was approved by the Institutional Review Board of the University Medical Center at El Paso, TX, USA, and complied with Health Insurance Portability and Accountability Act regulations.

Each procedure was performed in a hospital endoscopy unit and each patient was placed under either general anesthesia or monitored anesthesia care. Preprocedural prophylaxis antibiotics were given. A linear Olympus GF-UC140P echoendoscope (Olympus America Inc., Center Valley, PA, USA) with a ProSound SSD 5000 processor (Aloka, Wallingford, CT, USA) was used to identify the desired access point for EUS-BD. Color Doppler was used to identify intervening blood vessels. Extrahepatic versus intrahepatic access was at the discretion of the endoscopist. A 19-gauge flexible FNA needle Expect (Boston Scientific Natick, MA, USA) was used to puncture the bile duct at the desired location. Bile was aspirated and contrast medium injected for cholangiography (Figure 2). An angled tip guide wire was then inserted through the needle and passed across the ampulla of Vater into the duodenum in anterograde fashion under fluoroscopic guidance. Guide wires used were the 0.025 in × 450 cm VisiGlide (Olympus America Inc., Center Valley, PA, USA), 0.035 in × 480 cm Tracer Metro (Cook Medical, Bloomington, IN, USA), or the 0.035 in × 450 cm Dreamwire or Jagwire (Boston Scientific, Marlborough, MA, USA) per operator preference. The echoendoscope was then removed over the guide wire and a TJV-Q180V duodenoscope (Olympus America Inc., Center Valley, PA) was advanced parallel to the guide wire until it was adjacent to the ampulla. Depending on the operator preference, a standard sphincterotome was used to cannulate the CBD alongside the RV wire or the intraluminal free end of the guide wire was then grasped with forceps and brought through the working channel of the duodenoscope. After that, ERCP was performed per conventional fashion, including biliary sphincterotomy, stone extraction,

TABLE 1: Baseline characteristics of study population.

Characteristics	EUS-RV ($n = 25$)
Age, y, mean (±SD)	69.1 (±16.8)
Female, number (%)	15 (60)
Race	
Hispanic, number (%)	15 (60)
White, number (%)	8 (32)
Other, number (%)	2 (8)
BMI (±SD)	27.4 (±6.5)
Indications	
Malignant obstruction, number (%)	13 (52)
Benign obstruction, number (%)	10 (40)
Bile leak, number (%)	1 (4)
Biliary dilation, number (%)	1 (4)
Inpatient, number (%)	18 (72)
Outpatient, number (%)	7 (28)

stent placement, and/or stricture dilation as indicated and EUS-RV was deemed technically successful. A single expert endoscopist performed all procedures (MO).

Each patient's demographics, indications for procedure, sedation methods, procedure time, and procedural outcomes, including procedure related complications, were collected in the database. Severity of adverse events such as pancreatitis, cholangitis, or hemorrhage is defined as outlined by Schmit et al. [20]. Data is reported in descriptive statistics where applicable and categorical variables were compared using chi squared tests.

3. Results

Our database included 25 patients who met the inclusion criteria with mean age of 69.1 ± 16.8 years (range 22–97 years) of which 15 (60%) were females. Baseline characteristics of the study are summarized in Table 1. The indications for the procedure were malignant obstruction of the bile ducts in 13 patients (52%), benign obstruction of the bile ducts (stone/benign stricture) in 10 patients (40%), bile leak in 1 patient (4%), and biliary dilation in 1 patient (4%).

Per protocol, all 25 patients had a previously failed ERCP; reasons for failure were deformed ampulla in 8 patients (32%), failure to cannulate in 6 patients (24%), deformed duodenum in 4 patients (16%), periampullary diverticula in 4 patients (16%), and biliary stricture in 3 patients (12%).

Mean procedure time, including EUS-RV after failed conventional ERCP in a single session, was 103 ± 38 minutes. VisiGlide guide wire was used in 13 (52%) procedures with the balance of the procedures using other guide wires detailed above. Procedures using the VisiGlide guide wire had a success rate of 92.3% (12 of 13 cases) while procedures using other guide wires had a success rate of 67.85 (8 of 12 cases). This difference was not statistically significant ($P = 0.11$). There was also no statistically significant difference in success rates between cases performed for benign (10/12, 83.3%) versus malignant indications (10/13, 77%, $P = 0.69$) or between inpatients (13/18, 72%) and outpatients (7/7, 100%, $P = 0.11$).

TABLE 2: Clinical outcomes.

	Success, number (%)	P value
Overall	20/25 (80)	
Extrahepatic access	20/24 (83.3)	
Intrahepatic access	0/1 (0)	
Benign	10/12 (83.3)	
Malignant	10/13 (77)	0.69
Inpatient	13/18 (72)	
Outpatient	7/7 (100)	0.11
VisiGlide guidewire	12/13	
Other guidewires	8/12	0.11

Successful EUS guided biliary access and cholangiogram were achieved in all the 25 patients. Successful EUS-RV was achieved in 20 of 25 patients (80%), including 20 of 24 patients (83.3%) in which extrahepatic biliary access was attempted (Table 2). The impossibility to guide the wire into the direction of the distal common bile duct was the reason for failure in the above-mentioned four cases. All procedures were done in the long scope position.

One unsuccessful attempt at EUS-RV via intrahepatic access was made in a patient with a malignant biliary obstruction of the proximal common bile duct. In this case, puncture of the intrahepatic bile duct was successful but the guide wire could not be advanced past the common bile duct stricture and the patient was referred for PTC. This was also the only patient who had a postsurgical anatomy as she had a roux-en-y choledochojejunostomy for prior bile duct injury. The remaining patients all had normal bowel continuity.

Of the 4 patients with failed EUS-RV via extrahepatic access, 1 patient had a severe duodenal deformity of benign etiology which precluded identification of the ampulla, 1 patient had a severe duodenal deformity arising from a large head of the pancreas adenocarcinoma that prevented passage of the guide wire, 1 patient had a large cystic neoplasm in the head of the pancreas that prevented passage of the guide wire, and 1 patient had a large periampullary diverticulum. All 4 of these patients were referred for PTC.

Complications were reported in 4 (16%) patients. Three patients (12%) had mild acute pancreatitis. One patient had cholangitis (4%). All complications were resolved within 3 days after the procedure. There was no periprocedural mortality.

4. Discussion

Interventional EUS is one of the leading fronts of endoscopic innovation and EUS-BD is an apt example of the potential for innovative, less costly, and less invasive endoscopic alternatives to traditional management techniques for high mortality gastrointestinal illness. From its first description in 1996 by Wiersema et al. [21] of EUS guided transluminal cholangiography, this technique has been advanced to direct EUS guided transluminal biliary drainage, which was first described by Giovannini et al. in 2001 [22], and subsequently to EUS-RV by Mallery et al. [23]. The specific role of EUS guided transmural drainage and EUS-RV, both with

Table 3: Outcomes of EUS-RV Studies > 15 Patients; a: 5 patients with failed intrahepatic access subsequently underwent extrahepatic access.

Study	Method	Needle size	Extrahepatic access Success rate, % (*n*)	Intrahepatic access Success rate, % (*n*)	Overall Success rate, % (*n*)	Adverse events Rate, % (*n*)	Adverse events details
Kahaleh et al. [24] (2006)	RS	19- or 22-gauge	70 (7/10)	61 (11/18)	78 (18/23)[†]	17 (4/23)	Pneumoperitoneum 2, bile leak 1, bleeding 1
Shah et al. [25] (2012)	RS	19- or 22-gauge	NS	NS	74 (37/50)	12 (6/50)	Pancreatitis 4, bile leak 1, duodenal perforation 1
Artifon et al. [26] (2012)	RS	19-gauge	98 (57/58)	NS	98 (57/58)	3 (2/58)	Pericholedochal contrast leak 2
Iwashita et al. [27] (2012)	RS	19-gauge	81 (25/31)	44 (4/9)	73 (29/40)	13 (5/40)	Pancreatitis 2, abdominal pain 1, pneumoperitoneum 1, sepsis/death within four days of procedure 1
Park et al. [28] (2013)	PS	19-gauge	93 (13/14)[†]	50 (3/6)	80 (16/20)	14 (2/14)	Pancreatitis 1, bile peritonitis 1
Dhir et al. [29] (2013)	RS	19-gauge	94 (16/17)	100 (18/18)	97 (34/35)	23 (8/35)	Pain alone 4, bile leak 2, pneumoperitoneum 2
Dhir et al. [30] (2014)	RS	19-gauge	NS	NS	100 (20/20)	15 (3/20)	NS
Current study	RS	19-gauge	83.3 (20/24)	0 (0/1)	80 (20/25)	16 (4/25)	Pancreatitis 3, cholangitis 1

[†]5 patients with failed intrahepatic access subsequently underwent successful extrahepatic access.
NS, not specified; RS, retrospective; PS, prospective.

respect to each other and to non-EUS guided drainage modalities, remains to be clarified. EUS-RV seems to perform favorably compared to EUS guided transmural drainage, with retrospective studies having shown no difference in technical success or adverse event rates [13].

Our retrospective study demonstrated the efficacy and safety of a nitinol covered 19-gauge flexible FNA needle in the performance of EUS-RV. Khashab et al. [13] reported on the use of the Expect 19-gauge flex needle in a retrospective study protocol but did not specify the proportion of procedures using this needle versus conventional 22-gauge FNA needles in attempted EUS-RV. To our knowledge, the current study is the first to specifically report the performance of this flexible needle for EUS-RV.

The current study included patients with both benign and malignant indications for biliary intervention who had prior failed ERCP for a multiple reasons. We achieved successful EUS guided biliary access in 100% of patients and completed rendezvous with subsequent completion ERCP in 84% of our patients. Though we only had one patient who underwent intrahepatic biliary access, the focus on extrahepatic access was consistent with the anticipated advantage of the more flexible needle in allowing both long and short echoendoscope positioning. The flexibility of the needle allowed for 100% success in gaining biliary access and obtaining cholangiogram. Our complication rate was 16% with 3 of the 4 instances being mild acute pancreatitis. These results are consistent with a review of previous published moderate and large scale retrospective studies of EUS-RV (Table 3).

Though there has not been a published prospective study of EUS-RV methods, a randomized controlled trial comparing EUS guided hepaticogastrostomy (EUS-HPG, intrahepatic) versus EUS guided choledochoduodenstomy (EUS-CD, extrahepatic) in patients with malignant biliary stricture enrolled 9 patients who had unsuccessful EUS-RV out of 30 cases attempted in total, yielding an EUS-RV success rate of 70% (21/30). No statistically significant differences were found between the two techniques, with technical success rate of 96% for EUS-HPG and 91% for EUS-CD [31]. This is in contrast to a previously published retrospective study in which intrahepatic access route was an independent risk factor for increased complications from EUS-BD [32].

Other retrospective studies have shown no difference in complication rates between EUS-RV and EUS guided transluminal biliary drainage [13]. When compared with a historical cohort of patients who had precut papillotomy, EUS-RV resulted in better technical success without increase in complications [33].

As seen in recent study protocols, EUS-RV is starting to occupy a rational spot along the escalation of biliary access techniques between precut papillotomy and EUS guided direct transluminal biliary drainage [13, 31]. Direct transluminal drainage has been shown to be equivalent to PTC in success and complication rates when utilized after failed EUS-RV [26] and EUS-BD appears to be equivalent to ERCP for short term outcomes in relief of malignant distal CBD obstruction [32].

Our study has several limitations. It was a retrospective study at a single institution of procedures performed by a single endoscopist and therefore subject to selection bias and limiting generalizability. In addition, we did not directly compare the flexible 19-gauge FNA needle with conventional access needles used in EUS-BD. We also used different types of angle tipped guide wires in our series though technical success rates did not differ between wire types. Finally, our study included only short term periprocedural follow-up. Even so, our study fills an important need for published experience with refined EUS-BD techniques and devices in line with other recent reports [34, 35].

As with development of therapeutic ERCP a generation ago, EUS-BD will benefit from further studies to identify its place within the armamentarium of gastrointestinal interventions [36]. Because of the relative rarity of failed ERCP cannulation, future randomized trials may necessarily be multicentered. For example, EUS guided antegrade transpapillary drainage has not been directly compared with transmural drainage; such a study may be important since EUS-RV is not feasible if the papilla cannot be reached due to surgically altered anatomy or luminal obstruction. With further refinement of technique, formalization of protocol, and development of dedicated devices, EUS-BD may yet become an effective solution to the knotty problem of biliary drainage after failed ERCP.

Additional Points

Successful completion of EUS guided rendezvous biliary drainage is dependent on accurate puncture of the bile duct and precise guide wire manipulation across the ampulla of Vater. A flexible nitinol covered 19-gauge needle for biliary access can be safe and effective when used to perform EUS guided rendezvous biliary drainage.

Competing Interests

The authors disclose no competing interests.

Authors' Contributions

The manuscript has been read and approved by all the authors, the requirements for authorship have been met, and each author believes that the manuscript represents honest work.

References

[1] T. H. Baron, "Endoscopic management of biliary disorders: diagnostic and therapeutic," *Surgical Clinics of North America*, vol. 94, no. 2, pp. 395–411, 2014.

[2] A. T. Debenedet, B. J. Elmunzer, S. T. McCarthy, G. H. Elta, and P. S. Schoenfeld, "Intraprocedural quality in endoscopic retrograde cholangiopancreatography: a meta-analysis," *American Journal of Gastroenterology*, vol. 108, no. 11, pp. 1696–1704, 2013.

[3] F. Lella, F. Bagnolo, E. Colombo, and U. Bonassi, "A simple way of avoiding post-ERCP pancreatitis," *Gastrointestinal Endoscopy*, vol. 59, no. 7, pp. 830–834, 2004.

[4] S. Maeda, H. Hayashi, O. Hosokawa et al., "Prospective randomized pilot trial of selective biliary cannulation using pancreatic guide-wire placement," *Endoscopy*, vol. 35, no. 9, pp. 721–724, 2003.

[5] E. Goldberg, M. Titus, O. Haluszka, and P. Darwin, "Pancreatic-duct stent placement facilitates difficult common bile duct cannulation," *Gastrointestinal Endoscopy*, vol. 62, no. 4, pp. 592–596, 2005.

[6] T. Rabenstein, T. Ruppert, H. T. Schneider, E. G. Hahn, and C. Ell, "Benefits and risks of needle-knife papillotomy," *Gastrointestinal Endoscopy*, vol. 46, no. 3, pp. 207–211, 1997.

[7] J. J. Park, S. S. Kim, Y. K. Kim et al., "Biliary drainage by endoscopic choledochoduodenal fistulotomy in patients with papillary carcinoma," *Gastrointestinal Endoscopy*, vol. 55, no. 6, pp. 730–735, 2002.

[8] V. Cennamo, L. Fuccio, R. M. Zagari et al., "Can early precut implementation reduce endoscopic retrograde cholangiopancreatography-related complication risk? Meta-analysis of randomized controlled trials," *Endoscopy*, vol. 42, no. 5, pp. 381–388, 2010.

[9] P. M. Spanheimer, A. R. Cyr, J. Liao et al., "Complications and survival associated with operative procedures in patients with unresectable pancreatic head adenocarcinoma," *Journal of Surgical Oncology*, vol. 109, no. 7, pp. 697–701, 2014.

[10] A. Weber, J. Gaa, B. Rosca et al., "Complications of percutaneous transhepatic biliary drainage in patients with dilated and nondilated intrahepatic bile ducts," *European Journal of Radiology*, vol. 72, no. 3, pp. 412–417, 2009.

[11] P. R. Mueller, E. Van Sonnenberg, and J. T. Ferrucci Jr., "Percutaneous biliary drainage: technical and catheter-related problems in 200 procedures," *American Journal of Roentgenology*, vol. 138, no. 1, pp. 17–23, 1982.

[12] D. Prichard, "Endoscopic ultrasound guided biliary and pancreatic duct interventions," *World Journal of Gastrointestinal Endoscopy*, vol. 6, no. 11, pp. 513–524, 2014.

[13] M. A. Khashab, A. K. Valeshabad, R. Modayil et al., "EUS-guided biliary drainage by using a standardized approach for malignant biliary obstruction: rendezvous versus direct transluminal techniques (with videos)," *Gastrointestinal Endoscopy*, vol. 78, no. 5, pp. 734–741, 2013.

[14] S. Varadarajulu and R. H. Hawes, "EUS-guided biliary drainage: taxing and not ready," *Gastrointestinal Endoscopy*, vol. 78, no. 5, pp. 742–743, 2013.

[15] T. Iwashita, S. Doi, and I. Yasuda, "Endoscopic ultrasound-guided biliary drainage: a review," *Clinical Journal of Gastroenterology*, vol. 7, no. 2, pp. 94–102, 2014.

[16] S. Varadarajulu, J. Y. Bang, and S. Hebert-Magee, "Assessment of the technical performance of the flexible 19-gauge EUS-FNA needle," *Gastrointestinal Endoscopy*, vol. 76, no. 2, pp. 336–343, 2012.

[17] A. Larghi, E. C. Verna, S. N. Stavropoulos, H. Rotterdam, C. J. Lightdale, and P. D. Stevens, "EUS-guided trucut needle biopsies in patients with solid pancreatic masses: a prospective study," *Gastrointestinal Endoscopy*, vol. 59, no. 2, pp. 185–190, 2004.

[18] J. Iglesias-Garcia, J.-W. Poley, A. Larghi et al., "Feasibility and yield of a new EUS histology needle: results from a multicenter, pooled, cohort study," *Gastrointestinal Endoscopy*, vol. 73, no. 6, pp. 1189–1196, 2011.

[19] J. J. Vila, M. Pérez-Miranda, E. Vazquez-Sequeiros et al., "Initial experience with EUS-guided cholangiopancreatography for biliary and pancreatic duct drainage: a Spanish national survey," *Gastrointestinal Endoscopy*, vol. 76, no. 6, pp. 1133–1141, 2012.

[20] A. Schmit, G. Lazaraki, A. Hittelet, M. Cremer, O. Le Moine, and J. Devière, "Complications of endoscopic retrograde cholangiopancreatography during live endoscopy workshop demonstrations," *Endoscopy*, vol. 37, no. 8, pp. 695–699, 2005.

[21] M. J. Wiersema, D. Sandusky, R. Carr, L. M. Wiersema, W. C. Erdel, and P. K. Frederick, "Endosonography-guided cholangiopancreatography," *Gastrointestinal Endoscopy*, vol. 43, no. 2, pp. 102–106, 1996.

[22] M. Giovannini, V. Moutardier, C. Pesenti, E. Bories, B. Lelong, and J. R. Delpero, "Endoscopic ultrasound-guided bilioduodenal anastomosis: a new technique for biliary drainage," *Endoscopy*, vol. 33, no. 10, pp. 898–900, 2001.

[23] S. Mallery, J. Matlock, and M. L. Freeman, "EUS-guided rendezvous drainage of obstructed biliary and pancreatic ducts: report of 6 cases," *Gastrointestinal Endoscopy*, vol. 59, no. 1, pp. 100–107, 2004.

[24] M. Kahaleh, A. J. Hernandez, J. Tokar, R. B. Adams, V. M. Shami, and P. Yeaton, "Interventional EUS-guided cholangiography: evaluation of a technique in evolution," *Gastrointestinal Endoscopy*, vol. 64, no. 1, pp. 52–59, 2006.

[25] J. N. Shah, F. Marson, F. Weilert et al., "Single-operator, single-session EUS-guided anterograde cholangiopancreatography in failed ERCP or inaccessible papilla," *Gastrointestinal Endoscopy*, vol. 75, no. 1, pp. 56–64, 2012.

[26] E. L. A. Artifon, D. Aparicio, J. B. Paione et al., "Biliary drainage in patients with unresectable, malignant obstruction where ERCP fails: endoscopic ultrasonography-guided choledochoduodenostomy versus percutaneous drainage," *Journal of Clinical Gastroenterology*, vol. 46, no. 9, pp. 768–774, 2012.

[27] T. Iwashita, J. G. Lee, S. Shinoura et al., "Endoscopic ultrasound-guided rendezvous for biliary access after failed cannulation," *Endoscopy*, vol. 44, no. 1, pp. 60–65, 2012.

[28] D. H. Park, S. U. Jeong, B. U. Lee et al., "Prospective evaluation of a treatment algorithm with enhanced guidewire manipulation protocol for EUS-guided biliary drainage after failed ERCP (with video)," *Gastrointestinal Endoscopy*, vol. 78, no. 1, pp. 91–101, 2013.

[29] V. Dhir, S. Bhandari, M. Bapat, N. Joshi, S. Vivekanandarajah, and A. Maydeo, "Comparison of transhepatic and extrahepatic routes for EUS-guided rendezvous procedure for distal CBD obstruction," *United European Gastroenterology Journal*, vol. 1, no. 2, pp. 103–108, 2013.

[30] V. Dhir, E. L. A. Artifon, K. Gupta et al., "Multicenter study on endoscopic ultrasound-guided expandable biliary metal stent placement: choice of access route, direction of stent insertion, and drainage route," *Digestive Endoscopy*, vol. 26, no. 3, pp. 430–435, 2014.

[31] E. L. A. Artifon, F. P. Marson, M. Gaidhane, M. Kahaleh, and J. P. Otoch, "Hepaticogastrostomy or choledochoduodenostomy for distal malignant biliary obstruction after failed ERCP: is there any difference?" *Gastrointestinal Endoscopy*, vol. 81, no. 4, pp. 950–959, 2015.

[32] V. Dhir, T. Itoi, M. A. Khashab et al., "Multicenter comparative evaluation of endoscopic placement of expandable metal stents for malignant distal common bile duct obstruction by ERCP or EUS-guided approach," *Gastrointestinal Endoscopy*, vol. 81, no. 4, pp. 913–923, 2015.

[33] V. Dhir, S. Bhandari, M. Bapat, and A. Maydeo, "Comparison of EUS-guided rendezvous and precut papillotomy techniques for biliary access (with videos)," *Gastrointestinal Endoscopy*, vol. 75, no. 2, pp. 354–359, 2012.

[34] T. J. Song, S. S. Lee, D. H. Park, D. W. Seo, S. K. Lee, and M.-H. Kim, "Preliminary report on a new hybrid metal stent for EUS-guided biliary drainage (with videos)," *Gastrointestinal Endoscopy*, vol. 80, no. 4, pp. 707–711, 2015.

[35] W. H. Paik, D. H. Park, J.-H. Choi et al., "Simplified fistula dilation technique and modified stent deployment maneuver for EUS-guided hepaticogastrostomy," *World Journal of Gastroenterology*, vol. 20, no. 17, pp. 5051–5059, 2014.

[36] C. Fabbri, C. Luigiano, A. Lisotti et al., "Endoscopic ultrasound-guided treatments: are we getting evidence based—a systematic review," *World Journal of Gastroenterology*, vol. 20, no. 26, pp. 8424–8448, 2014.

27

The Role of EUS-BD in the Management of Malignant Biliary Obstruction: The Indonesian Perspective

Dadang Makmun, Achmad Fauzi, Murdani Abdullah, and Ari Fahrial Syam

Division of Gastroenterology, Department of Internal Medicine, Faculty of Medicine, Universitas Indonesia, Cipto Mangunkusumo National General Hospital, Jakarta Pusat, Jakarta 10430, Indonesia

Correspondence should be addressed to Dadang Makmun; dadangmakmun1959@gmail.com

Academic Editor: Tony C. K. Tham

Aims. To evaluate the success rate and related factors of endoscopic ultrasound guided-biliary drainage (EUS-BD). *Material and Methods.* We conducted a retrospective study among 24 patients with malignant biliary obstruction who underwent EUS-BD after failed ERCP from January 2015 to December 2016 in a tertiary health center. The bilirubin levels before and after the procedure were used to define the clinical success rate, while the stent deployment was used to define the technical success rate. We placed either transluminal biliary stents or transpapillary biliary stents. *Results.* Among 24 patients, choledochoduodenostomy technique was conducted in 23 patients (95.8%) and hepaticogastrostomy technique in 1 patient (4.2%). Transluminal stent placement was conducted in 23 patients, while transpapillary stent placement was conducted in 1 patient. The clinical success rate was 78.2% (18) in choledochoduodenostomy route and 100% (1) in hepaticogastrostomy route. EUS-BD was 2.37 times and 2.11 times more likely to be successful in reducing the bilirubin level in patients with tumor of the head of pancreas and periampullary tumor, respectively, but not in cholangiocarcinoma. *Conclusions.* EUS-BD is an effective and efficient procedure to achieve biliary drainage among patients with malignant biliary obstruction after ERCP failure.

1. Introduction

Obstructive jaundice occurs when there is an obstruction to the passage of bile from the liver to the duodenum. The cause of this condition varies from benign conditions to malignant conditions in the biliary system. Obstructive jaundice is not a definitive diagnosis; it requires additional examinations and diagnostic procedures to determine the primary disease. The mortality and morbidity of obstructive jaundice depend on the cause of the obstruction [1].

Currently, endoscopic retrograde cholangiopancreatography (ERCP) is the main therapeutic procedure used in the management of biliary obstruction. For many decades, percutaneous transhepatic biliary drainage (PTBD) and surgical interventions have been the alternative procedures when ERCP failed to achieve biliary drainage, but those methods have been related to high-risk complications and prolonged hospitalization [2, 3].

Endoscopic ultrasonography (EUS), which was developed in the early 1980s, has become a valuable imaging modality to visualize the gastrointestinal luminal wall and its surrounding structures, including the pancreatobiliary system. The large channel echo endoscopes of EUS have allowed for the therapeutic application of EUS by combining real-time ultrasound and fluoroscopy imaging of ERCP to carry out an EUS-biliary drainage (EUS-BD). EUS-BD can be used as a less invasive alternative procedure instead of PTBD and surgical intervention. The superiority of EUS-BD compared to ERCP and PTBD includes the possibility of accessing the bile duct system through many routes. Wiersema et al. were the first to report on EUS-guided diagnostic cholangiography in 1996, and in 2001 Giovannini et al. reported the first EUS-BD using transduodenal stenting to create a choledochoduodenal fistula with a needle knife. After this initial report, many studies reported modifications of the techniques and expanding indications for EUS-BD. EUS is relatively new in Indonesia and it was firstly introduced in our hospital, Cipto Mangunkusumo National General Hospital, a top national referral hospital, in 2013. In 2015 our experienced endoscopists started to develop EUS-BD after being trained from several endoscopy training centers in Asia such as India and Thailand. Until today, only seven among more than 2,000 hospitals in our country provide EUS facilities. For EUS-BD procedure, the most frequently used stent is plastic stent due to the price and its availability. Recently, EUS-BD is one of the treatments of choice to perform biliary drainage when ERCP has failed [2, 4–7].

EUS-BD techniques are divided into two categories, a rendezvous technique and a direct access technique. In the rendezvous technique for EUS-BD, a temporary fistula at the stomach or the bulb is created followed by placement of a guidewire through the biliary duct and the ampulla into the duodenum; then, ERCP is reperformed using the EUS-guided placed wire. The direct access technique includes EUS-guided choledochoduodenostomy (EUS-CDS), EUS-guided hepaticogastrostomy (EUS-HGS), and EUS-guided gallbladder drainage (EUS-GBD) [8, 9].

This study aimed to retrospectively evaluate the primary diseases, access route, and success rate of stent placement and related factors among patients with malignant biliary obstruction who underwent EUS-BD after failed ERCP at a top national referral hospital.

2. Materials and Methods

2.1. Patient Characteristics. This study was conducted among patients with malignant biliary obstruction who underwent EUS-BD after failed ERCP from January 2015 to December 2016 ($n = 24$) at a top national referral hospital. We collected data from 755 patients who underwent ERCP, and 241 among them were diagnosed with malignant biliary obstruction such as tumor of head of pancreas, periampullary tumor, cholangiocarcinoma, and Klatskin tumor. From the 241 patients, we excluded patients who had a successful ERCP procedure, resulting in 24 patients who required an alternative technique for biliary drainage due to failed ERCP.

All patients enrolled in this study were diagnosed as having inoperable malignant obstructive jaundice based on clinical symptoms (jaundice, dark-colored urine, and pale stool), laboratory examinations (elevated bilirubin levels, alkaline phosphatase levels, and gamma glutamyl transferase levels), and imaging examinations including transabdominal ultrasound, computed tomography (CT) scan of the abdomen, magnetic resonance cholangiopancreatography (MRCP), and EUS.

2.2. Access Routes and Drainage Route. The EUS-BD procedure was performed by experienced endoscopists who have performed over 100 EUS procedures. EUS-CDS was performed through the transluminal route from the duodenal bulb into the bile duct in 23 patients (transduodenal access), and EUS-HGS was performed through the transluminal route from the stomach into the bile duct in 1 patient (transhepatic access) where insertion of the scope into the duodenum failed.

We used an Olympus GF type UCT 180 linear echoendoscope. The scope was introduced into the stomach or the duodenum. After visualization of the dilated bile duct, the scope was manipulated until an appropriate puncture route was identified. The stomach or the duodenal wall was then punctured with a 19-G needle (EchoTip Ultra; Cook Medical) into the bile duct. After that, a guidewire was inserted, and the fistula was dilated with an electrical needle knife (Zimmon papillotomy knife or Cystotome; Cook Medical) to facilitate stent placement. We placed a 10 Fr Cotton-Leung plastic stent in 21 patients and a fully covered self-expandable metallic stent (SEMS) with diameter of 10 mm in 3 patients. All stents were inserted in either an antegrade direction or retrograde direction (rendezvous technique). The insertion in the antegrade direction was performed after creating a tract from the stomach or duodenum into the bile duct, and the stent was placed following guidewire insertion. The insertion in retrograde direction was performed by inserting a guidewire into the bile duct and maneuvering it across the papilla into the duodenum. After that, the echoendoscope was withdrawn, leaving the guidewire. Then, the duodenoscope was inserted parallel to the guidewire until it was in front of the papilla. The guidewire was then caught with a snare through the working channel of the duodenoscope, and finally the stent was placed using a conventional ERCP procedure. The procedure of EUS-BD in a patient with a periampullary tumor is shown in Figure 1.

The results of the EUS-BD procedures were assessed using the technical success rate and clinical success rate. The technical success rate was defined as the success of deployment of the stent at the end of the procedure. The clinical success rate was defined as a 30% decrease in the bilirubin level one week after the procedure [10].

2.3. Data Collection. We retrospectively collected the data of the enrolled patients by reviewing the medical records of our hospital, including demographic data (age, gender, and body mass index (BMI)), EUS-BD technique (hepaticogastrostomy or choledochoduodenostomy), laboratory data (bilirubin levels, alkaline phosphatase levels, and gamma glutamyl transferase levels), primary disease (tumor of head of pancreas, periampullary tumor, or cholangiocarcinoma), EUS-BD indication, and complications. The collected data were then classified based on published literature to make them easier to analyze.

The patients were divided into groups based on demographic data such as age and BMI. The patients were divided by age in the group < 60 years and the group ≥ 60 years, while for the BMI data we used the World Health Organization (WHO) recommendation for Asian criteria of BMI classification to interpret the results. The patients were divided into those with difficult cannulation and those with unidentifiable ampulla based on the EUS-BD indication data. The laboratory data included the bilirubin level before the procedure and one week after the procedure. Complications that were observed included all complications that occurred during or after the EUS-BD procedure, such as bleeding, perforation, pneumoperitoneum, cholangitis, bile leakage, and death.

2.4. Statistical Analysis. All collected data were analyzed using univariate analysis to evaluate the correlation between the independent variables and dependent variables. The independent variables included age, gender, BMI, primary

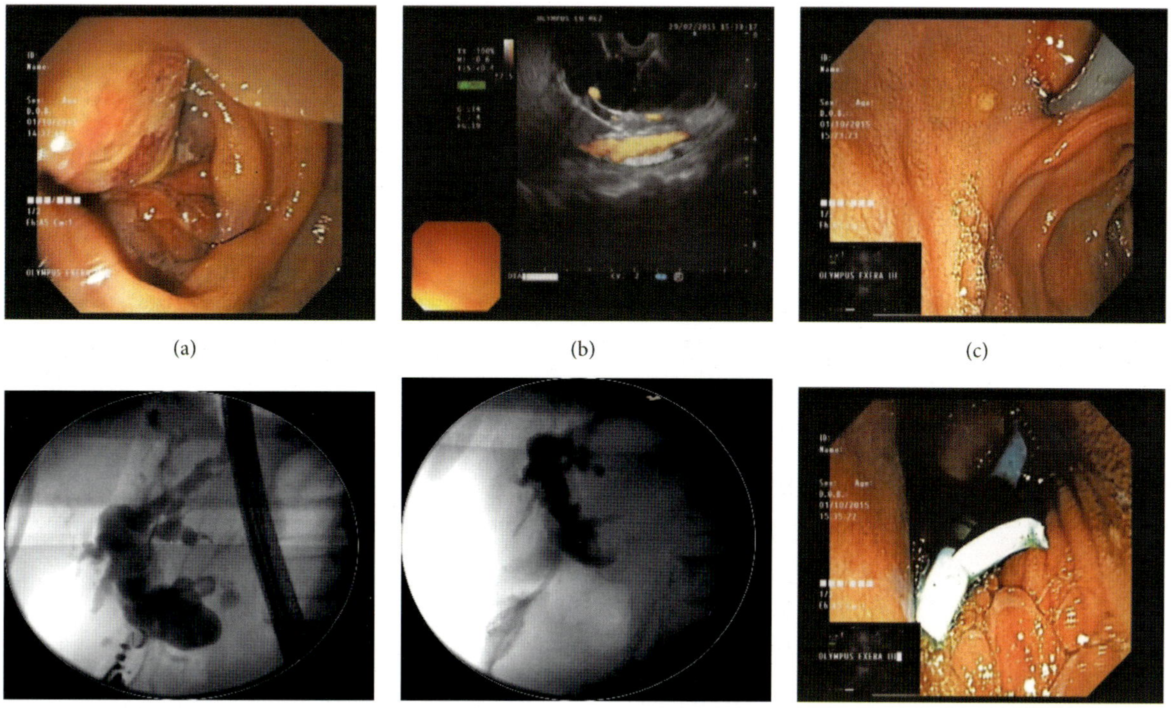

FIGURE 1: EUS-BD in a patient with a periampullary tumor with unidentifiable ampulla and failed ERCP: (a) endoscopy view of the periampullary tumor; (b) EUS imaging of the puncture into dilated CBD; (c) puncture point enlargement using Cystotome; (d) dilated intra- and extrahepatic CBD; (e) transduodenal plastic biliary stent placement; (f) bile drainage through the stent.

disease, EUS-BD indication, and EUS-BD complications. The dependent variable was the clinical success rate of all enrolled patients.

The Chi-square test method was used to examine the statistical significance of the correlation between dependent and independent variables. The required conditions for the Chi-square tests were that the value of the expected count inside the 2×2 table should be more than 5, and if the value was less than 5, we used the Fisher's exact test. The result was considered significant when p value < 0.05, and if the p value > 0.05, it was considered to be insignificant. Data analysis was done using SPSS computer software version 23.0 (version 23.0; IBM SPSS, IBM Corp., Armonk, NY, USA).

3. Results

Among the 24 patients who underwent EUS-BD, 54.2% were male, and 45.8% were female. The age of the patients ranged from 37 to 80 years with 54.2% aged < 60 years and 45.8% aged ≥ 60 years. According to BMI criteria, 29.2% were underweight, 45.8% were normoweight, and 25% were preobese. Primary diseases affecting the patients included tumor of the head of pancreas (54.2%), periampullary tumor (41.6%), and cholangiocarcinoma (4.2%). We also found that the most widely used EUS-BD technique was choledochoduodenostomy (95.8%). The indication of EUS-BD among all patients included difficult cannulation (66.7%) and unidentifiable ampulla (33.3%). Among 23 patients who underwent EUS-CDS, 20 received plastic stent and 3 received fully covered SEMS. One patient who underwent EUS-HGS received plastic stent. Stent placement in all patients was facilitated with electrical needle knife (Cystotome). Complications were developed in 4 patients (16.7%). Pneumoperitoneum caused by perforation during the procedure was found in 1 patient, and cholangitis was found in 3 patients. As a result, all 4 patients died within one week after the procedure. The causes of death included general peritonitis which occurred shortly after perforation and septic shock due to cholangitis. The characteristic of all subjects is summarized in Table 1.

In this study, stent placement could be achieved among patients who underwent EUS-BD procedure. The analysis showed that the technical success rate for both techniques of EUS-CDS and EUS-HGS was 100%. Based on the 30% bilirubin level reduction one week after the procedure, the clinical success rate for both techniques was 79.1%. The clinical success rates for the choledochoduodenostomy approach and the hepaticogastrostomy approach were 78.2% and 100%, respectively. One week after the procedure, 19 patients achieved successful biliary drainage, and the remaining 5 patients were unable to achieve biliary drainage. The outcome of EUS-BD procedures is described in Table 2. Among the 4 patients who died, 2 showed a decrease in the bilirubin level of more than 30% within one week after the procedure, indicating successful biliary drainage. The bilirubin level of all subjects before and after the procedure is shown in Table 3.

Statistical analysis showed that the demographic data of the patients including gender, age, and BMI had no significant

TABLE 1: Patient characteristics.

Characteristics	Frequency (n)	Percentage (%)
Gender		
Male	13	54.2
Female	11	45.8
Age (mean ± 59)		
<60 years	13	54.2
≥60 years	11	45.8
BMI (mean ± 20.36, median ± 19.25)		
Underweight	7	29.2
Normal	11	45.8
Preobese	6	25
Primary disease		
Tumor of the head of pancreas	13	54.2
Periampullary tumor	10	41.6
Cholangiocarcinoma	1	4.2
Technique		
Choledochoduodenostomy (CDS)	23	95.8
Hepaticogastrostomy (HGS)	1	4.2
EUS-BD indication		
Difficult cannulation	16	66.7
Unidentifiable ampulla	8	33.3
Stents		
Plastic stent	21	87.5
SEMS	3	12.5
Complications		
Cholangitis	3	12.5
Pneumoperitoneum	1	4.1

TABLE 2: Outcome of EUS-BD procedures.

Outcome	Frequency (n)	Percentage (%)
Technical success		
Choledochoduodenostomy	23/23	100
Hepaticogastrostomy	1/1	100
Clinical success		
Choledochoduodenostomy	18/23	78.2
Hepaticogastrostomy	1/1	100
Overall clinical outcome		
Successful	19/24	79.1
Unsuccessful	5/24	20.9

correlation with the clinical success rate of EUS-BD, p value > 0.05 (Table 4).

We found that EUS-BD was 2.37 times and 2.11 times more likely to be successful in reducing the bilirubin level in patients with tumor of the head of the pancreas and periampullary tumor, respectively. There was no association between clinical success rate of EUS-BD and cholangiocarcinoma (RR = 1, CI 0.949–1.174). In this study, the clinical success rate of EUS-BD did not reach statistical significance due to a small sample size. Only tumor of the head of pancreas and periampullary tumor had p value < 0.05. Factors related to the clinical success rate of EUS-BD are described in Table 5.

4. Discussion

This study found that patients with malignant biliary obstruction who required the EUS-BD procedure after failed ERCP were more often male than female, with the proportions being 54.2% and 45.8%, respectively. Similar results were reported in the study by Park et al. and Khashab et al. Park et al. reported that, among the 57 patients enrolled in their study, 35 patients (60.3%) were male [11]. Another multicenter prospective study involving 12 tertiary centers by Khashab et al. showed that, among the 96 patients enrolled in the study, 53 patients were male (55%) [12]. As of yet, there is no explanation regarding the tendency of malignant biliary obstructions that require a EUS-BD procedure after failed ERCP to affect males more than females. This topic requires more specific research with a larger sample population to evaluate the correlation between gender and the incidence of malignant biliary obstructions that require alternative biliary drainage after failed ERCP.

When examining age, our study found that the incidence of malignant biliary obstructions that required a EUS-BD procedure was more common in patients < 60 years (54.2%) than in patients ≥ 60 years (45.8%), with a mean age of 59 years. Another study by Khashab et al. reported that the incidence of malignant biliary obstructions that required EUS-BD occurred at a mean age of 66 years, while Kawakubo et al. found that the incidence of this circumstance occurred at a mean age of 72 years. Both of these studies revealed that the older age group is more commonly affected by malignant biliary obstructions that ultimately require EUS-BD for bile drainage after ERCP failure [10, 11]. Compared to the other studies by Khashab et al. and Kawakubo et al., the present study revealed a slight tendency of malignant biliary obstructions requiring EUS-BD to affect younger patients, with a mean age of 59 years. This discrepancy might be caused by the sample size, which in our study was smaller than that in the other studies. The present study was conducted in a tertiary center with 24 patients. In contrast, Khashab et al. conducted their study in 12 tertiary centers with 96 enrolled patients, and Kawakubo et al. also conducted their study in multiple centers with 64 enrolled patients [12, 13]. Another reason for this discrepancy is the different age range of patients in each study. The study by Kawakubo et al. included patients in the age range of 66–79 years, while our study included patients in the age range of 37–80 years, therefore resulting in a different mean age. Similar to this situation, a study conducted by Makmun et al. in Indonesia showed that there is a changing trend of gastrointestinal malignancy affecting people at a younger age, especially in the age group of 40–60 years [14].

The statistical analysis showed that there was no correlation between demographic characteristics and the clinical success rate of EUS-BD. Gender, as one of the analyzed variables, showed no significant correlation with the clinical success rate of EUS-BD (p value = 0.590). We also found no

Table 3: Patient characteristics and bilirubin levels before and after the procedure.

Patient	Gender	Age (years)	BMI	Primary disease	Total/direct bilirubin (TB/DB) before procedure (mg/dL)	Total/direct bilirubin (TB/DB) one week after the procedure (mg/dL)
(1)	Male	73	27.3	Periampullary tumor	25.75/22.4	8.71/7
(2)	Male	43	17.3	Tumor of head of pancreas	24.46/20.27	18.72/15.53
(3)	Female	58	21.4	Tumor of head of pancreas	37.85/29.85	13.22/11.71
(4)	Female	66	10.5	Periampullary tumor	16.02/13.99	10.86/9.42
(5)	Male	75	28.51	Tumor of head of pancreas	30.02/24.45	14.75/12.87
(6)	Male	77	25.71	Tumor of head of pancreas	18.25/15.65	14.41/10.89
(7)	Male	54	18.37	Tumor of head of pancreas	3.89/2.8	1.41/1.09
(8)	Female	63	15.62	Periampullary tumor	23.87/20.23	15.83/14,46
(9)	Female	63	18.73	Tumor of head of pancreas	9.9/9.3	13.9/12.79
(10)	Male	41	19.5	Tumor of head of pancreas	20.6/18.8	15.06/13.52
(11)	Female	76	17.5	Tumor of head of pancreas	15.28/14.53	13.75/12.33
(12)	Female	43	18.7	Periampullary tumor	13.88/12.90	4.45/3.98
(13)	Female	59	19	Periampullary tumor	14.21/12.48	10.11/8.35
(14)	Female	78	21.22	Periampullary tumor	21/18	4.67/3.23
(15)	Female	64	25.7	Periampullary tumor	9.15/8.06	6.4/5.3
(16)	Male	54	19.92	Tumor of head of pancreas	18.4/17.06	9.11/5.8
(17)	Male	37	17.3	Periampullary tumor	8.7/6.6	6.03/4.79
(18)	Male	58	19.53	Periampullary tumor	29.4/21.75	21.53/19.08
(19)	Male	63	21.30	Periampullary tumor	22.06/19.91	3.6/3.5
(20)	Male	53	25.34	Tumor of head of pancreas	25.64/23.08	20.22/17.42
(21)	Male	46	17.93	Tumor of head of pancreas	29.32/22.75	6.63/5.58
(22)	Female	80	18.73	Cholangiocarcinoma	29.13/25.83	16.74/15.34
(23)	Female	45	26.03	Tumor of head of pancreas	28.26/25.4	14.08/12.1
(24)	Male	52	17.5	Tumor of head of pancreas	13.69/11.02	11.36/9.52

Table 4: Correlation between demographic data and the clinical success rate of EUS-BD.

Variables	Clinical success rate				
	N	%	RR	95% CI	*p* value
Gender					
Male	13	54.2	1.140	0.496–2.623	0.585
Female	11	45.8	0.844	0.261–2.730	1.0
Age					
<60 years	13	54.2	0.091	0.221–2.160	0.415
≥60 years	11	45.8	1.425	0.586–3.466	0.630
BMI					
Underweight	7	29.2	1.520	0.410–5.639	0.462
Normoweight	11	45.8	0.380	0.063–2.309	0.215
Preobese	6	25	1.900	0.477–7.569	0.366

significant correlation with age or BMI (p value = 0.590, p value = 0.586, resp.). Hence, from the statistical analysis, there was no correlation between the clinical success rate of EUS-BD and gender, age, or BMI.

In a case report from Obana and Yamasaki of an obese patient (BMI: 35.1 kg/m^2) who underwent EUS-BD with the indication of difficult cannulation during ERCP, the bilirubin level clearly decreased from 14.1 mg/dL (before the procedure) to 2.3 mg/dL (after the procedure). The authors reported that EUS-BD could be performed successfully in this obese patient to achieve biliary drainage [15]. There have been no reports regarding the correlation of age or gender with the clinical success rate of the EUS-BD procedure.

The most common primary disease in our study was tumor of the head of pancreas (54.2%), and the remaining primary diseases were periampullary tumor (41.6%) and cholangiocarcinoma (4.2%). Other studies reporting similar findings include those conducted by Dhir et al., Khashab et al., and Kawakubo et al. These studies also found that tumor of the head of pancreas was the most common diagnosis in malignant biliary obstructions that require the EUS-BD procedure [7, 12, 13]. On the other hand, a study conducted by Panpimanmas and Ratanachu-Ek in Thailand found that the most common diagnosis in malignant biliary obstructions that required EUS-BD was cholangiocarcinoma [16]. Another report by Kuberan et al. found that periampullary carcinoma

TABLE 5: Factors related to the clinical success rate of EUS-BD.

Variables	Clinical success rate				
	N	%	RR	95% CI	p value
Primary disease					
Tumor of the head of pancreas	13	54.2	2.375	1.402–4.025	0.030
Periampullary tumor	10	41.6	2.111	1.314–3.391	0.047
Cholangiocarcinoma	1	4.2	1.056	0.949–1.174	0.792
Technique					
Choledochoduodenostomy	23	95.8	0.739	0.580–0.942	0.750
Hepaticogastrostomy	1	4.2	1.353	1.061–1.725	1.0
EUS-BD indication					
Difficult cannulation	16	66.7	1.0	0.613–1.632	0.698
Unidentifiable ampulla	8	33.3	1.0	0.230–4.349	1.0

was more common than carcinoma of the head of pancreas as a cause of malignant biliary obstructions that required EUS-BD after failed ERCP [17]. The various results of the abovementioned studies need to be investigated thoroughly. The differences in study methods and sample size might have contributed to the discordant results.

In this study, tumor of the head of pancreas and periampullary tumor are 2.37 times and 2.11 times more likely to be successful in reducing bilirubin level after EUS-BD. In patient with cholangiocarcinoma, the likelihood of EUS-BD clinical success rate was 1.05. These results might be due to the involvement of the proximal biliary tract among patients with cholangiocarcinoma, which causes difficulty in achieving biliary drainage compared to patients with tumor of the head of pancreas and periampullary tumor. Currently, no other published studies have evaluated the correlation between the primary disease and the clinical success rate among patients with malignant biliary obstruction who required EUS-BD as an alternative for bile drainage after failed ERCP.

Another analyzed related factor in this study was the EUS-BD technique used. We used two EUS-BD techniques in this study (EUS-CDS and EUS-HGS), resulting in a 79.1% (19/24) clinical success rate of both techniques. The EUS-CDS technique was carried out in 23 patients, and this technique had technical and clinical success rates of 100% (23/23) and 78.2% (18/23), respectively.

This result is inconsistent with the study conducted by Ikeuchi and Itoi, which reported that the average technical success rate of EUS-CDS was 91.8% (312/348) and the clinical success rate was 94.5% (223/236) [18]. Another review article by Artifon reported that the success rate of EUS-BD among patients with malignant biliary obstruction was above 70% [19]. A study conducted by Ogura and Higuchi involving more than 200 patients who underwent EUS-HGS reported that the technical and clinical success rates ranged from 65% to 100% and 87% to 100%, respectively [20]. On the other hand, Ikeuchi et al. reported that the average technical success rate of EUS-HGS was 95.4% (146/153), and the clinical success rate was 90.9% (100/110) [18, 19]. There have been no recent guidelines for the selection of EUS-BD techniques. Many endoscopists use EUS-CDS as their first choice of procedure due to the lower rate of complications compared to EUS-HGS [18, 21]. Therefore, the selection of the EUS-BD procedure is based on the patient's condition (patients with gastric obstruction, the site of the biliary obstruction, and patients with Roux-en-Y anastomosis), availability of equipment, and the decision of the endoscopist [21, 22]. Several studies have reported that there is no significant difference in the success rate, clinical success rate, or complications between EUS-CDS and EUS-HGS [21, 23, 24]. However, a retrospective multicenter study conducted by Dhir et al. found that complications from EUS-BD were more common in EUS-HGS than EUS-CDS [7].

Electrical needle knife (Cystotome), catheter dilator, and balloon dilator could be used to facilitate stent placement during EUS-BD procedures. In our study the stent placement could be facilitated with Cystotome only. Among 23 patients who underwent EUS-CDS, plastic stents with the diameter of 10 Fr were placed in 20 patients, and in the remaining 3 patients we used fully covered SEMS with diameter of 10 mm. Our study used more plastic stents than fully covered SEMS due to the price of the stent and the availability at the time the procedure was performed. In 5 patients, stent placement could not decrease the bilirubin level by 30% within a week after the procedure. It might be due to clogging of the stent or tumor infiltration. In our study, EUS-CDS could not be performed in 1 patient due to tumor ingrowth into the duodenal bulb which caused the failure of the scope insertion into the duodenum. Hence, the endoscopists used EUS-HGS as an alternative procedure. Based on the experience in our study, EUS-CDS could be used as the first method of choice to be performed among patients who required EUS-BD after failed ERCP.

In terms of EUS-BD indication, our study showed two indications, including difficult cannulation (66.7%) and unidentifiable ampulla (33.3%). The EUS-BD indication resulting from this study was different than those from another study conducted by Kim et al., which showed EUS-BD indications including periampullary tumor obstruction as the most common EUS-BD indication, followed by difficult cannulation, high-grade stricture, high-grade left-sided hilar stricture, duodenal stenosis due to a previous duodenal ulcer, and tumor obstruction of the duodenum [25].

Our study also reported complications that occurred after the procedure, including pneumoperitoneum (1 patient) and cholangitis (3 patients). A review article by Ikeuchi and Itoi involving 38 studies reported that the most common complication of EUS-CDS procedures was peritonitis, and other complications included pneumoperitonitis, bleeding, bile leakage, perforation, abdominal pain, biloma, cholangitis, pancreatitis, hemobilia, and stent misplacement. The other 21 studies reported that the complications associated with EUS-HGS included cholangitis, bleeding, stent migration, biloma, bile leakage, pneumoperitonitis, peritonitis, stent misplacement, abdominal pain, metal stent shrinkage, and ileus [18]. In our study, among all patients who underwent EUS-BD there was no case of biliary leak. We cannot evaluate the correlation between the techniques used and the complications occurred during or after the procedure, because almost all enrolled patients underwent EUS-CDS and only 1 patient underwent EUS-HGS.

5. Conclusions

In conclusion, patients with tumor of the head of pancreas and periampullary tumor had higher clinical success rates for EUS-BD than patients with cholangiocarcinoma among those with malignant biliary obstructions that required EUS-BD after failed ERCP. There was no correlation between the clinical success rate of EUS-BD and the patients' demographic characteristics, EUS-BD technique, or EUS-BD indication. When the ERCP procedures fail, EUS-BD is an effective and efficient procedure to achieve biliary drainage, and EUS-CDS could be used as the first method of choice.

Disclosure

This topic is already presented in poster session during World Congress of GI Endoscopy 2017 (ENDO 2017) which was held in Hyderabad, India, in February 2017.

Acknowledgments

The authors would like to thank R. Agung Suryoputro, M.D., Tasha Farhana Dahlan, M.D., and Arinna Irianti, M.D., for their great assistance in this study.

References

[1] T. Constantin, "Jaundice obstructive syndrome," *Current Health Sciences Journal*, vol. 37, no. 2, 2011.

[2] D. Chavalitdhamrong and P. V. Draganov, "Endoscopic ultrasound-guided biliary drainage," *World Journal of Gastroenterology*, vol. 18, no. 6, pp. 491–497, 2012.

[3] K. Hara, K. Yamao, Y. Niwa et al., "Prospective clinical study of EUS-guided choledochoduodenostomy for malignant lower biliary tract obstruction," *American Journal of Gastroenterology*, vol. 106, no. 7, pp. 1239–1245, 2011.

[4] M. J. Wiersema, D. Sandusky, R. Carr, L. M. Wiersema, W. C. Erdel, and P. K. Frederick, "Endosonography-guided cholangiopancreatography," *Gastrointestinal Endoscopy*, vol. 43, no. 2, pp. 102–106, 1996.

[5] M. Giovannini, V. Moutardier, C. Pesenti, E. Bories, B. Lelong, and J. R. Delpero, "Endoscopic ultrasound-guided bilioduodenal anastomosis: a new technique for biliary drainage," *Endoscopy*, vol. 33, no. 10, pp. 898–900, 2001.

[6] K. Yamao, K. Hara, N. Mizuno et al., "EUS-guided biliary drainage," *Gut and Liver*, vol. 4, supplement 1, pp. S67–S75, 2010.

[7] V. Dhir, E. L. A. Artifon, K. Gupta et al., "Multicenter study on endoscopic ultrasound-guided expandable biliary metal stent placement: choice of access route, direction of stent insertion, and drainage route," *Digestive Endoscopy*, vol. 26, no. 3, pp. 430–435, 2014.

[8] T. Iwashita, S. Doi, and I. Yasuda, "Endoscopic ultrasound-guided biliary drainage: a review," *Clinical Journal of Gastroenterology*, vol. 7, no. 2, pp. 94–102, 2014.

[9] H. Imai, M. Kitano, S. Omoto et al., "EUS-guided gallbladder drainage for rescue treatment of malignant distal biliary obstruction after unsuccessful ERCP," *Gastrointestinal Endoscopy*, vol. 84, no. 1, pp. 147–151, 2016.

[10] X.-Q. Zhao, J.-H. Dong, K. Jiang, X.-Q. Huang, and W.-Z. Zhang, "Comparison of percutaneous transhepatic biliary drainage and endoscopic biliary drainage in the management of malignant biliary tract obstruction: a meta-analysis," *Digestive Endoscopy*, vol. 27, no. 1, pp. 137–145, 2015.

[11] D. H. Park, J. W. Jang, S. S. Lee, D.-W. Seo, S. K. Lee, and M.-H. Kim, "EUS-guided biliary drainage with transluminal stenting after failed ERCP: predictors of adverse events and long-term results," *Gastrointestinal Endoscopy*, vol. 74, no. 6, pp. 1276–1284, 2011.

[12] M. Khashab, S. Van der Merwe, R. Kunda et al., "Prospective international multicenter study on endoscopic ultrasound-guided biliary drainage for patients with malignant distal biliary obstruction after failed endoscopic retrograde cholangiopancreatography," *Endoscopy International Open*, vol. 04, no. 04, pp. E487–E496, 2016.

[13] K. Kawakubo, H. Isayama, H. Kato et al., "Multicenter retrospective study of endoscopic ultrasound-guided biliary drainage for malignant biliary obstruction in Japan," *Journal of Hepato-Biliary-Pancreatic Sciences*, vol. 21, no. 5, pp. 328–334, 2014.

[14] D. Makmun, M. Simadibrata, M. Abdullah et al., "Changing trends in gastrointestinal malignancy in Indonesia: the jakarta experience," *Journal of Cancer Research and Therapy*, vol. 2, no. 9, pp. 160–168, 2014.

[15] T. Obana and S. Yamasaki, "A case of malignant biliary obstruction with severe obesity successfully treated by endoscopic ultrasonography-guided biliary drainage," *Case Reports in Medicine*, vol. 2016, 5 pages, 2016.

[16] S. Panpimanmas and T. Ratanachu-Ek, "Endoscopic ultrasound-guided hepaticogastrostomy for advanced cholangiocarcinoma after failed stenting by endoscopic retrograde cholangiopancreatography," *Asian Journal of Surgery*, vol. 36, no. 4, pp. 154–158, 2013.

[17] K. Kuberan, R. Vijayalakshmi, G. Chandrasekar, and A. S. Kumar, "A prospective study on etiology and management of obstructive jaundice due to extra hepatic biliary obstruction," *Stanley Medical Journal*, vol. 3, no. 1, pp. 22–30, 2016.

[18] N. Ikeuchi and T. Itoi, "Endoscopic ultrasonography-guided biliary drainage: an alternative to percutaneous transhepatic puncture," *Gastrointestinal Intervention*, vol. 4, no. 1, pp. 31–39, 2015.

[19] E. L. A. Artifon, "Endoscopic ultrasound-guided biliary drainage," *Endoscopic Ultrasound*, vol. 2, no. 2, pp. 61–63, 2013.

[20] T. Ogura and K. Higuchi, "Technical tips for endoscopic ultrasound-guided hepaticogastrostomy," *World Journal of Gastroenterology*, vol. 22, no. 15, pp. 3945–3951, 2016.

[21] T. Ogura and K. Higuchi, "Does endoscopic ultrasound-guided biliary drainage really have clinical impact?" *World Journal of Gastroenterology*, vol. 21, no. 4, pp. 1049–1052, 2015.

[22] S. Mukai and T. Itoi, "How should we use endoscopic ultrasonography-guided biliary drainage techniques separately?" *Endoscopic Ultrasound*, vol. 5, no. 2, pp. 65–68, 2016.

[23] J. Guo, S. Sun, X. Liu, S. Wang, N. Ge, and G. Wang, "Endoscopic ultrasound-guided biliary drainage using a fully covered metallic stent after failed endoscopic retrograde cholangiopancreatography," *Gastroenterology Research and Practice*, vol. 2016, Article ID 9469472, 6 pages, 2016.

[24] K. Hara, K. Yamao, N. Mizuno et al., "Endoscopic ultrasonography-guided biliary drainage: Who, when, which, and how?" *World Journal of Gastroenterology*, vol. 22, no. 3, pp. 1297–1303, 2016.

[25] T. H. Kim, S. H. Kim, H. J. Oh, Y. W. Sohn, and S. O. Lee, "Endoscopic ultrasound-guided biliary drainage with placement of a fully covered metal stent for malignant biliary obstruction," *World Journal of Gastroenterology*, vol. 18, no. 20, pp. 2526–2532, 2012.

28

Extended Cystogastrostomy with Hydrogen Peroxide Irrigation Facilitates Endoscopic Pancreatic Necrosectomy

Mohamed O. Othman,[1] Sherif Elhanafi,[2] Mohammed Saadi,[2] Christine Yu,[2] and Brian R. Davis[3]

[1] *Gastroenterology and Hepatology Division, Baylor College of Medicine, Houston, TX, USA*
[2] *Department of Medicine, Texas Tech University Health Sciences Center, Paul L. Foster School of Medicine, El Paso, TX, USA*
[3] *Department of Surgery, Texas Tech University Health Sciences Center, Paul L. Foster School of Medicine, El Paso, TX, USA*

Correspondence should be addressed to Mohamed O. Othman; mohamed.othman@bcm.edu

Academic Editor: Jean Marc Dumonceau

Introduction. Walled-off pancreatic necrosis (WOPN) is a major complication of acute pancreatitis. We hypothesized that an extended (2 cm) cystogastrostomy opening combined with hydrogen peroxide irrigation can increase the success of endoscopic necrosectomy and decrease the number of required endoscopic interventions. The aim of the study is to assess the safety and feasibility of the technique in the management of WOPN. *Methods.* This is a retrospective chart review of all cases that underwent EUS with extended cystogastrostomy and hydrogen peroxide irrigation prior to necrosectomy in a tertiary referral medical center. Clinical success was defined as complete resolution of the cyst cavity or a cyst cavity less than 2 cm in size on follow-up imaging. *Results.* 19 patients satisfied the inclusion criteria. The mean size of the walled-off cavity was 11 + 0.9 cm. Technical success of the procedure was 100%. The median number of necrosectomy sessions was 2 (range 1 to 7). Cavity resolution was noted in 18 out of 19 patients resulting in a clinical success of 94.7%. The median follow-up period was 12 months. The adverse events rate in our cohort was 15.7%. *Conclusion.* Extended cystogastrostomy coupled with hydrogen peroxide irrigation of WOPN cavity is safe and feasible.

1. Introduction

Walled-off pancreatic necrosis (WOPN) or infected pancreatic necrosis may develop in 40–70% of patients with pancreatic fluid collections following attacks of acute necrotizing pancreatitis [1]. Infected necrosis is frequently responsible for the late occurrence of multiple organ failure and sepsis and remains the major life-threatening complication of acute pancreatitis (mortality rate up to 30%). Median mortality rate of open surgical approaches can be up to 25% (range 12–56%) according to a recent systematic review [2]. High morbidity and mortality of laparotomy-based surgical intervention have necessitated the development of alternative therapies for the treatment of infected pancreatic necrosis.

Despite the overall success and application of endoscopic transmural techniques for pancreatic pseudocyst drainage, initial reports listed evidence of pancreatic necrosis as a contraindication for endoscopic intervention [3, 4]. Contrary to this belief, courageous investigators with surgical collaboration have evolved the endoscopic procedure to become widely applicable in patients with infected pancreatic necrosis. Baron et al. described the first reported experience of endoscopic treatment in pancreatic necrosis ($n = 11$) describing complications in up to 45% and recurrence at two years in 60% of the reported cohort after using stent drainage with nasocystic irrigation (mean procedure number = 2.7) [5].

Direct transmural endoscopic necrosectomy was first described by Seifert et al. in 2000 [6]. Nine years later, the same group published a large series from a multicenter trial ($n = 93$) which described an 84% success rate in the treatment of symptomatic pancreatic necrosis. This series described intervention over three procedures starting with initial transmural access and stent insertion and then balloon dilation (15–20 mm), followed by a third procedure for endoscopic removal of necrotic debris using forceful irrigation, suction, snares, forceps, and stone removal baskets. Repeated sessions were performed at intervals of 1–4 days until all necrotic material had been removed. Initial clinical success was 80% followed by sustained clinical improvement in 84% of included patients [7]. These serial treatments necessitate an extreme commitment of resources and expertise to treat each patient effectively.

Advances in endoscopic techniques and ultrasound guidance have made endoscopic cystogastrostomy and pancreatic necrosectomy the preferred options for treatment of infected pancreatic pseudocyst or walled-off pancreatic necrosis. Limitations of successful endoscopic drainage in these situations include the small size of the gastrostomy and the large amount of necrotic material within the cyst or abscess cavity. In this study we describe our technique of creating a large cystogastrostomy (2 cm) followed by hydrogen peroxide irrigation to facilitate drainage and necrosectomy. We propose that the use of extended gastrostomy and hydrogen peroxide may increase the success of direct endoscopic debridement and decrease the number of required endoscopic interventions for resolution of the abscess or necrosis cavity safely.

2. Methods

2.1. Study Design. This study represents a retrospective case series of patients referred to a single gastroenterologist and surgeon team at the University Medical Center of El Paso for management of acute pancreatitis complications. All patients with infected pseudocyst or walled-off pancreatic necrosis (WOPN) with or without infection who underwent Endoscopic Ultrasound (EUS) guided cyst necrosectomy with hydrogen peroxide irrigation were included (from August 2011 to April 2015). Patient with mature cavity wall and distance of less than 1 cm between the stomach wall and the cavity underwent this technique. Indications for endoscopic drainage in our cohort were infected pseudocyst or WOPN and symptomatic, noninfected WOPN which is larger than 6 cm and present with abdominal pain, gastric outlet obstruction, or jaundice. The clinical definition of acute pancreatitis complications was based on the revised Atlanta classification of acute pancreatitis [8]. The electronic database system (ProVation®, Minneapolis, MN) was used to identify the indication for the procedure, type of placed stent, number of sessions required for each patient, and adverse events. The electronic medical record was searched for patient demographics, imaging studies, and time for resolution of WOPN. The study was approved by the Institutional Review Board (IRB) of Texas Tech University Health Science Center.

2.2. Technique. This case series demonstrates a modified EUS-guided cystogastrostomy and necrosectomy technique. This technique involves the creation of an extended cystogastrostomy by single-stage dilation of the gastrostomy up to 2 centimeters if the EUS shows no blood vessels within the puncture site and the CT scan demonstrates a mature cyst wall. All procedures were performed by a single endoscopist (MO), who had performed more than 2000 EUS procedures at the time of the study. A linear Olympus GF-UC140P echoendoscope (Olympus America Inc., Center Valley, PA, USA) with a ProSound SSD 5000 processor (Aloka, Wallingford, CT, USA) was utilized in all cases. A 19-gauge flexible FNA needle Expect™ (Boston Scientific Natick, MA, USA) was advanced to the WOPN along the posterior wall of the stomach after ruling out intervening blood vessels using color Doppler. The stylet was then removed and cyst fluid was aspirated. A 0.035 in × 450 cm Jagwire (Boston Scientific, Marlborough, MA, USA) was then advanced through the needle and allowed to coil several times within the cyst under fluoroscopic guidance. The 19-gauge needle was then removed over the wire and needle knife (Boston Scientific, Marlborough, MA, USA) was introduced over the wire to create the cystogastrostomy using pure cut current. The gastrostomy was then dilated up to 20 mm using the scope CRE™ balloon dilator (Boston Scientific, Marlborough, MA, USA) (Figure 1). The echoendoscope was then removed over the guidewire and therapeutic gastroscope GIF-H180 (Olympus America Inc., Center Valley, Pa) was introduced alongside the wire and across the cystogastrostomy to the WOPN. Direct endoscopic examination of the cavity was done followed by hydrogen peroxide irrigation of the cavity using 30 cc of hydrogen peroxide mixed with 30 cc of water (1 to 1 concentration). Debridement of adherent necrotic tissue was done using several endoscopic retrieval devices such as nets, rat tooth forceps, and snares (Figures 2, 3, and 4). The final step included placement of two 10 French double pig tail stents or VIABIL® fully covered metal stent (CONMED, Utica, NY) based on the preference of the endoscopist to keep the gastrostomy tract open. The procedure was performed under general anesthesia administered by an anesthesiologist. Follow-up CT scan was done 2 to 4 weeks after the initial intervention. Endoscopic Retrograde Cholangiopancreatography (ERCP) was performed prior to cystogastrostomy if disconnected pancreatic duct was suspected on prior imaging. Stent removal was performed after confirmation of cavity resolution by an imaging study within 3 to 6 months from the initial debridement.

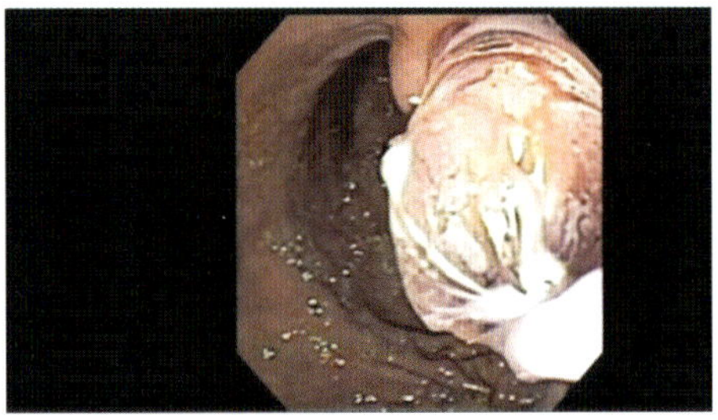

FIGURE 1: Balloon dilation of cystogastrostomy up to 20 mm.

2.3. Statistical Analysis. Continuous data were reported with a mean and standard deviation or median with averages. Categorical data were reported as proportions. Technical success was defined as the ability to perform the previously described technique without failure in any of the described

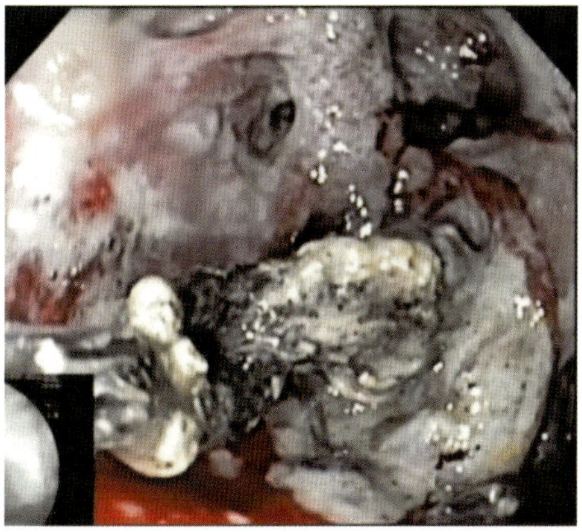

FIGURE 2: Removal of necrotic tissue after hydrogen peroxide irrigation.

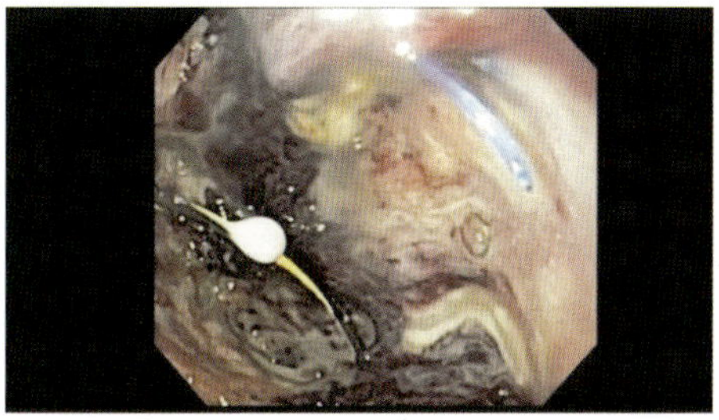

FIGURE 3: Surgical suture of distal pancreatectomy within pancreatic abscess bed.

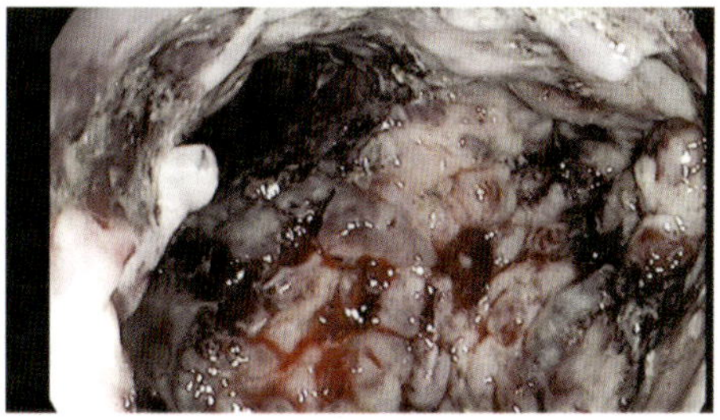

FIGURE 4: Walled-off pancreatic necrosis cavity after hydrogen peroxide irrigation and debridement.

steps. Clinical success was defined as cyst cavity less than 2 cm in size on follow-up imaging.

3. Results

3.1. Patients Characteristics. A total of 19 cases (13 males and 6 females) satisfied the inclusion criteria with a mean age of 50 (±2.6) years. Etiology of the pancreatitis was gallstone in 12 patients, alcohol in 5 patients, and postsurgical (distal pancreatectomy) abscess and idiopathic in 1 patient each. The mean number of weeks from the index acute pancreatitis to the intervention was 9 (±2.2) weeks (range 2 to 52). Cases in this series were categorized as walled-off necrosis (WON) (7), infected WON (8), infected pseudocysts (3), and postpancreatectomy pancreatic abscess (1). Three patients had splenic vein thrombosis with extensive gastric varices on imaging. Three patients had multiorgan failure prior to the planned cystogastrostomy and necrosectomy (Table 1).

TABLE 1: Patients characteristics.

Sex	Males: 13 Females: 6
Age (mean ± SD)	50 (±2.6) years
Ethnicity	NHW: 11 Hispanics: 8
Etiology of pancreatitis	Alcohol: 5 Gallstone: 12 Idiopathic: 1 Postsurgical abscess: 1
Time from index AP to intervention (mean weeks ± SD)	9 (±2.2)
Type of fluid collected	WOPN: 7 Infected WOPN: 8 Infected pseudocyst: 3 Pancreatic abscess: 1
Approach	Transgastric: 19

3.2. Procedure Characteristics. All cases were performed via a transgastric approach. The mean size of the walled-off cavity was 11 + 0.9 cm. Cystogastrostomy was created in 18 patients and it was dilated up to 20 mm. One patient had a wide open gastric fistula communicating with the WON and it was utilized for necrosectomy without the need for cystogastrostomy creation. ERCP was performed as a part of the evaluation for disconnected pancreatic duct in 9 patients (47.3%). Pancreatic duct stenting was done in 1 out of 9 patients for evidence of a pancreatic duct leak.

3.3. Study Outcomes. Technical success of the procedure was 100%. Median number of necrosectomy sessions was 2 (range 1 to 7). Cavity resolution was noted in 18 out of 19 patients resulting in a clinical success of 94.7%. The median follow-up period was 12 months (range 2 to 32 months). Radiological confirmation of cavity resolution in less than 3 months of the cystogastrostomy and necrosectomy was noted in 12 patients (63%). Among 18 patients who had cavity resolution, one patient required additional percutaneous drainage of paracolic gutter abscess. One patient died 5 days after the procedure from multiple organ failure (started prior to the procedure). As a result, the mortality rate of our series is 4.7%. Immediate adverse events were noted in one patient: bleeding from the gastrostomy site. Bleeding stopped after an epinephrine injection and fully covered stent placement. Delayed adverse events in the form of sepsis and recurrent cavity infection were seen in 2 patients. The two patients were treated with repeat cystogastrostomy and necrosectomy with hydrogen peroxide irrigation without any further adverse events. It was believed that cystogastrostomy blockage with a large amount of necrotic tissue was the culprit for recurrent infection in these patients. The complication rate in our cohort was 15.7% (3 out of 19 patients). One

Table 2: Study outcomes.

Technical success (%)	100%
Clinical success (cavity resolution)	95.2 (18/19)
Median number of sessions (range)	2 (1–7)
Follow-up period (median, range)	12 (2–32)
Cavity resolution within 3 months	63%
Mortality rate	4.7% (1/19)
Adverse events rate	15.7 (3/19)

patient had a recurrence of fluid collection 18 months after cavity resolution. The fluid collection was 5 cm in size and it contained clear fluid. The fluid collection resolved with EUS and aspiration of the cavity fluid without further recurrence up to 30 months. No other cases of cyst recurrence were noted in our cohort (Table 2).

4. Discussion

In this manuscript, we illustrated our modified technique of creating extending cystogastrostomy followed by hydrogen peroxide irrigation for management of WOPN. The technique was successful in 100% of patients with complete cavity resolution noted in 95% of the cohort.

Necrotizing pancreatitis is complicated with serial episodes of sepsis and multiorgan failure. Attempts at open necrosectomy have demonstrated high morbidity and mortality necessitating the utilization of alternative techniques. The initial treatment or temporization of pancreatic necrosis with minimally invasive procedures such as percutaneous drainage (PCD), endoscopic necrosectomy (EN), and video assisted retroperitoneal debridement (VARD) has been reported as the Step-Up protocol in several multicenter trials to include the PANTER trial from the Dutch Group [9]. The PENGUIN trial demonstrated reduced complications in patients receiving endoscopic necrosectomy compared with open surgical debridement [10]. The American multicenter trial by Gardner et al. demonstrated similar results with reduced morbidity and mortality in the endoscopic debridement group [11]. The Dutch consensus group has developed the TENSION trial to directly compare outcomes from endoscopic drainage with alternative treatments to include PCD and VARD [12]. The preponderance of evidence demonstrates that endoscopic drainage has proven superior results to other therapeutic modalities in patient with walled-off pancreatic necrosis (WOPN). Recently, lumen opposing metal stent was proposed as a facilitator of endoscopic necrosectomy with great success in multiple series [13, 14]. In spite of the safety profile of the lumen opposing metal stents, life threating complications such as bleeding or perforation were reported in the literature [15].

The purpose of this study is to demonstrate that the creation of an extended cystogastrostomy at the initial endoscopic drainage followed by debridement assisted by hydrogen peroxide leads to reduced procedural interventions compared with techniques previously described in the literature. In our series, 63% of patients achieved complete resolution of WOPN within 3 months of the procedure in spite of the large size of the included WOPN. Hydrogen peroxide can work as a chemical debriding agent which aids in removing adherent necrotic tissue and irritates healthy tissue to induce the formation of granulation tissue and subsequent fibrosis with cavity resolution. The creation of a 2 cm cystogastrostomy opening facilitated the continuous drainage of the debrided necrotic tissue and accelerated the process of cavity resolution. Abdelhafez et al. reported similar outcomes for hydrogen peroxide irrigation in pancreatic debridement in a series of 10 cases. However, all cases in the above-mentioned series were performed without EUS guidance [16].

Oxygen embolism after hydrogen peroxide irrigation is reported in the literature [17]. However, most reported cases resulted from the hydrogen peroxide injection into closed cavities which leads to injection of hydrogen peroxide under high pressure forcing it to penetrate into capillaries and blood vessels [18]. We believe that we did not encounter any incident of oxygen embolism due to the creation of a large cystogastrostomy opening which prevented the injection of hydrogen peroxide under high pressure.

In our series, only one patient had cyst recurrence after complete endoscopic drainage. Disconnected pancreatic duct syndrome is a common cause for pancreatic fluid collection recurrence. Permeant transmural stenting was associated with a decrease in pancreatic fluid collection recurrence in this category of patients [19].

Challenges to the validity of this study include the retrospective nature of the study. There was no ability to achieve randomization since these patients were referred primarily for the presence of WOPN. This study was unable to determine the benefits of endoscopic debridement compared with surgical debridement since most patients had survived the first four weeks of necrotizing pancreatitis prior to arrival at the referral hospital. The majority of patients in our study had mature cyst wall with abutment to the stomach with a distance between the stomach and cyst wall of no more than one centimeter.

In conclusion, the creation of an extended cystogastrostomy followed by hydrogen peroxide irrigation was safe and feasible in endoscopic necrosectomy of WOPN and infected pseudocysts.

Authors' Contributions

Mohamed O. Othman was responsible for study concept and design, acquisition of data, analysis and interpretation of data, drafting of the manuscript, statistical analysis, obtaining funding, and technical or material support. Sherif Elhanafi contributed to study concept and design and analysis and interpretation of data. Mohammed Saadi contributed to study concept and design and analysis and interpretation of data. Brian R. Davis contributed to study concept and design, acquisition of data, analysis and interpretation of data, drafting of the manuscript, critical revision of the manuscript for important intellectual content, and technical support.

References

[1] W. Uhl, A. Warshaw, C. Imrie et al., "IAP guidelines for the surgical management of acute pancreatitis," *Pancreatology*, vol. 2, no. 6, pp. 565–573, 2002.

[2] M. G. H. Besselink, T. J. Verwer, E. J. P. Schoenmaeckers et al., "Timing of surgical intervention in necrotizing pancreatitis," *Archives of Surgery*, vol. 142, no. 12, pp. 1194–1201, 2007.

[3] M. Hariri, A. Slivka, D. L. Carr-Locke, and P. A. Banks, "Pseudocyst drainage predisposes to infection when pancreatic necrosis is unrecognized," *The American Journal of Gastroenterology*, vol. 89, no. 10, pp. 1781–1784, 1994.

[4] R. A. Kozarek, "Endoscopic management of pancreatic necrosis: not for the uncommitted," *Gastrointestinal Endoscopy*, vol. 62, no. 1, pp. 101–104, 2005.

[5] T. H. Baron, W. G. Thaggard, D. E. Morgan, and R. J. Stanley, "Endoscopic therapy for organized pancreatic necrosis," *Gastroenterology*, vol. 111, no. 3, pp. 755–764, 1996.

[6] H. Seifert, T. Wehrmann, T. Schmitt, S. Zeuzem, and W. F. Caspary, "Retroperitoneal endoscopic debridement for infected peripancreatic necrosis," *Lancet*, vol. 356, no. 9230, pp. 653–655, 2000.

[7] H. Seifert, M. Biermer, W. Schmitt et al., "Transluminal endoscopic necrosectomy after acute pancreatitis: a multicentre study with long-term follow-up (the GEPARD Study)," *Gut*, vol. 58, no. 9, pp. 1260–1266, 2009.

[8] P. A. Banks, T. L. Bollen, and C. Dervenis, "Classification of acute pancreatitis—2012: revision of the Atlanta classification and definitions by international consensus," *Gut*, vol. 62, no. 1, pp. 102–111, 2013.

[9] H. C. van Santvoort, M. G. Besselink, O. J. Bakker et al., "A step-up approach or open necrosectomy for necrotizing pancreatitis," *The New England Journal of Medicine*, vol. 362, pp. 1491–1502, 2010.

[10] O. J. Bakker, H. C. van Santvoort, S. van Brunschot et al., "Endoscopic transgastric vs surgical necrosectomy for infected necrotizing pancreatitis: a randomized trial," *The Journal of the American Medical Association*, vol. 307, no. 10, pp. 1053–1061, 2012.

[11] T. B. Gardner, P. Chahal, G. I. Papachristou et al., "A comparison of direct endoscopic necrosectomy with transmural endoscopic drainage for the treatment of walled-off pancreatic necrosis," *Gastrointestinal Endoscopy*, vol. 69, no. 6, pp. 1085–1094, 2009.

[12] S. van Brunschot, H. van Santvoort, M. Boermeester et al., "Endoscopic transluminal step-up approach versus surgical step-up approach in patients with infected necrotizing pancreatitis (TENSION): design and rationale of a randomized controlled multicenter trial," *BMC Gastroenterol*, vol. 13, p. 161, 2013.

[13] J. B. Gornals, C. F. Consiglieri, J. Busquets et al., "Endoscopic necrosectomy of walled-off pancreatic necrosis using a lumen-apposing metal stent and irrigation technique," *Surgical Endoscopy and Other Interventional Techniques*, vol. 30, no. 6, pp. 2592–2602, 2016.

[14] R. Z. Sharaiha, A. Tyberg, M. A. Khashab et al., "Endoscopic therapy with lumen-apposing metal stents is safe and effective for patients with pancreatic walled-off necrosis," *Clinical Gastroenterology and Hepatology*, vol. 14, no. 12, pp. 1804-1805, 2016.

[15] R. Patil, M. A. Ona, C. Papafragkakis, S. Anand, and S. Duddempudi, "Endoscopic ultrasound-guided placement of axios stent for drainage of pancreatic fluid collections," *Annals of Gastroenterology*, vol. 29, no. 2, pp. 168–173, 2016.

[16] M. Abdelhafez, M. Elnegouly, M. S. Hasab Allah, M. Elshazli, H. M. S. Mikhail, and A. Yosry, "Transluminal retroperitoneal endoscopic necrosectomy with the use of hydrogen peroxide and without external irrigation: a novel approach for the treatment of walled-off pancreatic necrosis," *Surgical Endoscopy and Other Interventional Techniques*, vol. 27, no. 10, pp. 3911–3920, 2013.

[17] G. Haller, E. Faltin-Traub, D. Faltin, and C. Kern, "Oxygen embolism after hydrogen peroxide irrigation of a vulvar abscess," *British Journal of Anaesthesia*, vol. 88, no. 4, pp. 597–599, 2002.

[18] P. M. Jones, S. H. Segal, and A. W. Gelb, "Venous oxygen embolism produced by injection of hydrogen peroxide into an enterocutaneous fistula," *Anesthesia and Analgesia*, vol. 99, no. 6, pp. 1861–1863, 2004.

[19] J. Y. Bang, C. M. Wilcox, U. Navaneethan et al., "Impact of disconnected pancreatic duct syndrome on the endoscopic management of pancreatic fluid collections," *Annals of Surgery*, 2016.

29

Use of 4-Fr versus 6-Fr Nasobiliary Catheter for Biliary Drainage: A Prospective, Multicenter, Randomized, Controlled Study

Tomofumi Tsuboi,[1] Masahiro Serikawa,[1] Tamito Sasaki,[1,2] Yasutaka Ishii,[1] Yoshifumi Fujimoto,[3] Atsushi Yamaguchi,[4] Takashi Ishigaki,[5] Akinori Shimizu,[1] Keisuke Kurihara,[1] Yumiko Tatsukawa,[1] Eisuke Miyaki,[1] and Kazuaki Chayama[1]

[1] *Department of Gastroenterology and Metabolism, Applied Life Science, Institute of Biomedical & Health Science, Hiroshima University, Hiroshima, Japan*
[2] *Department of Gastroenterology, Hiroshima Prefectural Hospital, Hiroshima, Japan*
[3] *Department of Gastroenterology & Hepatology, JA Hiroshima General Hospital, Hiroshima, Japan*
[4] *Department of Gastroenterology, National Hospital Organization, Kure Medical Center and Chugoku Cancer Center, Kure, Hiroshima, Japan*
[5] *Department of Gastroenterology, National Hospital Organization Higashihiroshima Medical Center, Higashihiroshima, Japan*

Correspondence should be addressed to Tomofumi Tsuboi; tsuboitomo@hiroshima-u.ac.jp

Academic Editor: Tony C. K. Tham

Background and Aim. Endoscopic nasobiliary drainage (NBD) effects according to diameter remain unclear. We aimed to assess the drainage effects of the 4-Fr and 6-Fr NBD catheters. *Methods.* This prospective, multicenter, randomized, controlled study was conducted at Hiroshima University Hospital and related facilities within Hiroshima Prefecture. Endoscopic retrograde cholangiopancreatography (ERCP) in 246 patients revealed acute cholangitis, obstructive jaundice, and/or extrahepatic cholestasis; 4-Fr or 6-Fr NBD catheters were randomly allocated and placed in these patients. The primary endpoint was the efficacy of NBD based on the technical success rate and clinical success (rates of change in blood test and amount of bile output). Secondary endpoints included the spontaneous catheter displacement rate and nasal discomfort. *Results.* The technical success rate and clinical success did not differ significantly between groups. No spontaneous catheter displacement was noted in either group. Nasal discomfort due to catheter placement was significantly lower in the 4-Fr group versus the 6-Fr group (24 h after ERCP: 2.4 versus 3.5 cm, $P = 0.005$; 48 h after ERCP: 2.2 versus 3.1 cm, $P = 0.01$). *Conclusion.* The 4-Fr NBD catheter was not inferior to 6-Fr NBD catheter in terms of clinical success; the 4-Fr NBD catheter was useful to reduce nasal discomfort.

1. Introduction

The 3 methods of drainage treatment for acute cholangitis and obstructive jaundice include endoscopic drainage, percutaneous drainage, and surgical drainage [1]. A randomized controlled trial (RCT) that compared endoscopic drainage and surgical drainage for cholangitis showed that endoscopic drainage was safer and more effective in terms of the mortality rate and the complication rate [2]. Although no RCT has compared endoscopic drainage and percutaneous drainage in terms of invasiveness, frequency of complications, and length of hospital stay, endoscopic drainage is often considered as the preferred choice [3, 4]. In particular, endoscopic drainage can be performed via endoscopic nasobiliary drainage (NBD) and endoscopic biliary stenting (EBS). Although there is not any study to refer to with a head to head comparison of NBD to EBS with regard to clinical effectiveness, in East Asian countries such as Japan, NBD is preferred to EBS. The reasons for such a preference include monitoring the amount and quality of drained bile, identifying causative bacteria in cholangitis, and facilitating pathological examination. In contrast, NBD-induced obstructive pancreatitis, nose/throat discomfort, unacceptable esthetics, and self-removal by the patient are problems associated with NBD. We have previously reported that catheter diameter may be related to the occurrence of obstructive pancreatitis and throat discomfort [5]. At present, catheters of various sizes are available for NBD, ranging from 5-Fr to 7.5-Fr; however, the drainage results according to catheter size remain unclear. Here, we performed a multicenter RCT to verify whether the drainage results associated with the use of the 4-Fr NBD catheter are equivalent to those associated with the use of the 6-Fr NBD catheter (a widely applied catheter).

2. Materials and Methods

2.1. Study Design. In this multicenter, prospective, randomized controlled study, we compared and evaluated the clinical effectiveness of the 4-Fr catheter and the 6-Fr catheter in cases undergoing NBD.

The study was conducted at Hiroshima University and 11 affiliated hospitals.

The study protocol is available at the University Hospital Medical Information Network (UMIN) Clinical Trial Registry (UMIN000012677).

The protocol conformed to the Declaration of Helsinki and was approved by the institutional review board of Hiroshima University Hospital. Enrollment began in July 2013 and was completed in July 2015.

2.2. Patient Selection. We enrolled patients with obstructive jaundice, with acute cholangitis requiring biliary tract drainage, without jaundice, and with suspected cholestasis based on blood and imaging tests (bile duct diameter ≥ 10 mm on ultrasonography, computed tomography, and/or magnetic resonance imaging); all enrolled patients provided written informed consent for participation in the study.

Patients were excluded from the study if they were aged < 20 years; pregnant, breastfeeding, or possibly pregnant; had a history of endoscopic biliary sphincterotomy (EST) or endoscopic papillary balloon dilatation (EPBD); had acute pancreatitis or a serum pancreatic enzyme level ≥ 3 times the upper limit of normal prior to ERCP (pancreatic amylase or lipase values were preferred); had a history of sphincter of Oddi dysfunction; had pancreas divisum and malfusion of the pancreaticobiliary ducts; had a history of upper gastrointestinal tract reconstruction involving techniques other than Billroth 1 reconstruction, postoperative anatomy hindering endoscope from reaching the papilla; had undergone duodenal papilla procedures such as EST, EPBD, and papilla precutting; had prior or concurrent endoprosthesis other than the NBD used in the study (patients with concurrent biliary stents or multiple indwelling NBD catheters); were undergoing drainage of the right bile duct branch; had liver failure; or were allergic to polyurethane or ERCP contrast medium.

2.3. Randomization. A system was constructed on a server managed by a network management company, and each facility—which had been randomly allocated a specific catheter size to be used—entered data via the Internet. The facilities set obstructive jaundice as a stratification factor. The allocated catheter size was not communicated to the patient.

2.4. Sample Calculation and Statistical Analysis. We determined that the 4-Fr NBD catheter is as effective as the conventionally used 6-Fr NBD catheter. The efficacy of 4-Fr and 6-Fr NBD catheters is reportedly 92%. When the noninferiority limit was set to 10% (i.e., to verify whether the efficacy of the 4-Fr catheter is not <10% lower than that of the 6-Fr catheter), the α error was set to 0.05, and the power was set to 0.8, we found that each group would require 92 patients. Considering an expected 20% dropout rate, we concluded that 220 patients would be required overall (110 patients in each group); the 20% dropout rate accounted for the exclusion of certain patients after registration according to the exclusion criteria.

The Mann–Whitney U test was used to analyze the continuous variables, whereas the chi-squared test or Fisher's exact test was used to analyze categorical data (depending on the suitability). A P value of <0.05 was considered statistically significant.

2.5. NBD Catheter (Figure 1). A 4-Fr or 6-Fr polyurethane NBD catheter (260 cm; Gadelius Medical KK, Tokyo, Japan) was used for ERCP. The 4-Fr catheter had an internal diameter of 1.05 mm and an external diameter of 1.30 mm, whereas the 6-Fr catheter had an internal diameter of 1.30 mm and an external diameter of 2.00 mm. The ends were hooked to facilitate bile duct insertion in the lateral segment of the liver (B2 or B3). The catheters were tapered at a distance of 10 mm from the tip; 17 side-holes (0.8 mm in diameter) were created at 5 mm intervals in a spiral pattern, spanning 10–90 mm from the tip. The duodenal portion of both the 4-Fr and 6-Fr catheters was shaped into a loop.

2.6. Placement of the NBD Catheter. Intravenous anesthesia (midazolam or flunitrazepam or diazepam) was used for all patients during ERCP. The anesthesia was adopted by the physician. The deep bile duct cannulation method was not permitted, although bile duct cannulation was performed using the methods normally adopted at each facility. After bile duct cannulation, a guidewire was introduced into B2 or B3. Intraductal ultrasonography (IDUS), brushing cytology, and bile duct biopsy were then performed as needed, and the NBD catheter was placed carefully. A nasopancreatic drainage (NPD) tube or pancreatic stent was placed in patients considered to be at high risk of pancreatitis, at the discretion of the physicians at each facility.

2.7. Protocol. Informed consent was obtained for ERCP and for study participation. After consent was provided for study participation, the patient's information was entered into the system via the Internet, and the patient was randomly allocated a specific catheter size (4-Fr or 6-Fr). Except for catheter selection, the procedure was performed as usual. At least the NBD catheter was placed for 48 hours since the NBD catheter was inserted. After 48 hours of blood test and clinical

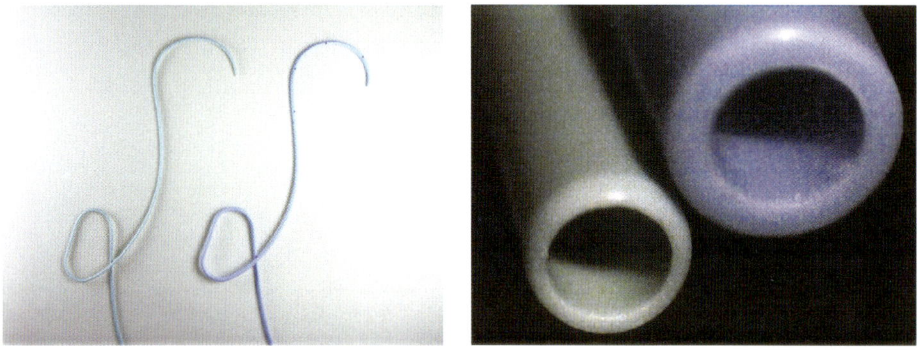

(a) (b)

Figure 1: Comparison of 4-Fr and 6-Fr nasobiliary drainage catheters. (a) Left, 4-Fr; right, 6-Fr. Both have the same looped configuration. (b) Cross-sectional view. Left, 4-Fr; right, 6-Fr.

symptoms improvement, the physician selected whether the patient continues to place the catheter or remove it. Blood was drawn within 24 hours prior to the test; at 24 and 48 hours after the test, blood was drawn again, abdominal radiography was performed, and nose/throat discomfort was evaluated on a visual analogue scale (VAS). The amount of bile output was measured by recording the time and the output volume from the start of the drainage until the removal of the catheter; the amount of bile output per hour was evaluated.

2.8. Study Endpoint. With regard to the primary endpoint, we compared the clinical success rate of the 4-Fr NBD catheter with that of the 6-Fr NBD catheter in patients with acute cholangitis and/or obstructive jaundice, without jaundice, and with findings of cholestasis. For the secondary endpoint, we compared nose/throat discomfort (based on the VAS score) associated with catheter placement and compared the frequency of spontaneous displacement of the catheter.

2.9. Subgroup Analysis. We compared the frequency of postoperative pancreatitis in patients with an indwelling NBD catheter (patients without concurrent pancreatic duct drainage with pancreatic duct stents or nasal pancreatic duct drainage) in the 4-Fr and 6-Fr groups.

2.10. Assessment of Blood Test Results. The rate of change in the blood test values was estimated as day 2 − day 0/day 0 × 100 (%) and was calculated for each patient. For instance, the rate of change in ALP levels was calculated as (ALP level on day 2 − ALP level on day 0)/ALP level on day 0 × 100 (%).

2.11. Definition of the Clinical Success Rate

2.11.1. Acute Cholangitis. An effective outcome was defined as a reduction in acute cholangitis-related fever and right hypochondriac pain, as well as an improvement in white blood cell count and hepatobiliary enzyme levels within 48 hours after NBD placement. Treatment was considered to be ineffective in patients who did not show any such improvement.

2.11.2. Obstructive Jaundice (T-Bil Level $\geq$ 3.0 mg/dL). An effective outcome was defined as a decrease in the T-bil level to below the baseline value (pretreatment value), as well as an improvement in the imaging findings that were suggestive of cholestasis or an improvement in hepatobiliary enzyme levels within 48 hours after NBD catheter placement. Treatment was considered to be ineffective in patients who did not show any such improvement.

2.11.3. Extrahepatic Cholestasis (T-Bil Level $\leq$ 3.0 mg/dL, Elevated Hepatobiliary Enzyme Levels, and Presence of Cholangiectasis, Clinically Indicative of Suspected Cholestasis). An effective outcome was defined as an improvement in the hepatobiliary enzyme findings and an improvement in the cholangiectasis findings on imaging tests within 48 hours after NBD catheter placement. Treatment was considered to be ineffective in patients who did not show any such improvement.

2.12. Definition of PEP. As reported by Cotton et al. [6], PEP was considered in cases that developed symptoms of pancreatitis within 24 hours after ERCP or that had serum pancreatic type amylase levels more than three times the normal value at 24 hours or 48 hours after ERCP.

3. Results

3.1. Patient Characteristics. Informed consent was obtained from 246 patients, and NBD catheter placement was performed in all of these cases (4-Fr group, 119; 6-Fr group, 127; Figure 2). Patient background, the procedure implemented, and the time required for the procedure did not differ significantly between groups (Table 1). NBD catheter placement was successful in 118 (99.1%) of the 119 patients in the 4-Fr group and in 121 (95.3%) of the 127 patients in the 6-Fr group. The reasons for unsuccessful catheter placement in all patients included difficulty of placement due to selective bile duct cannulation. Self-removal by the patient was noted in 6 patients (4-Fr group, $n = 5$; 6-Fr group: $n = 1$), whereas the NBD catheter was intentionally removed by the physician in

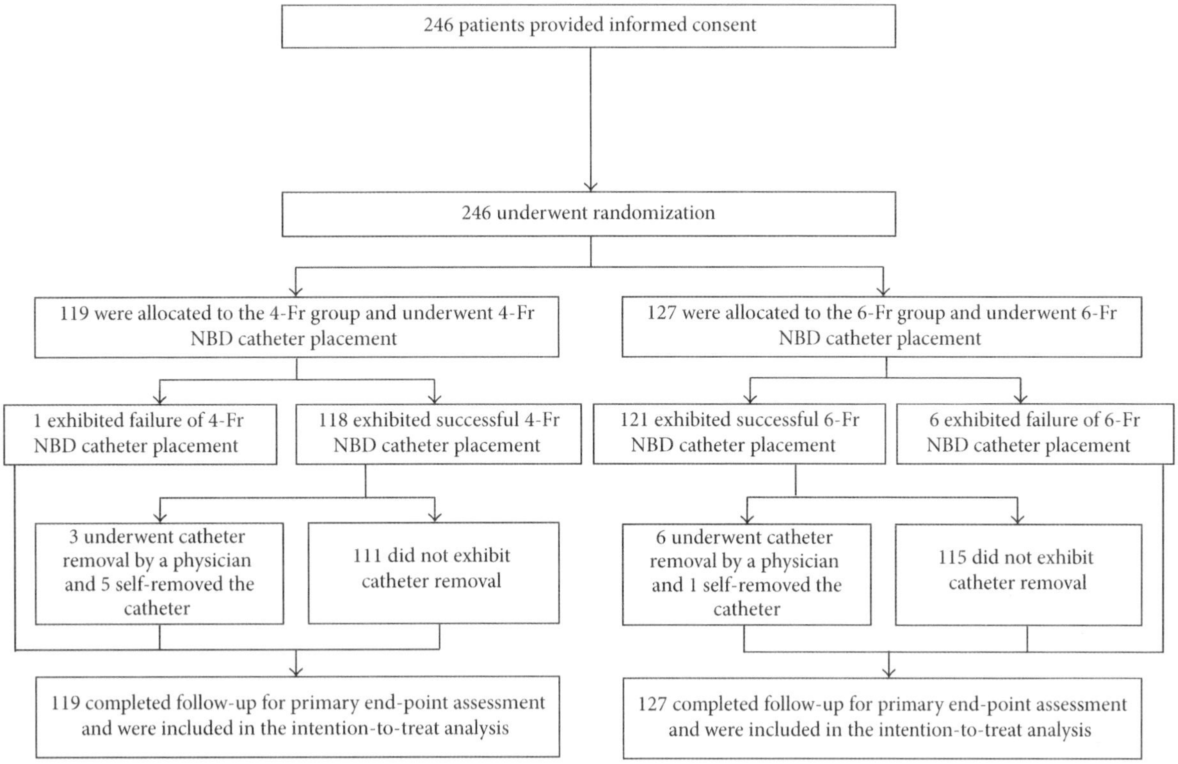

Figure 2: Study flowchart. Intention-to-treat analysis was performed. ERCP: endoscopic retrograde cholangiopancreatography; NBD: endoscopic nasobiliary drainage.

9 patients [4-Fr group: $n = 3$ (2 cases were pancreatitis and 1 case was poor drainage); 6-Fr group: $n = 6$ (5 cases were pancreatitis and 1 case was poor drainage)] due to procedural accidents associated with NBD. Cases for which placement was unsuccessful, cases of self-removal by the patient, and cases for which the catheter was intentionally removed by the physician were included in the intention-to-treat (ITT) analysis.

3.2. Primary Outcome Measurements. The NBD clinical success rates did not differ significantly between the groups (4-Fr group: 91.6%; 6-Fr group: 89.8%; $P = 0.78$). The rates of change in the ALP levels were $-18.6 \pm 13.6\%$ in the 4-Fr group and $-18.3 \pm 14.5\%$ in the 6-Fr group ($P = 0.51$), whereas the rates of change in the γ-GTP levels were $-23.9 \pm 13.6\%$ in the 4-Fr group and $-25.5 \pm 22.9\%$ in the 6-Fr group ($P = 0.10$). The amount of bile output was 22.4 ± 4.4 mL/h in the 4-Fr group and 22.6 ± 3.5 mL/h in the 6-Fr group; this value did not differ significantly between groups ($P = 0.32$; Table 2). With regard to the T-bil level, 74 patients in the 4-Fr group and 84 patients in the 6-Fr group had a T-bil level ≥ 3 mg/dL. Moreover, the rate of change in the T-bil level was $-37.2 \pm 25.6\%$ in the 4-Fr group and $-36.3 \pm 31.3\%$ in the 6-Fr group; this value did not differ significantly between groups ($P = 0.52$; Table 3).

3.3. Secondary Outcome Measurements. Spontaneous displacement and kinking of the catheter were not observed in either group. Nose/throat discomfort was assessed in 216 patients, excluding cases for which NBD catheter placement was unsuccessful, cases with NPD catheter placement, cases of self-removal by the patient, and cases for which the catheter was intentionally removed by the physician. Nose/throat discomfort was 2.4 ± 2.2 cm in the 4-Fr group and 3.5 ± 2.6 cm in the 6-Fr group on day 1 ($P = 0.005$) and 2.2 ± 2.2 cm in the 4-Fr group and 3.1 ± 2.4 cm in the 6-Fr group on day 2 ($P = 0.01$); the VAS scores showed a significant reduction in the 4-Fr group (Table 2).

3.4. Subgroup Analysis. Four patients in the 4-Fr group and 9 patients in the 6-Fr group had concurrent NPD placement and pancreatic stent placement, whereas 115 patients in the 4-Fr group and 118 patients in the 6-Fr group underwent only NBD catheter placement.

The incidence of pancreatitis was 3.5% (4/115) in the 4-Fr group and 7.6% (9/118) in the 6-Fr group ($P = 0.31$), which was not significantly different. With regard to PEP severity, 4 mild cases were noted in the 4-Fr group, and 6 mild, 2 moderate, and 1 severe cases were noted in the 6-Fr group (Table 4).

4. Discussion

In 1979, Cotton et al. [6] developed NBD as a technique for transnasal bile duct catheterization during ERCP. NBD is performed for biliary drainage in obstructive jaundice, the treatment of acute cholangitis, cytodiagnosis of bile duct neoplastic lesions, and the treatment of postoperative bile

Table 1: Baseline characteristics and ERCP procedures.

	4Fr group (n = 119)	6Fr group (n = 127)	P value
Age (y), mean (SD)	70.4 (12.6)	71.5 (11.6)	0.51
Sex			
Male, n (%)	64 (53.4)	77 (60.6)	0.33
Female, n (%)	55 (46.6)	50 (39.4)	
Body mass index (kg/m^2), mean (SD)	22.4 (4.3)	22.6 (3.5)	0.31
Indication (overlapping)			
Obstructive jaundice, n (%)	74 (62.2)	84 (66.1)	0.51
Acute cholangitis, n (%)	32 (26.9)	42 (33.1)	0.29
Extrahepatic cholestasis, n (%)	87 (73.1)	94 (74.0)	0.98
Diagnosis			
Choledocholithiasis, n (%)	39 (32.8)	38 (30.0)	0.63
Pancreatic cancer, n (%)	30 (25.2)	33 (26.0)	0.89
Cholangiocarcinoma, n (%)	21 (17.6)	22 (17.3)	0.95
Carcinoma of the papilla of Vater, n (%)	7 (5.9)	5 (3.9)	0.68
Gallbladder cancer, n (%)	5 (4.2)	5 (3.9)	0.83
Chronic pancreatitis, n (%)	2 (1.7)	0 (0)	
Others, n (%)	15 (12.6)	24 (18.9)	0.18
ERCP procedures			
Pancreatic duct injection, n (%)	67 (61.0)	75 (55.4)	0.66
Brushing of pancreatic duct, n (%)	2 (1.7)	2 (1.6)	0.66
Endoscopic pancreatic stent, n (%)	2 (1.7)	3 (2.3)	0.94
Endoscopic nasopancreatic drainage, n (%)	2 (1.7)	6 (4.7)	0.32
Biliary intraductal ultrasonography, n (%)	40 (33.6)	40 (31.5)	0.82
Brushing of bile duct, n (%)	26 (21.8)	29 (22.8)	0.85
Biopsy of bile duct, n (%)	3 (2.5)	2 (1.6)	0.94
Procedure time (min), mean (SD)	30.6 (14.6)	29.4 (14.1)	0.50

ERCP, endoscopic retrograde cholangiopancreatography; SD, standard deviation.
P value not significant for all comparisons.

leak after bile duct surgery [2, 7–10]. Catheters of various types and sizes can be used for drainage, and the selection of a specific catheter depends on the particular facility. In a previous study, we found that the use of the 4-Fr NBD catheter significantly reduced the onset of PEP and nose/throat discomfort [5]. Thus, the use of a catheter with a small diameter reduces the burden on the patient, and if such catheters have good drainage efficacy, then these smaller catheters should be the first choice for treatment. Several reports have described the effectiveness of ENBD for acute cholangitis and obstructive jaundice [11–14]; however, only a few studies have investigated the drainage effects according to NBD catheter diameter. Many studies have assessed the drainage effects of biliary stents based on the stent diameter. Sharma et al. investigated the placement and drainage results of 7-Fr and 10-Fr biliary stents in patients with cholangitis and/or obstructive jaundice [14–16] and reported that there was no significant difference between the 2 groups. Kadakia and Starnes [17] also reported that there was no significant difference in the drainage effects between 10-Fr and 11.5-Fr biliary stents [15]. However, the lengths of biliary stents and NBD catheters differ, and hence, it is difficult to conclude whether the effects of biliary stent drainage would be applicable to NBD catheter placement. Fujisawa et al. described the biliary drainage effects of NBD catheters of 5-Fr and 7-Fr diameters in cases with obstructive jaundice [18]; the authors found that the rate of reduction in bilirubin levels (day 0 − day 4/day 0 × 100) was significantly better with the 7-Fr NBD catheter than with the 5-Fr NBD catheter. However, the success rate of jaundice improvement was 98% with the 7-Fr NBD catheter and 88% with the 5-Fr NBD catheter, which was not significantly different. Furthermore, the drainage output (mL/day) did not differ significantly between the 7-Fr NBD catheter and the 5-Fr NBD catheter. Approximately 80% of the patients in that study had undergone EPBD and/or EST, and hence, these findings cannot be completely reflective of the drainage effects of an NBD catheter. The findings of the present study indicated that the rate of change in the ALP and γ-GTP levels and the amount of bile output (mL/h) did not differ significantly between the 4-Fr NBD catheter and the 6-Fr NBD catheter groups and that the clinical success rate did not differ significantly, either. Thus, we noted that the drainage effects of the 4-Fr NBD catheter and the 6-Fr NBD catheter are equivalent.

TABLE 2: Outcomes.

	4Fr group ($n = 119$)	6Fr group ($n = 127$)	P value
Technical success rate (%)	118 (99.1)	121 (95.3)	*0.15*
Clinical success rate (%)	109 (91.6)	114 (89.8)	*0.78*
ALP (IU/L)			
Before biliary drainage	1217 (865)	1168 (908)	*0.49*
After biliary drainage	963 (673)	932 (681)	*0.51*
ALP decreasing rate (%), mean (SD)	18.6 (13.6)	18.3 (14.5)	*0.51*
γ-GTP (IU/L)			
Before biliary drainage	673 (511)	679 (542)	*0.52*
After biliary drainage	504 (377)	496 (412)	*0.51*
γ-GTP decreasing rate (%), mean (SD)	23.9 (13.6)	25.5 (22.9)	*0.1*
Amount of bile output (mL/hour), mean (SD)	22.4 (4.4)	22.6 (3.5)	*0.32*
Displacement			
Willful removal by the doctor, n (%)	3 (3.7)	6 (12.0)	0.56
Self-removal by the patient, n (%)	5 (3.7)	1 (1.2)	0.20
Spontaneous displacement, n (%)	0 (0.0)	0 (0.0)	
	4Fr group ($n = 109$)	6Fr group ($n = 107$)	
VAS score of discomfort (cm)			
24 h after ERCP, mean (SD)	2.4 (2.2)	3.5 (2.6)	0.005*
48 h after ERCP, mean (SD)	2.2 (2.2)	3.1 (2.4)	0.010*

SD, standard deviation; VAS, visual analog scale.
*Significant difference.
ALP: Alkaline phosphatase.
γ-GTP: Gamma-Glutamyl transpeptidase.

TABLE 3: In patients with obstructive jaundice.

	4Fr group ($n = 74$)	6Fr group ($n = 84$)	P value
Baseline serum total bilirubin (mg/dL), mean (SD)	8.3 (4.9)	9.1 (5.6)	0.41
Amount of bile output (mL/hour), mean (SD)	17.9 (9.8)	20.5 (18.1)	0.52
T-bil decreasing rate (%), mean (SD)	37.2 (25.6)	36.3 (31.3)	*0.52*

SD, standard deviation.
P value not significant for all comparisons.

TABLE 4: Subgroup analysis.

	4Fr group ($n = 115$)	6Fr group ($n = 118$)	P value
Pancreatitis, n (%)			
Total	4 (3.5)	9 (7.6)	0.31
Severity			
Mild	4 (3.5)	6 (5.1)	
Moderate	0 (0.0)	2 (1.7)	
Severe	0 (0.0)	1 (0.8)	

In the present study, we found that nasal discomfort—a major problem in NBD—was significantly reduced with the 4-Fr catheter as compared to that with the 6-Fr catheter. The VAS score for nasal discomfort with NBD catheter placement decreases as the placement time increases, suggesting that the patient becomes accustomed to the catheter. However, long-term catheter placement also increases the risk of self-removal by the patient; hence, unnecessary long-term placement should be avoided. The incidence of PEP associated with NBD catheter placement did not differ significantly between groups, although it was numerically lower in the 4-Fr NBD catheter group. In addition, the incidence of moderate or severe pancreatitis was 2.5% in the 6-Fr group, compared to 0% in the 4-Fr group. One reason for the lack of difference between groups in the incidence of PEP could be that concurrent placement of NPD and pancreatic stents was permitted in cases at high risk of developing PEP.

5. Conclusion

In conclusion, we found that the drainage effects did not differ between the use of the 4-Fr NBD catheter and the use of the 6-Fr NBD catheter. Moreover, we found that the 4-Fr NBD catheter was associated with reduced nasal discomfort. We believe that the 4-Fr NBD catheter should represent the first choice amongst NBD for treatment of patients with obstructive jaundice and acute cholangitis.

Acknowledgments

The authors would like to acknowledge NBD 4 Study Group: Yoshifumi Fujimoto M.D., Department of Gastroenterology & Hepatology, JA Hiroshima General Hospital; Atsushi Yamaguchi M.D., Department of Gastroenterology, National Hospital Organization, Kure Medical Center and Chugoku Cancer Center; Takashi Ishigaki M.D., National Hospital Organization Higashihiroshima Medical Center; Kenichi Kuwahara M.D., Department of Gastroenterology, Hiroshima City Asa Hospital; Tamito Sasaki M.D., Department of Gastroenterology, Hiroshima Prefectural Hospital; Shinichiro Sugiyama M.D., Saiseikai Hiroshima Hospital; Bunjiro Noma M.D., Kure Kyosai Hospital; Keiji Hanada M.D., Onomichi General Hospital; Yoshinari Furukawa M.D., Hiroshima Red Cross Hospital & Atomic-Bomb Survivors Hospital; Tomohiro Iiboshi M.D., Department of Gastroenterology, Akitsu Prefectural Hospital; Noriaki Eguchi M.D., KKR Hiroshimakinen Hospital.

References

[1] T. Tsuyuguchi, T. Takada, Y. Kawarada et al., "Techniques of biliary drainage for acute cholangitis: Tokyo Guidelines," *Journal of Hepato-Biliary-Pancreatic Surgery*, vol. 14, no. 1, pp. 35–45, 2007.

[2] E. C. S. Lai, F. P. T. Mok, E. S. Y. Tan et al., "Endoscopic biliary drainage for severe acute cholangitis," *The New England Journal of Medicine*, vol. 326, no. 24, pp. 1582–1586, 1992.

[3] M. Sugiyama and Y. Atomi, "Treatment of acute cholangitis due to choledocholithiasis in elderly and younger patients," *Archives of Surgery*, vol. 132, no. 10, pp. 1129–1133, 1997.

[4] S. C. Kadakia, "Biliary tract emergencies: acute cholecystitis, acute cholangitis, and acute pancreatitis," *Medical Clinics of North America*, vol. 77, no. 5, pp. 1015–1036, 1993.

[5] T. Ishigaki, T. Sasaki, M. Serikawa et al., "A comparative study of 4 Fr versus 6 Fr nasobiliary drainage catheters: a randomized, controlled trial," *Journal of Gastroenterology and Hepatology*, vol. 29, no. 3, pp. 653–659, 2014.

[6] P. B. Cotton, P. G. J. Burney, and R. R. Mason, "Transanasal bile duct catheterisation after endoscopic sphincterotomy. Method for biliary drainage, perfusion, and sequential cholangiography," *Gut*, vol. 20, no. 4, pp. 285–287, 1979.

[7] J. W. C. Leung and P. B. Cotton, "Endoscopic nasobiliary catheter drainage in biliary and pancreatic disease," *The American Journal of Gastroenterology*, vol. 86, no. 4, pp. 389–394, 1991.

[8] H. Yagioka, K. Hirano, H. Isayama et al., "Clinical significance of bile cytology via an endoscopic nasobiliary drainage tube for pathological diagnosis of malignant biliary strictures," *Journal of Hepato-Biliary-Pancreatic Sciences*, vol. 18, no. 2, pp. 211–215, 2011.

[9] N. Uchida, H. Kamada, M. Ono et al., "How many cytological examinations should be performed for the diagnosis of malignant biliary stricture via an endoscopic nasobiliary drainage tube?" *Journal of Gastroenterology and Hepatology*, vol. 23, no. 10, pp. 1501–1504, 2008.

[10] P. G. Foutch, J. R. Harlan, and M. Hoefer, "Endoscopic therapy for patients with a post-operative biliary leak," *Gastrointestinal Endoscopy*, vol. 39, no. 3, pp. 416–421, 1993.

[11] B. C. Sharma, R. Kumar, N. Agarwal, and S. K. Sarin, "Endoscopic biliary drainage by nasobiliary drain or by stent placement in patients with acute cholangitis," *Endoscopy*, vol. 37, no. 5, pp. 439–443, 2005.

[12] H. Sugiyama, T. Tsuyuguchi, Y. Sakai, T. Nisikawa, M. Miyazaki, and O. Yokosuka, "Preoperative drainage for distal biliary obstruction: endoscopic stenting or nasobiliary drainage?" *Hepato-Gastroenterology*, vol. 60, no. 121, pp. 231–234, 2013.

[13] H. Kawakami, M. Kuwatani, M. Onodera et al., "Endoscopic nasobiliary drainage is the most suitable preoperative biliary drainage method in the management of patients with hilar cholangiocarcinoma," *Journal of Gastroenterology*, vol. 46, no. 2, pp. 242–248, 2011.

[14] B. C. Sharma, N. Agarwal, P. Sharma, and S. K. Sarin, "Endoscopic biliary drainage by 7 Fr or 10 Fr stent placement in patients with acute cholangitis," *Digestive Diseases and Sciences*, vol. 54, no. 6, pp. 1355–1359, 2009.

[15] F. M. Pedersen, "Endoscopic management of malignant biliary obstruction is stent size of 10 french gauge better than 7 french gauge?" *Scandinavian Journal of Gastroenterology*, vol. 28, no. 2, pp. 185–189, 1993.

[16] P. Katsinelos, J. Kountouras, G. Paroutoglou et al., "A comparative study of 10-Fr vs. 7-Fr straight plastic stents in the treatment of postcholecystectomy bile leak," *Surgical Endoscopy*, vol. 22, no. 1, pp. 101–106, 2008.

[17] S. C. Kadakia and E. Starnes, "Comparison of 10 French gauge stent with 11.5 French gauge stent in patients with biliary tract diseases," *Gastrointestinal Endoscopy*, vol. 38, no. 4, pp. 454–459, 1992.

[18] T. Fujisawa, K. Kagawa, S. Watanabe et al., "Endoscopic nasobiliary drainage for obstructive jaundice using either a 5 Fr or 7 Fr catheter: a prospective, randomized trial," *BMC Gastroenterology*, vol. 14, no. 1, article no. 161, 2014.

30

Therapeutic Endoscopy Can Be Performed Safely in an Ambulatory Surgical Center: A Multicenter, Prospective Study

Shaffer R. S. Mok, Henry C. Ho, John P. Gaughan, and Adam B. Elfant

Division of Gastroenterology and Liver Diseases, Department of Medicine, Cooper Medical School of Rowan University, MD Anderson Cancer Center at Cooper, Mount Laurel, NJ, USA

Correspondence should be addressed to Shaffer R. S. Mok; sshropemok@aol.com

Academic Editor: Tony C. K. Tham

Background. Even amongst experienced endoscopists, endoscopic retrograde cholangiopancreatography (ERCP) and endoscopic ultrasound with fine needle aspiration (EUS-FNA) carry a potential risk for complications. These procedures are typically performed in a hospital-based endoscopy unit with general anesthesia. *Aims.* The goal of our study was to evaluate the feasibility of ERCP and EUS-FNA in an ambulatory surgical center (ASC). *Methods.* From June to November of 2014, we prospectively enrolled consecutive subjects undergoing ERCP and/or EUS-FNA in an ASC. An anesthesiologist, who was not involved in our study group, screened all subjects prior to their scheduled procedure. In order to monitor for adverse events (AE), all subjects received a telephone call at day 1 and 30 days after procedure. *Results.* 375 subjects (98 inpatients and 277 from an ASC) were enrolled. In the total population, a high proportion of subjects underwent procedures for neoplasms (21 (23.3%) inpatients versus 44 (17.1%) from an ASC) and for sphincter of Oddi dysfunction (SOD) (27 (27.5%) versus 48 (17.3%)) and had the American Society for Anesthesiologists (ASA) class ≥III (75 (76.5%) versus 140 (50.5%)) and high-risk features (17 (17.3%) versus 75 (27.1%)). Overall ERCP-related AE (10 (13.2%) versus 12 (7.5%), $p = 0.2$), pancreatitis (7 (9.2%) versus 11 (6.9%), $p = 0.6$), and hemorrhage (3.9% versus 0.6%, $p = 0.25$) were not different between inpatients and ASC subjects. There was also no difference between inpatients and ASC subjects' EUS-related AE (1 (4.5%) versus 4 (3.4%), $p = 0.6$), pancreatitis (1 (4.5%) versus 3 (2.6%), $p = 0.2$), and hemorrhage (0% versus 1 (0.9%), $p = 0.9$). *Conclusions.* ERCP and EUS can be performed in a higher risk population under the supervision of anesthesia in ASCs. Overall, the AE are equivalent between inpatients and ASC subjects.

1. Introduction

Endoscopic retrograde cholangiopancreatography (ERCP) and endoscopic ultrasound with fine needle aspiration (EUS-FNA) are useful techniques for a variety of pancreaticobiliary disorders. Despite their benefit, both procedures carry potential adverse events (AE), which may lead to substantial morbidity and mortality [1, 2]. In a climate of rising health costs, several authors have evaluated the safety of performing ERCP in the outpatient setting with mixed results [3–18]. Among these studies, most were retrospective and only one study evaluated EUS-FNA [3–11, 18]. Additionally, there is paucity of data to evaluate individuals undergoing ERCP/EUS-FNA in an ambulatory surgical center (ASC) and, in particular, those with cancer, elevated American Society of Anesthesiologists (ASA) class, and sphincter of Oddi dysfunction (SOD) and those determined to be at high risk [5, 19–27].

The aim of this study was to evaluate the 30-day AE of inpatient versus ASC ERCP or EUS in a multicenter, prospective cohort in high-risk subjects. We evaluated the epidemiologic and procedural risk factors for AE, as well as costs related to these procedures. Our hypothesis was that there would be no significant difference in 30-day AE when comparing the inpatient group with the ASC group.

2. Materials and Methods

2.1. Study Design. This prospective multicenter study was approved by our Institutional Review Board (IRB 14-046EX) and was performed in accordance with the Declaration of Helsinki. From June 2014 until November 2014, we prospectively enrolled consecutive subjects from three medical centers (one tertiary care center (Cooper University Hospital), two community centers (Our Lady of Lourdes Medical Center in Camden and Burlington, New Jersey) (NJ)), their subsequent ASCs (1 tertiary care endoscopy unit (Cooper University Hospital Digestive Health Institute in Mount Laurel, NJ), and 2 community-based units (Our Lady of Lourdes Medical center in Camden and Burlington, NJ)). The ASC for Cooper University Hospital was located 10 miles from its tertiary care center and the ASCs for Our Lady of Lourdes were located 1 mile away from each community hospital location. All advanced endoscopy rooms were staffed with 2 skilled endoscopy nurses and 1 skilled endoscopy technician. Informed consent was obtained from all participants for our study and no substituted consent was used.

2.2. Study Population. Both men and women ≥ 18 years of age were included in this study. All subjects were undergoing ERCP and/or EUS for various indications. Inpatients and ASC subjects who completed all data points and follow-up were included. We excluded pregnant women and subjects with missing data from this study.

Demographic data was then obtained from all participants and included age, sex, ethnicity, relevant comorbid conditions (i.e., cardiovascular disease (acute coronary syndrome, stroke, and systolic congestive heart failure with ejection fraction under 45%), pulmonary disease (obstructive sleep apnea, chronic obstructive pulmonary disease, etc.), cirrhosis, end-stage renal disease on dialysis), and surgical history (i.e., endoscopic interventions). A medication history was obtained to evaluate the use of anticoagulants and antiplatelet agents at the time of advanced endoscopy. All subjects received baseline liver enzymes, an amylase, and lipase to determine whether pancreatitis was present prior to the procedure [1, 28, 29].

Subjects were deemed to be at high risk by standard criterion (see supplemental appendix 1 in Supplementary Material available online at http://dx.doi.org/10.1155/2016/7168280) [1, 25]. Major criterion included one of the following: suspicion for sphincter of Oddi dysfunction (SOD) (see supplemental appendix 2), a personal history of PEP, more than 8 cannulation attempts, precut sphincterotomy, endoscopic papillary balloon dilation (EPBD) of an intact sphincter, endoscopic pancreatic duct sphincterotomy (EPS), and ampullectomy [25]. Moderate risk was defined by the following minor criterion: female sex and usage under 50 years, personal history of recurrent acute pancreatitis, pancreatic duct (PD) injection leading to opacification of acinar cells or over 3 PD injections, and PD cytology acquisition.

On the day of the examination, the indication(s) for the intervention were recorded. Then, assessment of ASA class and Mallampati score were evaluated using standard means (defined in supplemental appendix 3) [19–23]. We then elicited baseline pain scores from subjects utilizing a ten-point Likert pain scale (Appendix 4).

2.3. Intervention. At time zero, subjects were prospectively enrolled and given study identification using a random number generator. Prior to their procedure, an anesthesiologist determined the location of their ERCP/EUS based upon this randomization.

Three endoscopists participated in this study, all of whom had >5 years of endoscopy experience and have performed over 200 ERCPs and EUSs per year. Two postgraduate year 6 (PGY-6) fellows participated in all endoscopies performed at our tertiary care setting.

Anesthesia was administered using propofol-based monitored anesthesia care (MAC) for the duration of the procedure. No rectal indomethacin was used as prophylaxis during the study as was not the standard practice at our center during enrollment.

2.4. Outcomes. Presence of any AE was the primary outcome and each of the individual AE was among the secondary outcomes. AE were defined by the presence of any of the following: fever, worsening abdominal pain (based upon Likert score), gastrointestinal bleeding (GIB), infection, perforation, aspiration, need for intubation, cardiovascular arrest, acute coronary syndrome (ACS), arrhythmia, surgery, admission (if so, reason for admission, length of stay, and cost of stay), service call (if so, reason and number of calls), systemic inflammatory response syndrome (SIRS), sepsis, infection, multiorgan failure (MOF), and death (reason). Additional AE included the presence of post-ERCP pancreatitis (PEP) (see supplemental appendix 5), defined by the presence of (1) new or worsening abdominal pain that is clinically consistent with acute pancreatitis and (2) associated pancreatic enzymes elevation ≥ 3 times the upper limit of normal twenty-four hours after the procedure and (3) resultant or prolongation of existing hospitalization of ≥2 nights. Other secondary outcomes included the cost of each procedure along with subsequent AE-related costs (i.e., hospital admission and surgery) obtained using insurance data.

In order to monitor for these outcomes, data were obtained intraprocedurally and postprocedurally, as well as 1 and 30 days after endoscopy. During the procedure, hemodynamic measurements and endoscopic interventions were recorded (i.e., sphincterotomy and FNA). After their procedure, subjects were then brought to the recovery room and monitored in standard fashion. Once conscious, the ten-point pain assessment scale was again assessed. If there was a concern for AE, the subjects underwent hemodynamic monitoring and intravenous fluid (IVF) resuscitation with 1-2 liters of crystalloid and the endoscopist was then able to admit the subject to our institution if needed. If admitted, all subjects underwent basic lab work (chemistry, blood count, amylase, lipase, and liver function testing), as well as abdominal imaging if required.

To evaluate delayed complications, subjects were encouraged to return to the institution in which their procedure was performed. For comprehensive data collection, participants received a telephone call or in person encounter (when hospitalized) within 24 hours or 30 days from their procedure.

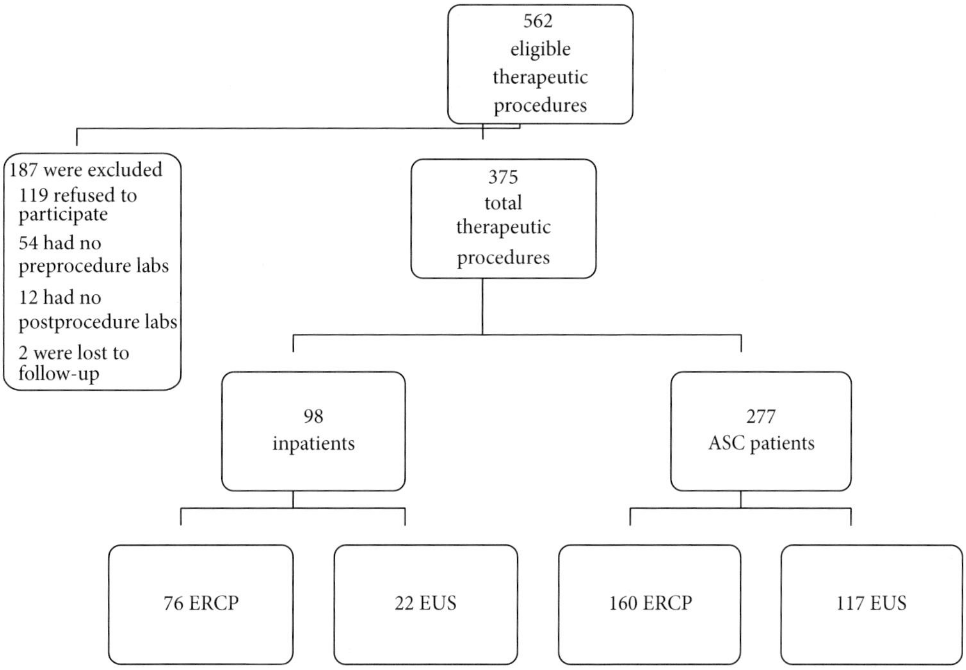

ERCP: endoscopic retrograde cholangiopancreatography; EUS: endoscopic ultrasound;
ASC: ambulatory surgical center.
Depicts the study schema for our study population

FIGURE 1: Study schema with group distribution and number/reason for exclusion in the study.

2.5. Statistical Methods. We determined 292 subjects would reach statistical significance. This is assuming 12% AE for ERCP and 3% for EUS with 5% risk of producing an alpha error to obtain 80% power.

Group and treatment comparisons were carried out using Fisher's exact test for categorical variables and ANOVA with contrasts for continuous variables. Outcomes were evaluated using single variable logistic regression with odds ratios and 99% confidence intervals. A p value of 0.01 was considered statistically significant. All analyses were carried out using SAS v9.4 software (SAS Institute, Cary, NC).

3. Results

3.1. Subjects. From June 2014 until November 2014, a total of 562 ERCP and EUS subjects were screened for study participation. Of those eligible for study participation, 375 agreed to participate in our study and were subsequently analyzed. Among this study sample, 98 procedures were inpatients and 277 were ASC subjects. Of these procedures, 76 were ERCP alone and 22 EUS alone were inpatients, while 160 ERCP and 117 EUS were ASC subjects (see our study schema, Figure 1). All procedures were completed and were technically successful.

Demographic and comorbid condition data did not demonstrate statistical significance between inpatients and ASC subjects (see Table 1). The mean preprocedural ASA classes were not significantly different among the inpatients as compared to the ASC population for ERCP (2.8 versus 2.3, resp.) and EUS (2.8 versus 2.6), as well as the summary of all procedures (2.8 versus 2.4, $p = 0.24$) (Table 1). Mean Mallampati scores also were not significantly different between the ERCP (1.7 versus 1.4), EUS (1.6 versus 1.5), and summary of all procedures (1.7 versus 1.5). No advanced airways were used nor was intubation performed during or prior to any of the therapeutic procedures.

Preprocedural risk factors, namely, "high-risk" components, were slightly variable among inpatients versus ASC ERCPs (22.3% versus 43.1%, resp., $p = 0.09$) and the total population (17.3% versus 27.1%, resp., $p = 0.1$) yet again did not reach statistical significance. There was no difference between high-risk features in the EUS group (0% inpatients versus 5.1% ASC subjects, $p = 0.99$). There was also no difference in moderate-risk features between the ERCP, EUS, and combined population. Table 1 demonstrated breakdown of each risk factor.

Among the inpatients versus ASC groups that underwent both ERCP and EUS, there were no significant differences in the indication. All indications can be summarized in Table 2. Evaluating indications that are considered to be at an increased risk of AE, there was no difference in procedures performed for SOD or palliation of a neoplasm. There were also a higher proportion of ASC procedures, in the total population, performed for the staging of neoplasms (11.2% versus 18.8%, $p < 0.0001$), but there was no difference in each subgroup (Table 2). Regarding findings, there were a significantly higher proportion of overall cancers (21.4% versus 15.9%, $p < 0.0001$) and pancreatic cancers (14.3% versus 13%,

TABLE 1: Demographic and risk data for inpatient versus ASC ERCP, EUS, and the total population.

	ERCP				EUS				Total			
	IN	ASC	ALL	p^* (95% CI)	IN	ASC	All	p^* (95% CI)	IN	ASC	ALL	p^* (95% CI)
Total cases	76	160	236		22	117	139		98	277	375	
Mean age (years)	61.8	60.2	62	0.54	64.2	67.6	63.5	0.62	62.7	63.8	63.5	0.85
Sex												
Male	31 (41%)	46 (29%)	77 (33%)	0.17	18 (82%)	56 (48%)	74 (53%)	0.13	49 (50%)	102 (37%)	151 (40%)	0.1
Female	45 (59%)	114 (71%)	159 (67%)		4 (18%)	61 (52%)	65 (47%)		49 (50%)	175 (63%)	224 (60%)	
Comorbid conditions												
Cardiovascular disease	35 (46%)	55 (34%)	90 (38%)	0.12	4 (18%)	57 (49%)	61 (44%)	0.22	39 (40%)	112 (40%)	151 (40%)	0.27
Pulmonary disease	17 (22%)	18 (11%)	35 (15%)	0.04	2 (9%)	17 (15%)	19 (14%)	0.53	19 (19%)	35 (13%)	54 (14%)	0.97
ESRD on dialysis	12 (16%)	27 (17%)	39 (17%)	0.70	1 (5%)	31 (27%)	32 (23%)	0.28	16 (16%)	62 (22%)	78 (21%)	0.03
Cirrhosis	5 (7%)	7 (4%)	12 (5%)	0.53	0	5 (4%)	5 (4%)	0.99	5 (5%)	13 (5%)	18 (5%)	0.98
Medications												
Anticoagulation	3 (4%)	6 (4%)	9 (4%)	1.00	1 (5%)	4 (3%)	5 (4%)	0.28	4 (4%)	10 (4%)	14 (4%)	0.55
Antiplatelet agent	16 (21%)	23 (14%)	39 (17%)	0.25	1 (5%)	25 (2%)	26 (19%)	0.43	17 (17%)	48 (17%)	65 (17%)	0.07
Endoscopic risk factors												
High risk features	17 (22%)	69 (43%)	86 (36%)	0.09	0	6 (5%)	6 (4%)	0.99	17 (17%)	75 (27%)	92 (25%)	0.1
History of SOD	4 (5%)	19 (12%)	23 (10%)	0.09	0	6 (5%)	6 (4%)	1.00	4 (4%)	25 (7%)	29 (6%)	0.72
History of post-ERCP pancreatitis	0	0	0	1.00	0	0	0	1.00	0	0	0	1.00
Pancreatic sphincterotomy	7 (9%)	37 (23%)	44 (19%)	0.03	NA			1.00	7 (7%)	37 (13%)	44 (12%)	0.01
Precut sphincterotomy	1 (1%)	1 (1%)	2 (1%)	0.62	NA			1.00	1 (1%)	1 (1%)	2 (1%)	1.00
>8 cannulation attempts	0	0	0	1.00	NA			1.00	0	0	0	1.00
Pneumatic dilation of an intact biliary sphincter	5 (7%)	9 (6%)	14 (6%)	0.84	NA			1.00	5 (5%)	9 (3%)	14 (4%)	1.00
Ampullectomy	0	3 (2%)	3 (1%)	0.95	NA			1.00	0	3 (1.1%)	3 (0.8%)	1.00
Moderate risk features	19 (25%)	68 (43%)	87 (37%)	0.10	0	7 (6%)	7 (5%)	0.98	19 (19%)	75 (27%)	94 (25%)	0.02
Age < 50 and female	9 (12%)	26 (16%)	35 (15%)	0.29	0	3 (3%)	3 (2%)	0.99	9 (9%)	29 (11%)	38 (10%)	0.09
History of recurrent pancreatitis	6 (8%)	7 (4%)	13 (6%)	0.38	0	4 (3%)	4 (3%)	0.99	6 (6%)	11 (4%)	17 (5%)	0.93
>3 injections to PD, 1 to tail	1 (1%)	11 (7%)	12 (5%)	1.00	NA			1.00	1 (1%)	11 (4%)	12 (3%)	1.00
Excessive injection PD contrast, leading to acini	0	0	0	1.00	NA			1.00	0	0	0	1.00
Acquisition of cytology from PD using brush	3 (4%)	5 (3%)	8 (3%)	0.30	NA			1.00	3 (3%)	5 (2%)	8 (2%)	0.30
Anesthesia risk												
Mean Mallampati score	1.7	1.4	1.5	0.09	1.6	1.5	1.5	0.93	1.7	1.5	1.5	0.02
Mean ASA score	2.8	2.3	2.5	0.12	2.8	2.6	2.6	0.38	2.8	2.4	2.5	0.24
1	2 (3%)	17 (11%)	19 (8%)		0	1 (1%)	1 (1%)		2 (2%)	18 (7%)	20 (5%)	
2	17 (22%)	74 (46%)	91 (39%)		4 (18%)	45 (39%)	49 (35%)		21 (21%)	119 (43%)	140 (37%)	
3	52 (68%)	69 (43%)	121 (51%)		18 (82%)	71 (61%)	89 (64%)		70 (71%)	140 (51%)	210 (56%)	
4	5 (7%)	0	5 (2%)		0	0	0		5 (5%)	0	5 (1%)	

ERCP: endoscopic retrograde cholangiopancreatography; EUS: endoscopic ultrasound; IN: inpatients; ASC: ambulatory surgical center patients; ALL: inpatients + ASC patients; CI: confidence interval; ESRD: end-stage renal disease; SOD: sphincter of Oddi dysfunction; PD: pancreatic duct; ASA: American society of anesthesia class.

*Note that $p < 0.01$ is significant.

Table 2: Indications, findings, and interventions for inpatient versus ASC ERCP, EUS, and the total population.

	ERCP				EUS				Total			
	IN	ASC	ALL	p^* (95% CI)	IN	ASC	ALL	p^* (95% CI)	IN	ASC	ALL	p^* (95% CI)
Indications												
Biliary												
Obstructive jaundice	39 (51%)	37 (23%)	76 (32%)	**0.0005**	10 (46%)	8 (7%)	18 (13%)	0.07	49 (50%)	45 (16%)	94 (25%)	**<0.0001**
SOD	24 (32%)	40 (25%)	64 (27%)	0.02	3 (14%)	8 (7%)	11 (8%)	0.98	27 (28%)	48 (17%)	75 (20%)	0.02
Dilated biliary ductal system	31 (41%)	25 (16%)	56 (24%)	**<0.0001**	4 (18%)	5 (4%)	9 (7%)	0.94	35 (36%)	30 (11%)	65 (17%)	**0.003**
Choledocholithiasis	19 (25%)	22 (14%)	41 (17%)	0.046	0	0	0	1.00	19 (19%)	22 (8%)	41 (11%)	0.55
Elevated LFT	17 (20%)	5 (3%)	22 (9%)	**0.0002**	3 (14%)	1 (1%)	4 (3%)	1.00	20 (20%)	6 (2%)	26 (7%)	**0.004**
Cholangitis	9 (12%)	0	9 (4%)	0.92	0	0	0	1.00	9 (9%)	10 (3%)	9 (2%)	1.00
Biliary stricture	3 (4%)	8 (5%)	11 (5%)	0.37	1 (5%)	1 (1%)	2 (1%)	0.99	4 (4%)	9 (3%)	13 (4%)	0.62
Stent extraction	9 (12%)	28 (18%)	37 (16%)	0.12	1 (5%)	0	1 (1%)	0.99	10 (10%)	28 (10%)	38 (10%)	0.03
Bile leak	10 (13%)	14 (9%)	24 (10%)	0.53	1 (5%)	0	1 (1%)	0.98	11 (11%)	14 (5%)	25 (7%)	0.35
Pancreatic												
Pancreatic mass	8 (11%)	10 (6%)	18 (8%)	0.09	6 (27%)	26 (22%)	32 (23%)	0.19	14 (14%)	36 (13%)	50 (13%)	**<0.0001**
Pancreatic cyst	0	6 (4%)	6 (3%)	0.96	1 (5%)	38 (33%)	39 (28%)	0.22	1 (1%)	44 (16%)	45 (12%)	**<0.0001**
Chronic pancreatitis	2 (3%)	16 (10%)	18 (8%)	0.11	1 (5%)	8 (7%)	9 (7%)	0.37	3 (3%)	24 (9%)	27 (7%)	0.48
Gall stone pancreatitis	11 (15%)	1 (1%)	12 (5%)	**0.003**	3 (14%)	3 (3%)	6 (3%)	0.02	14 (14%)	4 (1%)	18 (5%)	**0.009**
Pancreatic divisum	1 (1%)	10 (6%)	11 (5%)	0.11	0	2 (2%)	2 (1%)	0.99	1 (1%)	14 (5%)	15 (4%)	0.44
Neoplastic												
Any neoplasm	11 (15%)	12 (8%)	23 (10%)	0.10	3 (14%)	29 (25%)	32 (23%)	0.61	21 (21%)	44 (16%)	65 (17%)	**<0.0001**
Palliation neoplasm	5 (7%)	1 (1%)	6 (3%)	0.06	2 (9%)	0	2 (1%)	1.00	7 (7%)	1 (1%)	8 (2%)	0.50
Staging of neoplasm	6 (8%)	6 (4%)	12 (5%)	0.68	5 (23%)	46 (39%)	51 (37%)	0.98	11 (11%)	52 (19%)	63 (17%)	**<0.0001**
Generalized												
Chronic abdominal pain	8 (11%)	53 (33%)	61 (26%)	**0.0004**	0	6 (5%)	6 (3%)	0.99	8 (8%)	59 (21%)	67 (18%)	**<0.0001**
Intervention												
ERCP												
Biliary												
EBS	57 (75%)	108 (68%)	165 (70%)	**<0.0001**	NA			1.00	57 (58%)	108 (39%)	165 (44%)	**<0.0001**
Needle knife	1 (1%)	1 (1%)	2 (1%)	1.00	NA			1.00	1 (1%)	1 (1%)	2 (1%)	1.00
SEMS	12 (16%)	5 (3%)	17 (8%)	0.06	NA			1.00	12 (12%)	5 (2%)	17 (5%)	0.06
Plastic stent	23 (30%)	18 (11%)	41 (17%)	**0.003**	NA			1.00	23 (24%)	18 (7%)	41 (11%)	**0.003**
Cytology	11 (15%)	22 (14%)	33 (14%)	**0.0002**	NA			1.00	11 (1%)	22 (8%)	33 (9%)	**0.0002**
Cholangioscopy	4 (5%)	11 (7%)	15 (11%)	0.40	NA			1.00	4 (4%)	11 (4%)	15 (4%)	0.40
Manometry	2 (3%)	18 (11%)	20 (9%)	0.47	NA			1.00	2 (2%)	18 (7%)	20 (5%)	0.47
Pancreatic												
EPS	6 (8%)	30 (19%)	36 (15%)	0.03	NA			1.00	6 (6%)	30 (11%)	36 (10%)	0.03
Minor duct papillotomy	1 (1%)	8 (5%)	9 (4%)	0.92	NA			1.00	1 (1%)	8 (3%)	9 (2%)	0.92
PD Stent	21 (28%)	44 (28%)	65 (28%)	1.00	NA			1.00	21 (21%)	44 (16%)	65 (17%)	0.60
Ampullary biopsy	2 (3%)	13 (8%)	15 (6%)	0.13	0	1 (1%)	1 (1%)	1.00	3 (3%)	14 (5%)	17 (5%)	0.81
EUS												
FNA	NA			1.00	12 (55%)	77 (66%)	89 (64%)	**<0.0001**	12 (12%)	77 (28%)	89 (24%)	**<0.0001**

ERCP: endoscopic retrograde cholangiopancreatography; EUS: endoscopic ultrasound; IN: inpatients; ASC: ambulatory surgical center patients; ALL: inpatients + ASC patients; GI: gastrointestinal; LFT: liver function tests; SOD: sphincter of Oddi dysfunction; GIST: gastrointestinal stromal tumor; IPMN: intraductal papillary mucinous neoplasm; NE: neuroendocrine; EBS: endoscopic biliary sphincterotomy; EPS: endoscopic pancreatic sphincterotomy; SEMS: self-expanding metal stent; FNA: fine needle aspiration.

*Note that $p < 0.01$ is significant.

$p < 0.0001$) in the total inpatients population compared to ASC population. For these neoplasms, there were no significant differences in the ERCP or EUS groups.

Evaluating interventions at higher risk for AE (including needles knife sphincterortomy, manometry, ampullary biopsy, EPS, and minor duct papillotomy), we found no significant difference between inpatients and ASC subjects. There was also no significant difference in subjects who receive PD stents. All interventions are summarized in Table 2.

3.2. Outcomes. AE occurred in 7.2% of the study population. The overall AE rate of the total inpatient population (11.2%) was not significantly higher compared to the ASC population (5.8%, $p = 0.11$). There was also no increased risk in overall AE for ERCPs alone (13.2% inpatient versus 7.5% ASC, $p = 0.2$) or EUSs alone (4.5% versus 3.4%, $p = 0.6$).

When we evaluated each individual's procedure-related AE, no statistically significant differences in any groups or subpopulations were detected. Overall, 5.9% of subjects had PEP, among which there was no difference in the total inpatient versus ASC study population (8.2% versus 5.1%, $p = 0.4$). There was also no difference detected in the ERCP alone group (9% inpatients versus 7% ASC, $p = 0.6$). GIB occurred in 1% of the population; 3 occurred in the inpatients group, compared to two in the ASC group ($p = 0.3$). No differences were detected in the ERCP or EUS groups. No perforations or surgeries were required in our study sample and all outcomes are summarized in Table 3.

When evaluating 30-day mortality (3.2% overall), there was no significant difference among the total populations (9% versus 1%), ERCP (9% versus 1%), and EUS (5% versus 2%) (Table 3). Overall, there were 8 subjects who died in the inpatients group and 3 in the ASC group (9.2% versus 1.1%, $p = 0.09$). The time from procedure until death for the inpatients was 15.4 days (12, 18, 23, 30, 10, 5, and 25 days), compared with 20.7 days in ASC subjects (28, 25, and 27 days). All deaths, which occurred in this study, were the result of cancer-related mortality or while in a hospice and not from a procedure-related AE. Of the inpatient population, 2 of the cancer-related deaths were from nongastrointestinal septic shock, while another also developed respiratory compromise and cardiac arrest within 30 days. Among the ASC population, one subject developed combined septic/cardiogenic shock after surgery for their neoplasm. Another ASC subject developed respiratory failure and subsequent cardiac arrest within 30 days after having their procedures for neoplastic encasement. This subject had pancreatitis both before and after procedure.

We found no significant difference in service calls for any reason (Table 3). There was also no difference in the number of readmissions, ED visits, hospitalizations, or urgent care visits among any of the groups (Table 3). The patients undergoing readmission were not different in the ERCP group (11% versus 6), EUS group (5% versus 9%), or summary groups (19% versus 7%). Mean LOS was significantly longer in the total inpatient study population (8.7 days versus 0.8 days, $p < 0.0001$) and inpatient ERCP versus ASC groups (9.3 days versus 0.6 days, $p < 0.0001$, resp.). No significant difference in LOS was detected in the EUS group (Table 3).

Finally, mean procedural and total medical cost was evaluated. Mean procedural cost was significantly higher in the inpatient total population compared with the ASC population ($482.30 versus $423.20, $p < 0.0001$). No difference in cost was seen in the ERCP or EUS study groups. When evaluating mean total medical cost, both the total ($17,815.70 versus $2,026.90, $p < 0.0001$) and ERCP ($19,022.90 versus $1,574.30, $p < 0.0001$) inpatient populations were significantly larger than their ASC counterparts. The EUS group was not statistically different between the inpatient and ASC populations (Table 3).

4. Discussion

In this prospective, multicenter, observational study, we demonstrated no difference in overall or individual AE for subjects undergoing inpatient versus ASC advanced endoscopy. Our study population demonstrated a low AE rate, even with an increased incidence of high-risk procedural features and proportion with an ASA class ≥3.

At present, the American Society for Gastrointestinal Endoscopy (ASGE) has released two documents regarding quality indicators in therapeutic endoscopy [30, 31]. Within these documents are established rates of AE after advanced endoscopic procedures. Generally, it is estimated that ERCP-related AE occur in 5–8% of procedures, with relative mortality of 0.5–2% [1, 2, 7, 16, 30, 31]. Additionally, a similar risk of 0.5–2.9% has been estimated for EUS-FNA [2, 18, 31]. All in all, several prospective studies have been performed and a subsequent review of this topic yielded an overall vision of safety for ERCP in the ASC setting [3–18]. Despite this available evidence, there still exists the question of whether ASC therapeutic endoscopy is safe in a population at higher risk for AE or an ASA class ≥3.

Overall there is paucity of data regarding the safety of therapeutic endoscopy procedures in the ASC cancer population. Composite data from prior studies yielded low proportions of ampullary and pancreatic carcinomas when compared with our population [18]. Mehta et al.'s study did include ASC EUS which were performed for upper GI lesions and for luminal malignancies [7]. In addition to this study, Cvetkovski et al. evaluated this unique population in a retrospective chart review with low AE rates but with no data on postprocedural medical care or cost [5]. Yet the percentage of cancers in our population does appear to be larger than prior studies (17%, other studies, versus 18.7%, our study) [3–18].

Other than cancer subjects, another unique determination in our study is evaluation of AE in the ASC setting using this "higher risk" population. Freeman et al., among others, have evaluated various risk factors, which served to increase the risk of PEP, along with other AE after ERCP [1, 25]. Most other studies evaluating ASC therapeutic endoscopy occurred prior to the identification of high-risk features for post-ERCP AE [3–18]. Yet dissection of these studies included

Table 3: Outcomes and cost for inpatient versus ASC ERCP, EUS, and the total population.

	ERCP				EUS				Total			
	IN	ASC	ALL	p^* (95% CI)	IN	ASC	ALL	p^* (95% CI)	IN	ASC	ALL	p^* (95% CI)
Outcomes												
Postprocedural complications	10 (13%)	12 (8%)	18 (8%)	0.20	1 (5%)	4 (3%)	5 (4%)	0.60	11 (11%)	16 (6%)	27 (7%)	0.11
Pancreatitis	7 (9%)	11 (7%)	18 (8%)	0.60	1 (5%)	3 (3%)	4 (3%)	0.20	8 (8%)	14 (5%)	22 (6%)	0.43
Hemorrhage	3 (4%)	1 (1%)	4 (2%)	0.25	0	1 (1%)	1 (1%)	0.98	3 (3%)	2 (0.7%)	5 (1%)	0.92
Perforation	0	0	0	1.00	0	0	0	1.00	0	0	0	1.00
Mortality												
All-cause	7 (9%)[a,b]	1 (1%)[c]	8 (3%)	0.01	1 (5%)	2 (2%)[d]	3 (2%)	0.12	9 (9%)	3 (1%)	12 (3%)	0.09
Service call												
Fevers	7 (9%)	2 (1%)	9 (4%)	0.02	2 (9%)	2 (2%)	4 (3%)	1.00	9 (9%)	4 (1%)	13 (4%)	0.047
Nausea/vomiting	8 (11%)	17 (11%)	25 (11%)	0.87	0	7 (6%)	7 (5%)	0.98	8 (8%)	24 (9%)	32 (9%)	0.79
Abdominal pain	16 (21%)	37 (23%)	53 (23%)	0.41	2 (9%)	11 (9%)	13 (9%)	0.98	18 (18%)	48 (17%)	66 (18%)	0.13
Medical care												
ED	2 (3%)	5 (3%)	7 (3%)	0.60	0	2 (2%)	2 (%)	0.94	2 (2%)	7 (3%)	9 (2%)	0.70
Urgent care[e]	1 (1%)	2 (1%)	3 (1%)	1.00	0	0	0	1.00	1 (1%)	2 (1%)	3 (1%)	0.90
Hospitalization[f]	1 (1%)	4 (3%)	5 (2%)	0.32	0	2 (2%)	2 (1%)	0.94	1 (1%)	6 (2%)	7 (2%)	0.34
LOS	9.3	0.6	3.6	**<0.0001**	4.4	0.7	2.8	0.21	8.7	0.8	2.8	**<0.0001**
Readmission	8 (11%)	10 (6%)	18 (8%)	0.04	1 (5%)	10 (9%)	11 (8%)	0.80	9 (19%)	20 (7%)	29 (8%)	0.17
Cost												
Procedure	\$489.60	\$474.30	\$490.70	0.12	\$339.10	\$292.20	\$438.40	0.35	\$482.30	\$423.20	\$438.40	**<0.0001**
Total	\$19,022.90	\$1,574.30	\$7,662.80	**<0.0001**	\$9,196.30	\$1,668.90	\$6,082.20	0.21	\$17,815.70	\$2,026.90	\$6,082.20	**<0.0001**

ERCP: endoscopic retrograde cholangiopancreatography; EUS: endoscopic ultrasound; IN: inpatients; ASC: ambulatory surgical center patients; ALL: inpatients + ASC patients; ARDS: acute respiratory distress syndrome; CI: confidence interval; SIRS: systemic inflammatory response syndrome; MOF: multiple organ failure; MI: myocardial infarction; ED: emergency department; LOS: length of stay.

*Note that $p < 0.01$ is significant.

[a] Inpatient that suffered cardiac arrest or respiratory failure was found to have septic shock and mild pancreatitis on day 21 after ERCP.

[b] A second inpatient after cancer surgery died of septic shock.

[c] ASC admitted on day 28 with pancreatitis or respiratory failure was DNR/DNI but family desired to be made hospice.

[d] ASC admitted with septic/cardiogenic shock after surgery for cancer.

[e] Note that no urgent care visits were hospitalized.

[f] Note that all hospitalizations were sent from a call to the service or directly from the endoscopy unit to the ED.

a minimal percentage of subject characteristics determined to be high/moderate risk. Overall, our study was composed of a large proportion of high/moderate-risk subjects (24.5% and 25.1%, resp.). Of this high-risk population, we had 20% that underwent advanced endoscopic procedures for SOD (27% of ERCPs). The most recent study, evaluating ASC therapeutic endoscopy, was published by Rábago et al., with 3% of individuals undergoing ERCP for SOD, and in Mehta et al.'s study, the percentage was 14% [7, 13]. The aforementioned Mehta et al.'s study had 18.9% of ERCP performed for SOD, which is the highest among the studies performed for ASC therapeutic endoscopy [7]. Despite this, the average percentage of subjects included in prior studies for ASC therapeutic endoscopy with "higher risk features" was 9% of ASC subjects and 1% of inpatients with SOD, far lower than our population.

In addition to high-risk procedural factors, our study population did include a large proportion of subjects who had ASA classes greater than or equal to III (57.3% overall), determined to be high-risk from an anesthesia perspective. The ASA along with the ASGE has also expressed usage of ASA classes prior to endoscopic procedures [19–23, 32]. Within this document is the determination of ASA classes ≥III as high risk and subsequent need for anesthesia monitoring during endoscopy. This sentiment was examined by Coté et al. demonstrating significant risk for ASA scoring ≥3 predicting the need for airway maneuvers during advanced endoscopic procedures [33]. Other retrospective analyses have evaluated ASA scoring as a risk for serious AE in the setting of therapeutic endoscopy [34, 35]. As a result, most prior studies evaluating ASC therapeutic endoscopy either included a minimal number of individuals with ASA classes ≥III or excluded them entirely [3–18]. Among these studies, the highest percentages of ASA classes ≥III were seen in Mahnke et al. (17.5%) and Hui et al. (33.2%), with Mahnke et al. being the only prospective investigation [14, 18]. Again, these prior series have demonstrated lower incidence of ASA ≥3 when compared to our population.

At our institution, we utilize propofol-based anesthesia under the guidance of an anesthesiologist/Certified Registered Nurse Anesthetists (CRNA) for all endoscopic procedures. Using this care model, with no statistical difference in the mean ASA class in the inpatient population compared with the ASC population (2.8 inpatients versus 2.4 ASC subjects, $p = 0.24$), our study found no increased risk of overall postprocedural AE, PEP, hemorrhage, mortality, and so forth between these sample groups. Additionally, an elevated ASA class also led to additional 2.1 days in the hospital when admission was needed, but there was no increased risk for ED visit, hospitalization, urgent care visits, service calls, or readmissions. Thus, performance of ASC ERCP, EUS, or combined procedures in those with high-risk features, interventions, and an ASA class ≥III led to no increase in AE and medical disposition with a mild increase in LOS among inpatients.

Potential weakness could have included our cost analysis for procedures that may have been different between inpatients and ASC subjects because of the instruments utilized between procedures. However, standardized tools were utilized for all cases. Another potential risk may have been the large number of variables examined, which led to our statistical cut-off being $p < 0.01$ and not $p < 0.05$. This correction was used to eliminate errors from random chance and may have excluded some relevant findings. Points of strength of this paper included the prospective nature for which this study was performed and randomization of procedure location based upon a random number generator. We also methodically obtained postprocedure labs in all subjects and data with rigorous follow-up. To evaluate our study parameters, we also evaluated subjects in tertiary care centers as well as community centers; thus our information applied to both practice settings. Another point of strength was validating our data in a unique cohort of subjects described as having high-risk procedural and preprocedural risks, higher ASA classes, and a larger proportion of subjects with cancer. This allowed for more generalizable interpretation of our data. In future study, we hope to validate the safety of ASC AE in combined ERCP/EUS and therapeutic EUS and by incorporating prophylactic measures such as intravenous fluid strategy and rectal indomethacin.

In an age where healthcare costs continue to rise, the feasibility of performing both ERCP and EUS safely in the ASC setting has become of paramount importance. Also, with the publication of value-based metrics set forth by the ASGE, it has been integral for endoscopists to perform quality therapeutic procedures in a manner safe for subjects. In this prospective multicenter study, with 30-day follow-up, we determined that ERCP and EUS are safe and cost-effective procedures in the high-risk ASC population.

Abbreviations

ERCP:	Endoscopic retrograde cholangiopancreatography
EUS:	Endoscopic ultrasound
EUS-FNA:	Endoscopic ultrasound with fine needle aspiration
ASC:	Ambulatory surgical center
SOD:	Sphincter of Oddi dysfunction
ASA:	American Society for Anesthesiologists
NJ:	New Jersey
MAC:	Monitored anesthesia care
PGY:	Postgraduate year
BSC:	Boston Scientific Corporation, Incorporated
ACEI:	Angiotensin converting enzymes inhibitors
ARB:	Angiotensin II receptor blocker
IVF:	Intravenous fluids
ED:	Emergency department
PEP:	Post-ERCP pancreatitis
GIB:	Gastrointestinal bleeding
ACS:	Acute coronary syndrome
SIRS:	Systemic inflammatory response syndrome
MOF:	Multiple organ failure
ESRD:	End-stage renal disease
LOS:	Length of stay

ANOVA: Analysis of variance
SAS: Statistical analysis system
OR: Odds ratio
EBS: Endoscopic biliary sphincterotomy
EPS: Endoscopic pancreatic sphincterotomy
ASGE: American Society for Gastrointestinal Endoscopy
CRNA: Certified Registered Nurse Anesthetists.

Competing Interests

Shaffer R. S. Mok, Henry C. Ho, and John P. Gaughan have no competing interests. Adam B. Elfant is a consultant for Boston Scientific Corporation.

Acknowledgments

The authors would like to thank Tara L. Lautenslager and Jeffrey M. Costanzo for their assistance in this project and care of the subjects. They would also like to thank Krystal Hunter for providing additional statistical support. Finally, they would like to thank Samuel N. Giordano for allowing them to involve his subjects in this study.

References

[1] M. A. Anderson, L. Fisher, R. Jain et al., "Complications of ERCP," *Gastrointestinal Endoscopy*, vol. 75, no. 3, pp. 467–473, 2012.

[2] D. S. Early, R. D. Acosta, V. Chandrasekhara et al., "Adverse events associated with EUS and EUS with FNA," *Gastrointestinal Endoscopy*, vol. 77, no. 6, pp. 839–843, 2013.

[3] I. Podolsky, P. Kortan, and G. B. Haber, "Endoscopic sphincterotomy in outpatients," *Gastrointestinal Endoscopy*, vol. 35, no. 5, pp. 372–376, 1989.

[4] T. C. Tham, J. Vandervoort, R. C. Wong et al., "Therapeutic ERCP in outsubjects," *Gastrointestinal Endoscopy*, vol. 45, no. 3, pp. 225–230, 1997.

[5] B. Cvetkovski, H. Gerdes, and R. C. Kurtz, "Outpatient therapeutic ERCP with endobiliary stent placement for malignant common bile duct obstruction," *Gastrointestinal Endoscopy*, vol. 50, no. 1, pp. 63–66, 1999.

[6] P. Katsinelos, J. Kountouras, G. Chatzimavroudis et al., "Outpatient therapeutic endoscopic retrograde cholangiopancreatography is safe in patients aged 80 years and older," *Endoscopy*, vol. 43, no. 2, pp. 128–133, 2011.

[7] S. N. Mehta, E. Pavone, and A. N. Barkun, "Outpatient therapeutic ERCP: a series of 262 consecutive cases," *Gastrointestinal Endoscopy*, vol. 44, no. 4, pp. 443–449, 1996.

[8] M. H. Urban, "Endoscopic retrograde cholangiopancreatography. A diagnostic outpatient procedure," *AORN Journal*, vol. 50, no. 3, pp. 572–581, 1989.

[9] H. D. Duncan, L. Hodgkinson, M. Deakin, and J. R. B. Green, "The safety of diagnostic and therapeutic ERCP as a daycase procedure with a selective admission policy," *European Journal of Gastroenterology and Hepatology*, vol. 9, no. 9, pp. 905–908, 1997.

[10] C. Kyriakides, Y. Service, D. E. F. Tweedle, and D. F. Martin, "Day-case transfer of inpatients for diagnostic and therapeutic endoscopic retrograde cholangiopancreatography," *British Journal of Surgery*, vol. 84, no. 9, pp. 1260–1263, 1997.

[11] S. M. Jeurnink, J. W. Poley, E. W. Steyerberg, E. J. Kuipers, and P. D. Siersema, "ERCP as an outpatient treatment: a review," *Gastrointestinal Endoscopy*, vol. 68, no. 1, pp. 118–123, 2008.

[12] A. B. Elfant, M. J. Bourke, R. Alhalel, P. P. Kortan, and G. B. Haber, "A prospective study of the safety of endoscopic therapy for choledocholithiasis in an outpatient population," *American Journal of Gastroenterology*, vol. 91, no. 8, pp. 1499–1502, 1996.

[13] L. Rábago, I. Guerra, M. Moran et al., "Is outpatient ERCP suitable, feasible, and safe? The experience of a Spanish community hospital," *Surgical Endoscopy and Other Interventional Techniques*, vol. 24, no. 7, pp. 1701–1706, 2010.

[14] C.-K. Hui, K.-C. Lai, W.-M. Wong et al., "Outpatients undergoing therapeutic endoscopic retrograde cholangiopancreatography: six-hour versus overnight observation," *Journal of Gastroenterology and Hepatology*, vol. 19, no. 10, pp. 1163–1168, 2004.

[15] C. J. Fox, R. A. Harry, and S. R. Cairns, "A prospective series of out-patient endoscopic retrograde cholangiopancreatography," *European Journal of Gastroenterology and Hepatology*, vol. 12, no. 5, pp. 523–527, 2000.

[16] M. L. Freeman, D. B. Nelson, S. Sherman et al., "Same-day discharge after endoscopic biliary sphincterotomy: observations from a prospective multicenter complication study," *Gastrointestinal Endoscopy*, vol. 49, no. 5, pp. 580–586, 1999.

[17] D. J. Bjorkman and J. Van Dam, "Outpatient therapeutic ERCP: cutting sphincters and cutting costs," *American Journal of Gastroenterology*, vol. 91, no. 8, pp. 1485–1486, 1996.

[18] D. Mahnke, Y. K. Chen, M. R. Antillon, W. R. Brown, R. Mattison, and R. J. Shah, "A prospective study of complications of endoscopic retrograde cholangiopancreatography and endoscopic ultrasound in an ambulatory endoscopy center," *Clinical Gastroenterology and Hepatology*, vol. 4, no. 7, pp. 924–930, 2006.

[19] S. R. Mallampati, S. P. Gatt, L. D. Gugino et al., "A clinical sign to predict difficult tracheal intubation: a prospective study," *Canadian Anaesthetists' Society Journal*, vol. 32, no. 4, pp. 429–434, 1985.

[20] A. Lee, L. T. Y. Fan, T. Gin, M. K. Karmakar, and W. D. N. Kee, "A systematic review (meta-analysis) of the accuracy of the mallampati tests to predict the difficult airway," *Anesthesia & Analgesia*, vol. 102, no. 6, pp. 1867–1878, 2006.

[21] M. Saklad, "Grading of patients for surgical procedures," *Anesthesiology*, vol. 2, no. 3, pp. 281–284, 1941.

[22] ASA, *ASA Relative Value Guide 2002*, Code 99140, American Society of Anesthesiologists, Park Ridge, Ill, USA, 2002.

[23] ASA, *ASA Physical Status Classification System*, American Society of Anesthesiologists, Park Ridge, Ill, USA, 2013.

[24] M. Yaghoobi, S. Rolland, K. A. Waschke et al., "Meta-analysis: rectal indomethacin for the prevention of post-ERCP pancreatitis," *Alimentary Pharmacology and Therapeutics*, vol. 38, no. 9, pp. 995–1001, 2013.

[25] M. L. Freeman, D. B. Nelson, S. Sherman et al., "Complications of endoscopic biliary sphincterotomy," *The New England Journal of Medicine*, vol. 335, no. 13, pp. 909–918, 1996.

[26] Rome Foundation, *Rome III Diagnostic Criteria for Functional Gastrointestinal Disorders*, Rome Foundation, 2014.

[27] D. N. Prajapati and W. J. Hogan, "Sphincter of Oddi dysfunction and other functional biliary disorders: evaluation and treatment," *Gastroenterology Clinics of North America*, vol. 32, no. 2, pp. 601–618, 2003.

[28] P. B. Cotton, G. Lehman, J. Vennes et al., "Endoscopic sphincterotomy complications and their management: an attempt at consensus," *Gastrointestinal Endoscopy*, vol. 37, no. 3, pp. 383–393, 1991.

[29] S. Tenner, J. Baillie, J. DeWitt et al., "American college of gastroenterology guideline: management of acute pancreatitis," *American Journal of Gastroenterology*, vol. 108, pp. 1400–1415, 2013.

[30] D. G. Adler, J. G. Lieb, J. Cohen et al., "Quality indicators for ERCP," *Gastrointestinal Endoscopy*, vol. 81, no. 1, pp. 54–66, 2015.

[31] S. Wani, M. B. Wallace, J. Cohen et al., "Quality indicators for EUS," *Gastrointestinal Endoscopy*, vol. 81, no. 1, pp. 67–80, 2015.

[32] D. R. Lichtenstein, S. Jagannath, T. H. Baron et al., "Sedation and anesthesia in GI endoscopy," *Gastrointestinal Endoscopy*, vol. 68, no. 5, pp. 815–826, 2008.

[33] G. A. Coté, R. M. Hovis, M. A. Ansstas et al., "Incidence of sedation-related complications with propofol use during advanced endoscopic procedures," *Clinical Gastroenterology and Hepatology*, vol. 8, no. 2, pp. 137–142, 2010.

[34] B. G. Goudra, P. M. Singh, and A. C. Sinha, "Outpatient endoscopic retrograde cholangiopancreatography: safety and efficacy of anesthetic management with a natural airway in 653 consecutive procedures," *Saudi Journal of Anaesthesia*, vol. 7, no. 3, pp. 259–265, 2013.

[35] B. K. Enestvedt, G. M. Eisen, J. Holub, and D. A. Lieberman, "Is the American Society of Anesthesiologists classification useful in risk stratification for endoscopic procedures?" *Gastrointestinal Endoscopy*, vol. 77, no. 3, pp. 464–471, 2013.

31

Endoscopic Ultrasound Elastography for Evaluation of Lymph Nodes: A Single Center Experience

Ahmed Youssef Altonbary,[1] **Hazem Hakim**,[1] **and Ahmed Mohamed El-Shamy**[2]

[1]*Department of Gastroenterology and Hepatology, Mansoura Specialized Medical Hospital, Mansoura University, Mansoura, Egypt*
[2]*Department of Anesthesia and Intensive Care, Mansoura University, Mansoura, Egypt*

Correspondence should be addressed to Ahmed Youssef Altonbary; a.tonbary@gmail.com

Academic Editor: Timothy A. Woodward

Background and Aim. The differentiation between malignant and benign lymph nodes (LNs) is important for tumor staging, for detection of prognosis, and for selection of the best treatment strategy in many cancers. On B-mode EUS, there are some known criteria that suggest the malignant nature of LNs; these criteria may be found in benign LNs. The aim of the work is to evaluate the effectiveness of elasticity score and SR to differentiate between benign and malignant LNs. *Patients and Methods.* The study was designed as a retrospective study that included 40 patients with abdominal or mediastinal LNs, either associated with primary masses or isolated, referred for EUS evaluation. Elasticity scores and SR were determined during the examination and finally, EUS-FNA was done at the end of the procedure. *Results.* In this 2-years study, 40 patients were enrolled (24 malignant; 16 benign). There were 23 males and 17 females. Their mean age was 52.5 years (range: 28–77). ES alone had a specificity of 87.5%, sensitivity of 41.7%, PPV of 83.3%, NPV of 50%, and accuracy of 60%. Based on the ROC curve analysis results, the best cut-off level of SR to obtain the maximum area under the curve (AUC) was 6.7 with a specificity of 99.9%, sensitivity of 57.1%, PPV of 99.9%, NPV of 64%, and accuracy of 77.5%. *Conclusion.* The use of elasticity score and SR increases the reliability of differentiation between benign and malignant LNs and can decrease the number of unnecessary biopsies.

1. Introduction

The differentiation between malignant and benign lymph nodes (LNs) is important for tumor staging, for detection of prognosis and for selection of the best treatment strategy in many cancers, as esophageal, stomach, bronchial, and pancreatic tumors. EUS can provide real time images of LNs close to the gastrointestinal tract, but the ability of EUS to differentiate between malignant and benign LNs remains a challenge [1]. On B-mode EUS, there are some known criteria that suggest the malignant nature of LNs (such as hypoechogenicity, rounded shape, sharp borders, and diameter more than 1 cm). However, some of these criteria may be found in benign LNs. Also, it should be considered that none of these typical criteria are found in the early stages of malignant LNs [2]. The accuracy and specificity of these criteria in diagnosis of malignant LNs are considered low [3, 4].

In the past 2 decades, EUS elastography has emerged as a noninvasive tool for estimating the mechanical characteristics of tissues [5]. This technique is used to assess tissue stiffness according to the degree of tissue distortion in response to an external power [6]. The strain ratio (SR), a semiquantitative elastography method, is measured by assessing the elastography pattern of the targeted LN in comparison to that of a nearby reference tissue [7].

In this study, we evaluate the effectiveness of elasticity score and SR to differentiate between benign and malignant LNs.

2. Patients and Methods

2.1. Patients. Of 309 EUS examinations performed over the 2 years study period from January 2016 to January 2018 at the EUS Unit of the Department of Gastroenterology of

Mansoura Specialized Medical Hospital, Mansoura University (Egypt), lymph nodes were detected in 50 patients and 40 of them were included in the study. Eight patients with missing data and two patients with inconclusive biopsy were excluded from the study.

The inclusion criteria were as follows: all patients with abdominal or mediastinal LNs, either associated with primary masses or isolated, referred for EUS evaluation. The exclusion criteria were as follows: patients with a contraindication to interventional endoscopy, as patients with coagulation disorders, or patients unfit for sedation, patients who refused to be involved in the study, and patients in whom the final diagnosis was not known. The study protocol was approved by our ethical committee and written consents were taken from all patients before the procedure.

2.2. Methods. The study was designed as a retrospective study to evaluate the effectiveness of elasticity score and SR in diagnosing LNs. On the day of the procedure, eligible patients were appointed to the endoscopy room for EUS examination under intravenous propofol sedation. EUS examination was done in all patients with a Pentax linear Echoendoscope EG3870UTK (PENTAX medical, Tokyo, Japan) attached to a Hitachi Avius ultrasound system (Hitachi Medical Systems, Tokyo, Japan). All EUS examinations were done by two endosonographers. After localization of the LN, elastography was applied to evaluate their hardness. Theoretically, the hardness of malignant LNs is greater than that of inflammatory ones. The hardness of the lesion is assessed by the degree of tissue distortion illustrated on a color map (from red to blue representing soft to hard areas, respectively). Elasticity scores and SR were determined during the examination and finally, EUS-FNA was done at the end of the procedure.

2.2.1. Elasticity Score and Strain Ratio. Elasticity score (ES) was defined as the following: ES 1 was given to homogeneous green and interpreted as normal tissue. ES 2 was given to heterogeneous green predominant and interpreted as inflammation or fibrosis. ES 3 was given to heterogeneous blue predominant and interpreted as indeterminate for malignancy. ES 4 was given to homogeneous blue and interpreted as malignant lesions (Figures 1 and 2).

SR was calculated as the following: two areas were selected, the region of interest selected as area (A) and the normal reference tissue selected as area (B) then dividing area (B) by area (A) (Figures 1 and 2). The final result for SR was calculated from the mean of repeated measures. Subsequently, the receiver operating characteristic (ROC) curve was used to determine the best cut-off value and to calculate the diagnostic value of the SR.

2.2.2. Statistical Analysis. IBM SPSS statistics for widows (version 24) was used for calculating the means of strain ratios, sensitivity, specificity, positive predictive value (PPV), negative predictive value (NPV), and accuracy. The best cut-off value was selected by comparing diagnosis made by elasticity score, SR, and final diagnosis obtained by the cytopathological examination of the EUS-FNA samples or

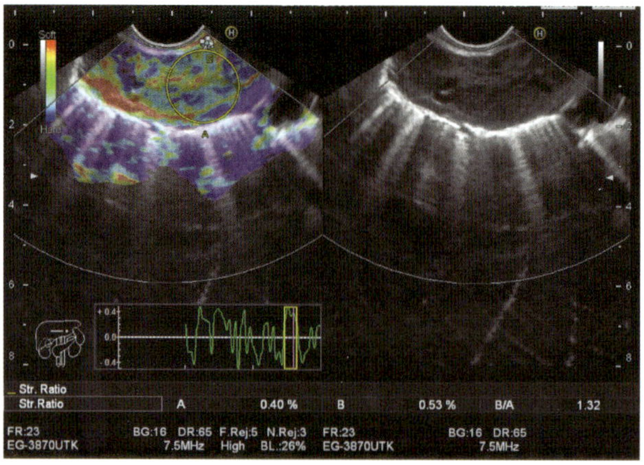

FIGURE 1: Benign lymph node with elasticity score (ES) 2 and strain ratio (SR) 1.32.

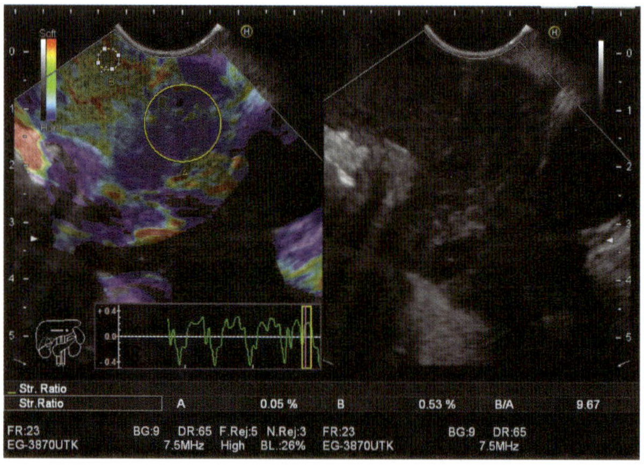

FIGURE 2: Malignant lymph node with elasticity score (ES) 3 and strain ratio (SR) 9.67.

after surgical excision using the receiver operating characteristic (ROC) curve and was used to calculate the diagnostic value. Shapiro-Wilk test was used to check the normality of data and Student t-test and Mann-Whitney Tests were used for parametric and nonparametric data, respectively, with 95% confidence interval (CI). P value ≤ 0.05 was considered statistically significant.

3. Results

In this 2-year study, 40 patients were enrolled (24 malignant, 16 benign). There were 23 males and 17 females. Their mean age was 52.5 years (range: 28-77). The size, site, final diagnosis of lymph nodes, SR, and elasticity score are shown in Tables 1–5.

ES 1 and 2 were deemed benign while ES 3 and 4 were deemed malignant. ES alone had a specificity of 87.5%, sensitivity of 41.7%, PPV of 83.3%, NPV of 50%, and accuracy of 60% (Table 6).

There was a significant statistical difference between the mean value of the SR for benign LNs (3) and the mean value of

TABLE 1: Location of the lymph nodes.

Location	Number of cases =40	
	Frequency	Percent
Mediastinum	16	40%
Portahepatis	8	20%
Para-aortic	8	20%
Perigastric	5	12.5%
Perirectal	2	5%
Paraesophageal	1	2.5%

TABLE 2: Size (cm) of the lymph nodes (n = 40).

	All lesions (n= 40)	Benign lesions (n= 16)	Malignant lesions (n= 24)	P value
Mean± SD	4.3±1.7	3.7±1.3	4.9±1.7	0.021
Median	4.0	3.5	5	
Range	1.1: 9.0	2.0: 6.0	1.1: 9.0	

TABLE 3: Diagnosis of the lymph nodes (n = 40).

Diagnosis		Frequency	Percent
Benign	Inflammatory	14	35%
	Thymoma	1	2.5%
	Sarcoidosis	1	2.5%
Malignant	Lymphoma	13	32.5%
	Undifferentiated carcinoma	7	17.5%
	Adenocarcinoma	3	7.5%
	Small cell carcinoma	1	2.5%

TABLE 4: Strain ratio of the lymph nodes.

Elastography	All lesions (n= 40)	Benign lesions (n= 16)	Malignant lesions (n= 24)	P value
Mean± SD	10.9±23.5	3±1.1	17±30	0.001
Median	3.4	2.7	9.5	
Range	1.7: 140	1.7: 5.4	2: 140	

TABLE 5: Elasticity score of the lymph nodes.

	All lesions (n= 40)		Benign lesions (n= 16)		Malignant lesions (n= 24)	
	Frequency	Percent	Frequency	Percent	Frequency	Percent
ES 2	28	70%	14	87.5%	14	58.3%
ES 3	12	30%	2	12.5%	10	41.7%

TABLE 6: Diagnostic values of ES and SR of the lymph nodes.

	ES	SR 6.7
Sensitivity	41.7%	57.1%
Specificity	87.5%	99.9%
PPV	83.3%	99.9%
NPV	50%	64%
Accuracy	60%	77.5%

the SR for malignant LNs (17) (p=0.001). Based on the ROC curve analysis results, the best cut-off level of SR to obtain the maximum area under the curve (AUC) was 6.7 with a specificity of 99.9%, sensitivity of 57.1%, PPV of 99.9%, NPV of 64%, and accuracy of 77.5% (Table 6).

4. Discussion

The present study provides evidence supporting EUS elastography as an accurate and useful tool for the differential diagnosis of LNs. Strain ratio (SR) adds important and objective information to EUS by providing a quantitative evaluation of tissue stiffness, which supports the benign or malignant nature of LNs.

Although EUS-FNA is considered as the gold standard for the diagnosis of malignant LNs, with PPV and specificity approaching 100%, FNA needs appropriate training and good experience and may be associated with many complications [8]. Recently, many studies showed that EUS elastography and SR are useful tools in assessing LNs and selecting the suspected nodes. Also, EUS elastography can be used to target the hardest area in the LN which is considered the most suspicious area of the node before tissue sampling. In case of multiple LNs, EUS elastography can increase the sensitivity of EUS-FNA by reducing the number of unnecessary biopsies. Moreover, in patients with negative EUS-FNA or in situations in which FNA cannot be done (technical difficulties or interposed blood vessel), EUS elastography can be used as a useful alternative to differentiate malignant from benign LNs [9, 10].

Okasha and his colleges evaluated the value of the SR in the differentiation between benign and malignant LNs. They examined 126 LNs, with a SR cut-off value of 4.6 for malignant LNs. The specificity, sensitivity, NPV, and PPV were 83.3%, 89.8%, 90.2%, and 82.5%, respectively [11].

Paterson and his colleges evaluated the value of the SR in the LN staging of esophageal and gastric tumors, using EUS-FNA cytology as the reference method. They examined 50 LNs, with a SR cut-off value of 7.5 for malignant LNs. The specificity, sensitivity, NPV, PPV, and accuracy were 96%, 83%, 86%, 95%, and 90%, respectively, compared to the values of 22–70%, 64–96%, 61–83%, 57–72%, and 60–75%, respectively, that were gained from different criteria of B-mode EUS [12].

Larsen and his colleges assessed the use of EUS elastography and SR in the evaluation of nodes present with upper gastrointestinal tract malignancies, using surgical pathology as the reference method. A total of 56 LNs were evaluated. For EUS elastography, the specificity, sensitivity, PPV, NPV, and accuracy were 85%, 55%, 71%, 74%, and 73%, respectively. And for the SR at a cut-off value of 4.5, the specificity, sensitivity, PPV, NPV, and accuracy were 82%, 55%, 67%, 74%, and 71%, respectively [13].

In our study, ES alone had a specificity of 87.5%, sensitivity of 41.7%, PPV of 83.3%, NPV of 50%, and accuracy of 60%. This was in contrast to the previous published study by Larsen et al. [13] that showed higher sensitivity, NPV, and accuracy. This may be attributed to the subjectivity of ES.

Many studies mentioned the SR with different cut-off levels to overcome the subjectivity and increase specificity of EUS elastography. We had a cut-off level of 6.7 that had specificity, sensitivity, PPV, NPV, and accuracy of 99.9%, 57%, 99.9%, 64%, and 77.5%, respectively. This was comparable to the study done by Paterson et al. [12] that identified a cut-off level of 7.5 that had specificity and PPV of 96% and 95%, respectively, but higher values of sensitivity, NPV, and accuracy of 83%, 86%, and 90%, respectively. Okasha et al. [11] and Larsen et al. [13] identified a lower cut-off value for SR of 4.6 and 4.5 that gave lower values in specificity and PPV of 83.3%, 82.5% and 82%, 67%, respectively.

The present study has some limitations as follows: EUS elastography and SR were used to evaluate different types of pathology in malignant nodes (e.g., mediastinal, pancreatic, perigastric, paraaortic, etc.) and benign nodes, which may cause divergence in the results due to different tissue heterogeneity. Also, relatively small number of patients are compared to other studies. On the other hand, the use of elasticity score and strain ratio may be useful alternative, in patients with negative EUS-FNA or in situations in which FNA cannot be done.

In conclusion, the use of elasticity score and SR increases the reliability of differentiation between benign and malignant LNs and can decrease the number of unnecessary biopsies.

References

[1] X.-W. Cui, J.-M. Chang, Q.-C. Kan, L. Chiorean, A. Ignee, and C. F. Dietrich, "Endoscopic ultrasound elastography: Current status and future perspectives," *World Journal of Gastroenterology*, vol. 21, no. 47, pp. 13212–13224, 2015.

[2] X. W. Cui, C. Jenssen, A. Saftoiu, A. Ignee, and C. F. Dietrich, "New ultrasound techniques for lymph node evaluation," *World Journal of Gastroenterology*, vol. 19, no. 30, pp. 4850–4860, 2013.

[3] J. Janssen, "EUS elastography: Current status and perspectives," *Zeitschrift für Gastroenterologie*, vol. 46, no. 6, pp. 572–579, 2008.

[4] M. S. Bhutani, R. H. Hawes, and B. J. Hoffman, "A comparison of the accuracy of echo features during endoscopic ultrasound (EUS) and EUS-guided fine-needle aspiration for diagnosis of malignant lymph node invasion," *Gastrointestinal Endoscopy*, vol. 45, no. 6, pp. 474–479, 1997.

[5] C. F. Dietrich, C. Jenssen, P. G. Arcidiacono et al., "Endoscopic ultrasound: Elastographic lymph node evaluation," *Endoscopic Ultrasound*, vol. 4, no. 3, pp. 176–190, 2015.

[6] J.-L. Gennisson, T. Deffieux, M. Fink, and M. Tanter, "Ultrasound elastography: Principles and techniques," *Diagnostic and Interventional Imaging*, vol. 94, no. 5, pp. 487–495, 2013.

[7] J. Iglesias-Garcia, B. Lindkvist, J. Lariño-Noia, and J. E. Domínguez-Muñoz, "Endoscopic ultrasound elastography," *Endoscopic Ultrasound*, vol. 1, no. 1, pp. 8–16, 2012.

[8] M. Hocke, A. Ignee, T. Topalidis, and C. F. Dietrich, "Back to the roots - Should gastroenterologists perform their own cytology?" *Zeitschrift für Gastroenterologie*, vol. 51, no. 2, pp. 191–195, 2013.

[9] C. F. Dietrich, "Real-time tissue elastography. Multiple clinical applications," *Multiple clinical solutions. Endo Heute*, vol. 8, 2011.

[10] C. F. Dietrich, M. Hocke, and C. Jenssen, "Ultrasound for abdominal lymphadenopathy," *Deutsche Medizinische Wochenschrift*, vol. 138, no. 19, pp. 1001–1018, 2013.

[11] H. Okasha, S. Elkholy, M. Sayed et al., "Ultrasound, endoscopic ultrasound elastography, and the strain ratio in differentiating benign from malignant lymph nodes," *Arab Journal of Gastroenterology*, vol. 19, no. 1, pp. 7–15, 2018.

[12] S. Paterson, F. Duthie, and A. J. Stanley, "Endoscopic ultrasound-guided elastography in the nodal staging of oesophageal cancer," *World Journal of Gastroenterology*, vol. 18, no. 9, pp. 889–895, 2012.

[13] M. H. Larsen, C. Fristrup, T. P. Hansen, C. P. Hovendal, and M. B. Mortensen, "Endoscopic ultrasound, endoscopic sonoelastography, and strain ratio evaluation of lymph nodes with histology as gold standard," *Endoscopy*, vol. 44, no. 8, pp. 759–766, 2012.

Unsuspected Small-Bowel Crohn's Disease in Elderly Patients Diagnosed by Video Capsule Endoscopy

Che-Yung Chao,[1,2] Carl Frederic Duchatellier,[1] and Ernest G. Seidman[1]

[1]*Division of Gastroenterology, McGill University Health Center, Montreal, QC, Canada*
[2]*Department of Gastroenterology and Hepatology, Princess Alexandra Hospital, Brisbane, QLD, Australia*

Correspondence should be addressed to Ernest G. Seidman; ernest.seidman@mcgill.ca

Academic Editor: Tony C. K. Tham

Background. Video capsule endoscopy (VCE) is increasingly performed among the elderly for obscure bleeding. Our aim was to report on the utility of VCE to uncover unsuspected Crohn's disease (CD) in elderly patients. *Methods.* Retrospective review of VCE performed in elderly patients (≥70 y) at a tertiary hospital (2010–2015). All underwent prior negative bidirectional endoscopies. CD diagnosis was based on consistent endoscopic findings, exclusion of other causes, and a Lewis endoscopic score (LS) > 790 (moderate-to-severe inflammation). Those with lower LS (350–790) required histological confirmation. Known IBD cases were excluded. *Results.* 197 VCE were performed (mean age 78; range 70–93). Main indications were iron deficiency anemia (IDA), occult GI bleeding (OGIB), chronic abdominal pain, or diarrhea. Eight (4.1%) were diagnosed as CD based on the aforementioned criteria. Fecal calprotectin (FCP) was elevated in 7/8 (mean 580 μg/g). Mean LS was 1824. Small-bowel CD detected by VCE led to a change in management in 4/8. One patient had capsule retention secondary to NSAID induced stricture, requiring surgical retrieval. *Conclusions.* VCE can be safely performed in the elderly. A proportion of cases may have unsuspected small-bowel CD despite negative endoscopies. FCP was the best screening test. Diagnosis frequently changed management.

1. Introduction

Video capsule endoscopy (VCE) is an advanced technology developed to provide noninvasive endoscopic assessment of the small bowel [1]. The capsule consists of an optical camera with light source, batteries, and wireless transmitter. Following ingestion, its movement is propelled by intestinal motility. Luminal images are captured and transmitted to the data recorder worn by the patient. Dedicated computer and software program are used for analysis of the image data.

The main clinical indications for VCE are occult GI bleeding (OGIB), iron deficiency anemia (IDA), suspected or follow-up of Crohn's disease (CD), suspected small-bowel tumor, surveillance of polyposis syndromes, refractory celiac disease, and protein losing enteropathy [2]. VCE is usually used in conjunction with standard esophagogastroduodenoscopy and colonoscopy. It may also be used in preference to other imaging modalities including computer tomography or magnetic resonance enterography or push or balloon assisted enteroscopy, depending on the clinical scenario [3, 4].

VCE is increasingly performed in the elderly population, particularly for IDA and OGIB, due to its superior diagnostic accuracy compared to cross-sectional imaging as well as its noninvasive nature when compared to enteroscopy in a population with significant comorbidities [5].

CD is a chronic relapsing inflammatory bowel disease involving any segment of the GI tract. The age of onset is ordinarily between 15 and 40 years. However, some studies suggested a bimodal peak at a later age [6]. It was recently reported that, compared with patients with adult-onset CD, patients with elderly onset CD were more likely to have isolated colonic disease and a nonstricturing, nonpenetrating phenotype but less likely to have perianal complications [7]. There is however very limited data on newly diagnosed CD in elderly patients uncovered by VCE, thus prompting this retrospective study evaluating the relevant clinical parameters and outcomes in this distinctive population.

TABLE 1: Lewis video capsule endoscopy scoring index.

Parameters	Number	Longitudinal extent	Descriptor
Villous appearance (separate score for each small bowel tertile)	Normal: 0 Edematous: 1	Short segment: 8 Long segment: 12 Whole tertile: 20	Single:1 Patchy:14 Diffuse:17
Ulcer (separate score for each small bowel tertile)	None: 0 Single: 3 Few: 5 Multiple: 10	Short segment: 5 Long segment: 10 Whole tertile: 15	<1/4—9 1/4–1/2—12 >1/2—18
Stenosis (for whole study only)	None: 0 Single: 14 Multiple: 20	Ulcerated: 24 Nonulcerated: 2	Traversed:7 Not traversed: 10

Total score: maximum tertile score {[(villous parameter × extent × descriptor) + (ulcer parameter × extent × size)] for tertile 1 or [(villous parameter × extent × descriptor) + (ulcer parameter × extent × size)] for tertile 2 or [(villous parameter × extent × descriptor) + (ulcer parameter × extent × size)] for tertile 3} + (stenosis number × ulcerated × traversed).

Reprinted with permission from Gralnek et al., Alimentary Pharmacology & Therapeutics, 2008 [8].

2. Patients and Methods

A retrospective review was performed on all patients who underwent VCE at the McGill University Health Centre between January 2010 and September 2015. All patients aged 70 or above without prior diagnosis of IBD were included in the study. All indications for VCE were acceptable other than for follow-up of CD. Furthermore, all included patients needed to have had prior and recent (within 1 year) negative bidirectional GI endoscopies.

The diagnosis of small-bowel CD was based on consistent endoscopic findings and exclusion of other potential causes of small-bowel inflammation such as infections, celiac disease, or drugs such as nonsteroidal anti-inflammatory drugs (NSAID) or telmisartan in the previous month. In addition, patients were included if the Lewis endoscopic severity score (LS, Table 1) [8] was >790 (indicating moderate-to-severe inflammation). For cases with a lower LS (350–790), histological confirmation of CD was necessary. Capsule retention was defined as delayed capsule excretion for more than 2 weeks, or requiring retrieval.

Patient demographics, clinical information, diagnostic results, and management outcomes were retrieved through their electronic medical records for analysis. Serum C-reactive protein (CRP) and fecal calprotectin (FCP) results prior to VCE were also collected, if available.

All VCE were performed with PillCam SB2/SB3 (Given Imaging Ltd., Yokneam, Israel) following standard 24-hour clear fluid diet and 2-liter polyethylene glycol based bowel preparation. Images were interpreted with the use of RAPID viewer (Given Imaging Ltd., Yokneam, Israel). LS was calculated with the integrated calculator in the RAPID viewer in accordance with previously validated criteria [8].

3. Results

A total of 197 VCE were performed for elderly patients aged 70 or above during this period. Eight patients (4.1%) were diagnosed with CD using the aforementioned criteria. Representative images are shown in Figure 1. The mean age in this elderly small-bowel CD (SBCD) group is 75 (range 70–87) with 6 females and 2 males. Three patients had IDA either alone, with chronic abdominal symptoms (pain and/or diarrhea), or with a history of ankylosing spondylitis (AS). Two patients had chronic abdominal pain and diarrhea. One patient was being investigated for overt OGIB. The remaining two patients were asymptomatic and had been referred to exclude SBCD in light of their clinical history of AS.

The mean FCP was 580 μg/g (range 15–818), with all but one patient having a value ≥600. Mean CRP was 3.9 mg/l (range 0.96–5.8) and mean white blood cell count (WBC) was 6.3×10^9 /L (range 5.1–8.6). The mean combined LS was 1824 (range 768–6680) with the majority of the patients having moderate-to-severe inflammation and one with strictures. One patient with LS < 790 had subsequent histological confirmation of CD following further endoscopic investigation with balloon assisted enteroscopy. CRP (Pearson correlation $r = 0.71$, $p = 0.29$), WBC ($r = 0.56$, $p = 0.92$), and FCP ($r = 0.38$, $p = 0.53$) were not statistically correlated to the LS. Cross-sectional imaging results prior to VCE were available in 3 of the 8 CD patients, all of which were standard computed tomography of the abdomen without a specific enterography protocol. Two of these patients had abdominal symptoms. No definitive findings of CD were found in all of the scans.

One patient had an incomplete study due to delayed capsule passage related to an inflammatory SB stenosis. The capsule was eventually passed within a few days, without the need for retrieval. No other complications were observed.

The VCE results led to therapeutic changes in 4 out of 8 SBCD patients. Ensuing treatments included methotrexate, adalimumab, budesonide, and 5-amino salicylic acid. A patient was continued on mycophenolate mofetil and cyclosporine for a previous renal transplant. One other patient was managed expectantly for her mild asymptomatic CD. Follow-up was not available for the remaining 2 patients (Table 2).

The non-CD group consists of 189 elderly patients with a mean age of 77 (range 70–93) and 51.9% were female. The majority of the patients (94.7%) were referred for investigation of IDA, OGIB, or a combination thereof (Table 3). 41.8% had a normal study. Otherwise, the most common findings

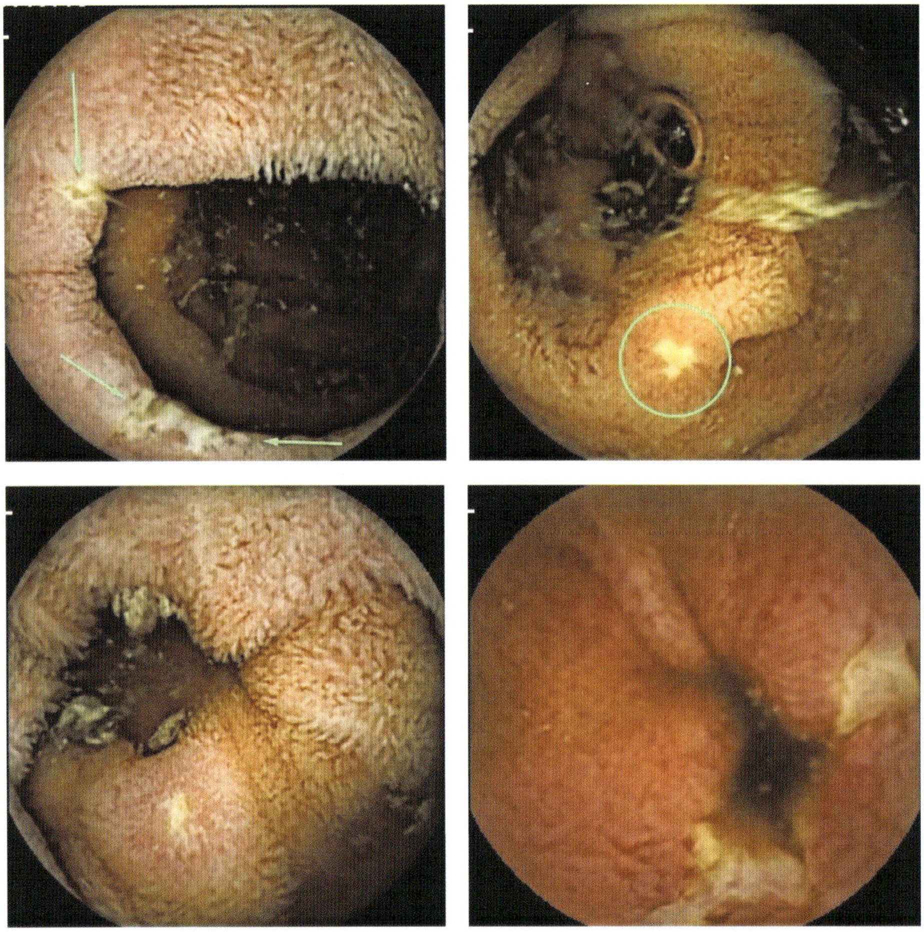

FIGURE 1: Representative video capsule endoscopy images of small-bowel Crohn's disease.

were angiodysplasia and minor nonspecific inflammatory changes (erythema, villous changes, aphthous ulcers, and edema) (Table 4).

One patient in the non-CD group had capsule retention due to a NSAID induced inflammatory stricture which required surgical retrieval. This patient did not undertake patency capsule testing priorly as there were no significant symptoms or risk factors suggestive of intestinal obstruction. Five patients had an incomplete study, two resulting from delayed gastric emptying and 3 from delayed intestinal transit without an obvious cause.

4. Discussion

This single center retrospective review showed that, despite negative bidirectional GI endoscopies, a small proportion of elderly patients may have unsuspected SBCD uncovered by VCE. Previous population studies have demonstrated that although only approximately 5% of CD cases are diagnosed in patients aged 60 and over, the incidence is increasing around the world [9, 10]. Accurate diagnosis based on VCE in this population remains challenging in light of other confounding factors such as NSAID use as well as the restricted capacity for invasive tissue confirmation. Nevertheless, this study highlights an important finding on VCE in the elderly population which is likely to rise in view of the widespread use of this technology in the aging population.

There has been a growing focus on issues relating to elderly IBD patients. However, often studies fail to distinguish patients with older-onset CD versus others who transition into older age following diagnosis at an earlier age, even though the prior group may exhibit different clinical phenotypes and natural history compared to their younger counterparts [7, 11]. A recent meta-analysis demonstrated that older-onset CD patients are more likely to have colonic disease (OR 2.56, 95% CI 1.88–3.48), inflammatory phenotype (OR 1.19, 95% CI 1.07–1.33), and a similar likelihood of stricturing disease (OR 0.90, 95% CI 0.67–1.20), but lower risk for penetrating phenotype (OR 0.48, 95% CI 0.33–0.69) and less perianal disease (0.64, 95% CI 0.56–0.80) [12]. A recent multicenter retrospective cohort study of patients with IBD also found that, compared with younger patients, those with elderly onset CD were more likely to have isolated colonic involvement, a nonstricturing, and nonpenetrating phenotype and less likely to have perianal complications or to receive immunosuppressants [7]. Rates of bowel resection, and both colonic and extracolonic malignancies, did not differ based on the age of IBD onset. It is notable that Ananthakrishnan et al. also observed that despite the lower rate of immunomodulator use (OR 0.44, 95% CI 0.33–0.57),

Table 2: Baseline demographics, indication for VCE, clinical parameters, and outcomes for elderly Crohn's cohort.

Elderly SBCD	8 patients
Age: mean ± SD/range (years)	72 ± 6 (70–87)
Gender	6 females : 2 males
IDA	1/8
OGIB	1/8
Abdominal symptoms	2/8
AS	2/8
IDA + abdominal symptoms	1/8
IDA + AS	1/8
Mean fecal calprotectin ± SD/range (μg/g)	580 ± 326 (15–818)
Mean CRP ± SD/range (mg/l)	3.9 ± 2.1 (0.96–5.8)
Mean Lewis score ± SD/range	1824 ± 1986 (768–6680)
Capsule retention	0
Other complications	1 (incomplete study)
Change in management	4/6 (5-amino salicylate acid/methotrexate/ adalimumab/budesonide)
Lost to follow-up	2/8

SBCD: small-bowel Crohn's disease; SD: standard deviation; *N*: number; IDA: iron deficiency anemia; OGIB: occult gastrointestinal bleeding; AS: ankylosing spondylitis.

Table 3: Indication for video capsule endoscopy in elderly patients.

Non-CD patients	189
Age: mean ± SD/range (years)	77 ± 5 (70–93)
Gender	91 females : 98 males
IDA	128 (67.7%)
Overt OGIB	32 (16.9%)
Abdominal symptoms	7 (3.7%)
AS	2 (1.1%)
IDA + abdominal symptoms	1 (0.5%)
IDA + overt OGIB	19 (10.1%)

CD: Crohn's disease; *N*: number; SD: standard deviation; IDA: iron deficiency anemia; OGIB: occult gastrointestinal bleeding; AS: ankylosing spondylitis.

Table 4: Diagnostic findings of video capsule endoscopy in elderly patients (excluding Crohn's disease cohort).

Non-CD patients	189
Normal	79 (41.8%)
Angiodysplasia	63 (33.3%)
Celiac disease	4 (2.1%)
Mass lesions	6 (3.2%)
Nonspecific changes	31 (16.4%)
Angiodysplasia/Polyp	5 (2.6%)
Angiodysplasia/Celiac	1 (0.5%)
Capsule retention	1 (0.5%)
Incomplete study	5 (2.6%) (2 due to gastroparesis)
Other complications	0

CD: Crohn's disease.

presumably due to age related concerns, the rate of surgery (OR 0.70, 95% CI 0.40–1.22) was similar compared to younger patients [12]. This suggests that the disease pattern in the elderly is no less benign than in their younger counterparts and that timely diagnosis along with appropriate treatment may prevent complications and need for surgery in the elderly population with more comorbidities.

The majority of patients in this study had moderate-to-severe inflammation on VCE and most required a change in management. Optimal therapeutic approach in the elderly CD population continues to be a contentious issue and is often based on expert opinion, with limited robust data. The main issues reside with the concerns relating to the risks of infection and malignancy along with other adverse effects in this population where existing risks associated with the medications are further compounded by advanced age [13–15]. In addition, elderly patients are generally excluded from clinical trials, rendering management expertise in this age group to be of lower quality. It is thus not uncommon to find a preferential use of medications such as budesonide and 5-amino salicylic acid in this population for their perceived lower side effect profile. No clear difference in efficacy nonetheless has been demonstrated with the use of thiopurine or methotrexate in the elderly [16]. However, the CESAME study showed that incidence rate of lymphoproliferative disorders in IBD patients aged over 65 with persisting thiopurine exposure was significantly increased [13].

The response and tolerance to antitumor necrosis factor alpha therapy have been reported to vary with age. Some studies have suggested similar long term response compared to younger patients whereas others have shown a lower response rate along with higher chance of discontinuation among elderly onset disease [17, 18]. Additionally, therapeutic options are also hindered by polypharmacy, drug interactions, and other pertinent issues in this cohort, such as heart failure [19]. Anti-TNF alpha therapy is contraindicated in patients with classes III-IV New York Heart Association heart failure [20]. These factors should be taken into consideration when forming a tailored and individualised approach to the management of elderly CD patients. Gut selective anti-integrin therapy such as vedolizumab may theoretically provide a superior safety profile in this higher risk population [21].

In this study, the majority of CD cases had a significantly elevated FCP, suggesting that this may serve as a helpful predictive biomarker for the presence of small-bowel inflammation on VCE in the elderly. Other serum biomarkers including CRP and WBC performed poorly. FCP is a well-established diagnostic test in detecting the presence of GI tract inflammation and is widely used as a screening test [22]. It is yet to be conclusively demonstrated whether there is a difference in its diagnostic accuracy when assessing for small bowel versus colonic CD, as previous studies have shown conflicting results [23, 24]. A recent meta-analysis involving

7 clinical studies with 463 patients examined the accuracy of FCP in detecting SBCD on VCE. At the cut-off level of 50 μg/g, the sensitivity, specificity, and diagnostic odds ratio were 0.89, 0.55, and 10.3, respectively, in patients suspected of SBCD. This suggests that the probability of SBCD below this cut-off is low and thus may be used as a screening tool to forego VCE use in those with negative bidirectional GI endoscopies in the right clinical context. Two additional studies published since also provided evidence in support of this notion [25, 26]. On the other hand, some studies have shown that the correlation between FCP and objective assessment of the SB inflammation such as the validated LS is equivocal or moderate at best [27, 28]. This may have been influenced by the retrospective nature of these studies or inherently within the LS itself, as the presence of a stricture without an associated inflammation will significantly increase the score but may not be associated with a corresponding increase in FCP. There are nevertheless no studies to date examining the use of FCP in the elderly population as a screening test prior to VCE. Variation in FCP with age was reported in healthy individuals [29]. Children aged 2–9 y had significantly higher concentrations than subjects aged $\geq$10 y. Adults $\geq$ 60 years had a higher concentration than those aged 10–59 y. Further prospective studies would be helpful in determining whether stratification with FCP may lead to improved outcomes and cost-effectiveness in the elderly.

Finally, this study demonstrates that the feasibility and safety of VCE in the elderly population are comparable to younger onset CD [30]. Only one non-CD patient with NSAID enteropathy experienced capsule retention, requiring intervention. The patency capsule was developed to assess intestinal patency prior to administration of VCE in an attempt to minimize capsule retention [31]. It is highly predictive of successful VCE completion, comparable to other cross-sectional imaging [32]. However, the decision to use a patency capsule varies between institutions. None of the patients in this study received patency testing as they did not exhibit any high-risk features predictive of retention. Currently, it is recommended to use a patency capsule in those with clinical or radiological features of SB stenosis, such as history of intestinal obstruction, surgery, or radiation, as well as those with established CD [33]. A recent study has challenged whether all CD patients need patency testing since the nonselective use of patency capsule in established CD patients did not improve retention rates in comparison with restricted patency testing in high-risk patients only [34].

The Korean Gut Image Study Group has developed guidelines for use of VCE in the following situations: diagnosis of OGIB, small-bowel preparation for VCE, diagnosis of CD, and diagnosis of small-bowel malignancy [35]. They concluded that VCE is the most sensitive diagnostic modality for detecting mucosal lesions in patients with suspected or established CD and that VCE is useful for diagnosing CD after negative colonoscopy and small-bowel radiology when there is a strong suspicion of CD. They recommended small-bowel radiology or the patency capsule test before VCE in patients with suspected or established CD. The European evidence-based consensus for endoscopy in IBD also recommends cross-sectional imaging or patency capsule testing before VCE in patients with established CD [36].

The main limitations of the study are those inherent within a retrospective study of which missing data, including potential confounding factors, and the relatively small SBCD sample size impact the ability to comprehensively characterize this patient cohort. In addition, most of the CD diagnosis was not confirmed by tissue sampling in light of the accessibility issues within the elderly population therefore potentially being exposed to misclassification bias. Nonetheless, this should be minimized by the inclusion criteria, including consistent VCE appearance of CD, exclusion of other differential diagnoses and moderate-to-severe inflammation, or tissue confirmation for those with only mild inflammation on VCE. Furthermore, VCE interpretation in this study was performed by an expert reader, thus reducing potential interobserver variations. The Lewis score was routinely used prospectively in assessing degree of small-bowel inflammation for all VCE performed at the McGill University Health Centre, which ensured all eligible cases were captured. Finally, although regular NSAID use was an exclusion criterion, 1 of 8 elderly patients with SBCD on VCE was on low dose ASA (80 mg/d).

5. Conclusions

Video capsule endoscopy can be safely performed in the elderly population where a proportion of these patients may have unsuspected SBCD despite negative conventional bidirectional GI endoscopies, resulting in change in management. Further studies in this unique group would assist with identifying predictive clinical and biochemical parameters for risk stratification.

Authors' Contributions

Che-Yung Chao and Ernest G. Seidman were involved in the design, implementation, and execution of the study and contributed to the authorship of this manuscript. Che-Yung Chao and Carl Frederic Duchatellier participated in data collection and interpretation of data.

Acknowledgments

Che-Yung Chao was supported by the Advanced Fellowship in IBD at McGill University. Ernest G. Seidman is supported by a Tier 1 Canada Research Chair in Immune Mediated Gastrointestinal Disorders and the Bruce Kaufman Chair in IBD at McGill University. The authors are grateful to Melissa Diamond for her administrative support (IRB approval, manuscript preparation).

References

[1] G. Iddan, G. Meron, A. Glukhovsky, and P. Swain, "Wireless capsule endoscopy," *Nature*, vol. 405, no. 6785, pp. 417-418, 2000.

[2] U. Kopylov and E. G. Seidman, "Clinical applications of small bowel capsule endoscopy," *Clinical and Experimental Gastroenterology*, vol. 6, no. 1, pp. 129–137, 2013.

[3] A. K. Hara, J. A. Leighton, V. K. Sharma, R. I. Heigh, and D. E. Fleischer, "Imaging of small bowel disease: Comparison of capsule endoscopy, standard endoscopy, barium examination, and CT," *RadioGraphics*, vol. 25, no. 3, pp. 697–711, 2005.

[4] R. Sidhu, D. S. Sanders, A. J. Morris, and M. E. McAlindon, "Guidelines on small bowel enteroscopy and capsule endoscopy in adults," *Gut*, vol. 57, no. 1, pp. 125–136, 2008.

[5] A. Muhammad, G. Vidyarthi, and P. Brady, "Role of small bowel capsule endoscopy in the diagnosis and management of iron deficiency anemia in elderly: A comprehensive review of the current literature," *World Journal of Gastroenterology*, no. 26, pp. 8416–8423, 2014.

[6] A. Ekbom, C. Helmick, M. Zack, and H.-O. Adami, "The epidemiology of inflammatory bowel disease: A large, population-based study in Sweden," *Gastroenterology*, vol. 100, no. 2, pp. 350–358, 1991.

[7] J. K. Hou, L. A. Feagins, and A. K. Waljee, "Characteristics and behavior of elderly-onset inflammatory bowel disease: a multicenter US study," *Inflammatory Bowel Diseases*, vol. 22, no. 9, pp. 2200–2205, 2016.

[8] I. M. Gralnek, R. Defranchis, E. Seidman, J. A. Leighton, P. Legnani, and B. S. Lewis, "Development of a capsule endoscopy scoring index for small bowel mucosal inflammatory change," *Alimentary Pharmacology & Therapeutics*, vol. 27, no. 2, pp. 146–154, 2008.

[9] J. P. Gisbert and M. Chaparro, "Systematic review with meta-analysis: inflammatory bowel disease in the elderly," *Alimentary Pharmacology & Therapeutics*, vol. 39, no. 5, pp. 459–477, 2014.

[10] S. Taleban, J.-F. Colombel, M. J. Mohler, and M. J. Fain, "Inflammatory bowel disease and the elderly: A Review," *Journal of Crohn's and Colitis*, vol. 9, no. 6, pp. 507–515, 2015.

[11] P. Stepaniuk, C. N. Bernstein, L. E. Targownik, and H. Singh, "Characterization of inflammatory bowel disease in elderly patients: A review of epidemiology, current practices and outcomes of current management strategies," *Canadian Journal of Gastroenterology and Hepatology*, vol. 29, no. 6, pp. 327–333, 2015.

[12] A. N. Ananthakrishnan, H. Y. Shi, W. Tang, C. C. Law, J. J. Sung, F. K. Chan et al., "Systematic review and meta-analysis: Phenotype and clinical outcomes of older-onset inflammatory bowel disease," *Journal of Crohn's & Colitis*, vol. 10, no. 10, pp. 1224–1236, 2016.

[13] L. Beaugerie, N. Brousse, A. M. Bouvier et al., "Lymphoproliferative disorders in patients receiving thiopurines for inflammatory bowel disease: a prospective observational cohort study," *The Lancet*, vol. 374, no. 9701, pp. 1617–1625, 2009.

[14] M. Naganuma, R. Kunisaki, N. Yoshimura, Y. Takeuchi, and M. Watanabe, "A prospective analysis of the incidence of and risk factors for opportunistic infections in patients with inflammatory bowel disease," *Journal of Gastroenterology*, vol. 48, no. 5, pp. 595–600, 2013.

[15] G. R. Lichtenstein, B. G. Feagan, R. D. Cohen et al., "Drug therapies and the risk of malignancy in crohn's disease: Results from the TREAT™ registry," *American Journal of Gastroenterology*, vol. 109, no. 2, pp. 212–223, 2014.

[16] J. H. del Val, "Old-age inflammatory bowel disease onset: A different problem?" *World Journal of Gastroenterology*, vol. 17, no. 22, pp. 2734–2739, 2011.

[17] T. Lobatón, M. Ferrante, P. Rutgeerts, V. Ballet, G. Van Assche, and S. Vermeire, "Efficacy and safety of anti-TNF therapy in elderly patients with inflammatory bowel disease," *Alimentary Pharmacology & Therapeutics*, vol. 42, no. 4, pp. 441–451, 2015.

[18] M. Cottone, A. Kohn, M. Daperno et al., "Advanced Age Is an Independent Risk Factor for Severe Infections and Mortality in Patients Given Anti-Tumor Necrosis Factor Therapy for Inflammatory Bowel Disease," *Clinical Gastroenterology and Hepatology*, vol. 9, no. 1, pp. 30–35, 2011.

[19] E. R. Hajjar, A. C. Cafiero, and J. T. Hanlon, "Polypharmacy in elderly patients," *American Journal of Geriatric Pharmacotherapy*, vol. 5, no. 4, pp. 345–351, 2007.

[20] E. Sinagra, G. Perricone, C. Romano, and M. Cottone, "Heart failure and anti tumor necrosis factor-alpha in systemic chronic inflammatory diseases," *European Journal of Internal Medicine*, vol. 24, no. 5, pp. 385–392, 2013.

[21] W. A. Bye, V. Jairath, and S. P. Travis, "Systematic review: the safety of vedolizumab for the treatment of inflammatory bowel disease," *Alimentary Pharmacology & Therapeutics*, vol. 46, no. 1, pp. 3–15, 2017.

[22] F. S. Lehmann, E. Burri, and C. Beglinger, "The role and utility of faecal markers in inflammatory bowel disease," *Therapeutic Advances in Gastroenterology*, vol. 8, no. 1, pp. 23–36, 2015.

[23] K. Stawczyk-Eder, P. Eder, L. Lykowska-Szuber et al., "Is faecal calprotectin equally useful in all Crohn's disease locations? A prospective, comparative study," *Archives of Medical Science*, vol. 11, no. 2, pp. 353–361, 2015.

[24] M. D. Jensen, J. Kjeldsen, and T. Nathan, "Fecal calprotectin is equally sensitive in Crohn's disease affecting the small bowel and colon," *Scandinavian Journal of Gastroenterology*, vol. 46, no. 6, pp. 694–700, 2011.

[25] M. F. Hale, K. Drew, M. E. McAlindon, and R. Sidhu, "The diagnostic accuracy of faecal calprotectin and small bowel capsule endoscopy and their correlation in suspected isolated small bowel Crohn's disease," *European Journal of Gastroenterology & Hepatology*, vol. 28, no. 10, pp. 1145–1150, 2016.

[26] J. Egea Valenzuela, A. Pereñíguez López, V. Pérez Fernández, F. Alberca de las Parras, and F. Carballo Álvarez, "Fecal calprotectin and C-reactive protein are associated with positive findings in capsule endoscopy in suspected small bowel Crohn's disease," *Revista Española de Enfermedades Digestivas*, vol. 108, 2016.

[27] A. Koulaouzidis, T. Sipponen, A. Nemeth et al., "Association Between Fecal Calprotectin Levels and Small-bowel Inflammation Score in Capsule Endoscopy: A Multicenter Retrospective Study," *Digestive Diseases and Sciences*, vol. 61, no. 7, pp. 2033–2040, 2016.

[28] P. A. S. Olsen, R. Fossmark, and G. Qvigstad, "Fecal calprotectin in patients with suspected small bowel disease - A selection tool for small bowel capsule endoscopy?" *Scandinavian Journal of Gastroenterology*, vol. 50, no. 3, pp. 272–277, 2014.

[29] S. Joshi, S. J. Lewis, S. Creanor, and R. M. Ayling, "Age-related faecal calprotectin, lactoferrin and tumour M2-PK concentrations in healthy volunteers," *Annals of Clinical Biochemistry*, vol. 47, no. 3, pp. 259–263, 2010.

[30] S. Mehdizadeh, G. C. Chen, L. Barkodar et al., "Capsule endoscopy in patients with Crohn's disease: diagnostic yield and safety," *Gastrointestinal Endoscopy*, vol. 71, no. 1, pp. 121–127, 2010.

[31] R. Eliakim, "Video capsule endoscopy of the small bowel," *Current Opinion in Gastroenterology*, vol. 29, no. 2, pp. 133–139, 2013.

[32] A. Yadav, R. I. Heigh, A. K. Hara et al., "Performance of the patency capsule compared with nonenteroclysis radiologic examinations in patients with known or suspected intestinal strictures," *Gastrointestinal Endoscopy*, vol. 74, no. 4, pp. 834–839, 2011.

[33] J. Panes, Y. Bouhnik, W. Reinisch, J. Stoker, S. A. Taylor, D. C. Baumgart et al., "Imaging techniques for assessment of inflammatory bowel disease: joint ECCO and ESGAR evidence-based consensus guidelines," *Journal of Crohn's & Colitis*, vol. 7, no. 7, pp. 556–585, 2013.

[34] A. Nemeth, U. Kopylov, A. Koulaouzidis et al., "Use of patency capsule in patients with established Crohn's disease," *Endoscopy*, vol. 48, no. 4, pp. 373–379, 2016.

[35] S. K. Park, B. D. Ye, and K. O. Kim, "Guidelines for video capsule endoscopy: emphasis on Crohn's disease," *Clinical Endoscopy*, vol. 48, no. 2, pp. 128–135, 2015.

[36] V. Annese, M. Daperno, M. D. Rutter et al., "European evidence based consensus for endoscopy in inflammatory bowel disease," *Journal of Crohn's and Colitis*, vol. 7, no. 12, pp. 982–1018, 2013.

Outcomes of the Use of Fully Covered Esophageal Self-Expandable Stent in the Management of Colorectal Anastomotic Strictures and Leaks

Chad J. Cooper,[1,2] Angel Morales,[3] and Mohamed O. Othman[2]

[1]*Department of Internal Medicine, Texas Tech University Health Sciences Center of El Paso, 4800 Alberta Avenue, El Paso, TX 79905, USA*
[2]*Division of Gastroenterology, Texas Tech University Health Sciences Center of El Paso, 4800 Alberta Avenue, El Paso, TX 79905, USA*
[3]*Department of General Surgery, Texas Tech University Health Sciences Center of El Paso, TX 79905, USA*

Correspondence should be addressed to Chad J. Cooper; chad.cooper@ttuhsc.edu

Academic Editor: Shai Friedland

Introduction. Colorectal anastomotic leak or stricture is a dreaded complication leading to significant morbidity and mortality. The novel use of self-expandable metal stents (SEMS) in the management of postoperative colorectal anastomotic leaks or strictures can avoid surgical reintervention. *Methods.* Retrospective study with particular attention to the indications, operative or postoperative complications, and clinical outcomes of SEMS placement for patients with either a colorectal anastomotic stricture or leak. *Results.* Eight patients had SEMS (WallFlex stent) for the management of postoperative colorectal anastomotic leak or stricture. Five had a colorectal anastomotic stricture and 3 had a colorectal anastomotic leak. Complete resolution of the anastomotic stricture or leak was achieved in all patients. Three had recurrence of the anastomotic stricture on 3-month flexible sigmoidoscopy follow-up after the initial stent was removed. Two of these patients had a stricture that was technically too difficult to place another stent. Stent migration was noted in 2 patients, one at day 3 and the other at day 14 after stent placement that required a larger 23 mm stent to be placed. *Conclusions.* The use of SEMS in the management of colorectal anastomotic leaks or strictures is feasible and is associated with high technical and clinical success rate.

1. Introduction

Anastomotic adverse events after partial colectomy include bleeding, leaks, fistulas, or strictures. Anastomotic leaks or strictures are a dreaded adverse event of colorectal surgery that can lead to a prolonged hospital stay and significant morbidity and mortality. An anastomotic leak is defined as a defect of the intestinal wall at the anastomotic site leading to a communication between the intra/extraluminal compartments [1]. The risk varies with the site of the anastomosis with those placed less than 5 centimeters (cm) from the anal verge being particularly vulnerable [2]. The incidence of an anastomotic leak depends on the location of the anastomosis with the highest incidence of 10–20% occurring with colorectal anastomosis [3]. The majority of patients suspected of having an anastomotic leak based on clinical assessment will undergo imaging studies to confirm the diagnosis. The usual approach for management of postoperative anastomotic leaks includes intravenous antibiotics, bowel rest, percutaneous drainage, parenteral nutrition, and surgical diversion [4]. The patient may require reoperation that consists of taking down the anastomosis and creation of an end colostomy. The distal portion of the bowel can be closed and left within the abdominal cavity or exteriorized as a mucous fistula. Postoperative patients with a colorectal anastomotic leak have a mortality rate of 25–35% [5].

The development of anastomotic strictures following colorectal surgery is a frequent problem, occurring in up to 30% of cases [6]. Anastomotic strictures eventually become symptomatic by presenting with signs of partial or complete intestinal obstruction. An anastomotic stricture is defined by the inability to pass a 12-millimeter (mm) diameter sigmoidoscope through the anastomosis [7].

The use of covered self-expandable esophageal metal stents (SEMS) has been described in the management of benign leaks, perforations, and fistulae of the esophagus, stomach, postsurgical anastomoses of the upper gastrointestinal (GI) tract, and the biliary tree [8]. Currently, CSEMS have been approved in the United States for use in the esophagus and bile ducts only. SEMS have been used for the treatment of malignant biliary obstruction or in malignant esophageal strictures [9]. The use of SEMS elsewhere in the GI tract and for other purposes warrants further investigation especially in the management of postoperative colorectal anastomotic leaks or strictures. In this case series, we present our experience with the temporary placement of covered esophageal SEMS in the nonoperative management of benign postoperative colorectal anastomotic leaks or strictures.

2. Specific Aims

The specific aim of this study was to evaluate the technical and clinical outcomes of fully covered SEMS placement for postoperative benign anastomotic leak or strictures that took place at a single endoscopic unit of tertiary university based hospital. This is a novel approach to the management of these anastomotic adverse events with limited existing literature on the topic.

3. Materials and Methods

A retrospective medical chart review was performed on all patients that had a covered self-expandable esophageal stent (CSEMS) placed for either a colorectal anastomotic stricture or leak at the Texas Tech University Health Sciences Center of El Paso Affiliated Hospital, University Medical Center of El Paso. This study was approved by the institutional review board (IRB) of Texas Tech University Health Sciences Center of El Paso, Texas, with the IRB number of E14044. Strict confidentiality and patient's privacy protection was maintained throughout the entire data collection process. At the time of the endoscopic procedure, the details of the procedure were explained to the patient and an informed consent was signed. However at the time of this study the procedure had already been performed. All patients were NPO after midnight and received 2 fleet enemas one day prior to the procedure. Depending on the postoperative clinical status of the patient, a liquid diet was given and advanced as tolerated.

3.1. Patient Population. Patients who underwent CSEMS for treatment of colorectal postoperative benign anastomotic leak or stricture from the period of January 1, 2011, through March 15, 2014, were included. The data collected pertained to patient demographics, type of postoperative anastomotic adverse events, characteristics of the stent placed, operative or postoperative adverse events, and clinical and technical outcomes.

3.1.1. Inclusion Criteria

(1) Males and females of age 18–70 years old.

(2) Abdominal surgery for colonic adenocarcinoma, diverticulosis, or diverticulitis with the creation of an end to end anastomosis.

(3) Diagnosis of a colorectal anastomotic stricture or leak based upon clinical manifestations and barium enema.

3.1.2. Exclusion Criteria

(1) A diagnosis of an anastomotic stricture or leak at a location other than the colorectal area.

(2) Previous endoscopic dilation of colorectal anastomotic stricture.

3.2. Procedure Details. Self-expandable metal stent (WallFlex Fully Covered Esophageal Stents, Boston Scientific, Natick, Mass.) was used in this case series. These stents were not dedicated (esophageal stent) with a slight different radial force compared with colonic stent. A barium enema was performed within 1 week before and after stent placement. We did not use the fluoroscopy because we were inserting the endoscope and we placed stents under endoscopic visualization. The CO_2 insufflator was used for all cases. An 18 mm stent diameter was used initially for stricture cases and 21 mm stent diameter was used for leak cases. In case of stent migration, 23 mm stent diameter was used for repeat stent placement. The choice of the stent length was dependent on stricture length.

A savory guidewire was placed endoscopically across the stricture of the leak (Figure 1(a)). The sigmoidoscope was then withdrawn and exchanged over the guidewire. The fully covered SEMS was then advanced over the guidewire and deployed under endoscopic visualization by advancing ultrathin endoscope (Olympus America Inc., Center Valley, PA) alongside the stent just below the stricture (Figure 1(b)). The stent was left at the anastomotic site for 40 to 50 days.

Endoscopic stent removal was performed with a rat tooth forceps (US Endoscopy, Mentor, OH) by grasping the distal end of the stent. Once the stent was removed a flexible sigmoidoscopy was performed to confirm healing of the leak or resolution of the stricture (Figure 1(c)). A final barium enema was performed within 3 months from stent removal to evaluate the status of the anastomotic defect before flexible sigmoidoscopy. A follow-up flexible sigmoidoscopy was performed between 3 to 4 months to evaluate recurrence of the defect. All flexible sigmoidoscopy procedures were performed under monitored anesthesia care (MAC) sedation.

4. Endpoints

Primary endpoints of the study were the clinical success that was quantified by the improvement in their quality of life, efficient bowel transit, and avoidance of surgical intervention. Each patient was followed up while hospitalized to evaluate their clinical status and postoperative pain. Further clinical and technical success was assessed as the resolution of the anastomotic leak or resolution of the anastomotic stricture as confirmed by flexible sigmoidoscopy at the time of stent removal and follow-up endoscopic and barium enema

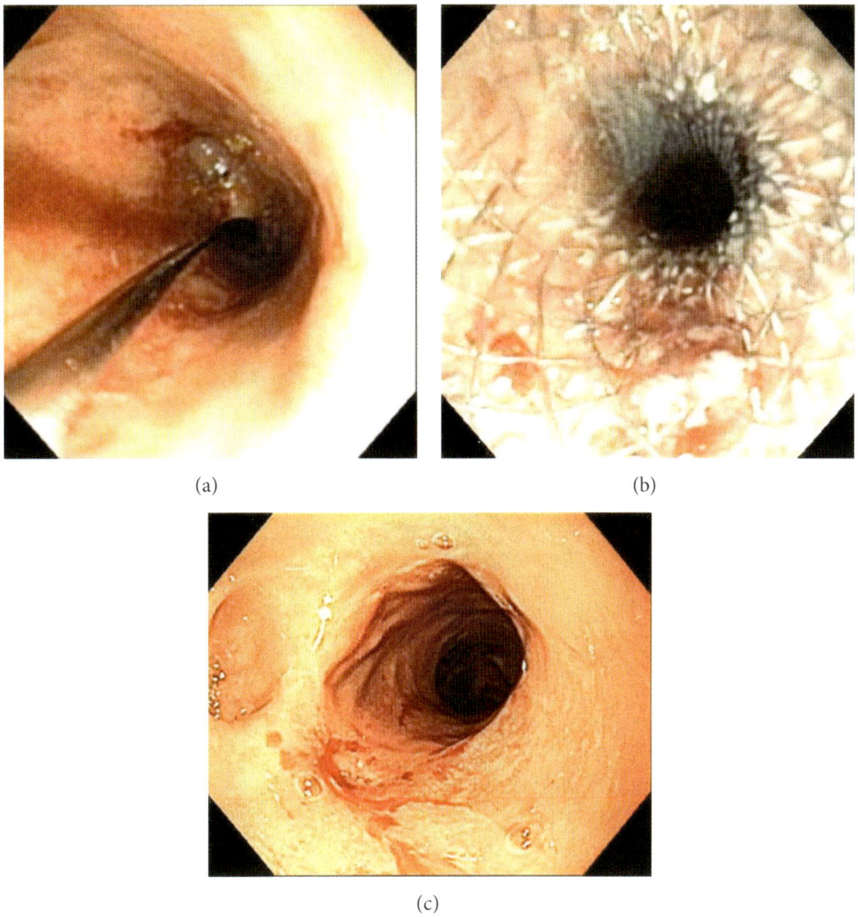

FIGURE 1: (a) Savory guidewire advanced through anastomotic stricture. (b) CSEMS deployment across the stricture. (c) Stricture resolution after stent removal.

evaluation 4 to 6 weeks afterwards. Other primary outcomes included the technical success of stent deployment and removal. Technical success was considered to be a success if the stent deployed and was placed at the appropriate location of the anastomotic adverse event. Technical success at the time of removal was considered to be successful if the whole stent was removed without adverse events such as perforation. Secondary endpoints included complications such as stent migration, excessive bleeding, bowel perforation, or anorectal pain. Both immediate and delayed (>30 days after the procedure) adverse events such as stent migration were noted.

4.1. Statistical Analysis. All results were expressed as mean or percentage. Descriptive statistics such as means and percentages were used for continuous and categorical data, respectively.

5. Results

A total of 8 patients (5 males and 3 females) underwent flexible sigmoidoscopic placement of a fully CSEMS for management of a postoperative colorectal anastomotic leak or stricture. The mean age of the patients was 55.8 years. Table 1 provides overall the patient demographics, anastomotic characteristics, stent characteristics, adverse events, and technical and clinical outcomes. The primary disease process included 5 patients with colorectal adenocarcinoma, 2 had diverticulitis, and 1 had diverticulosis. All 8 patients had a colorectal anastomosis. Five patients had a colorectal anastomotic stricture and 3 had a colorectal anastomotic leak. The SEMS were left in place for a mean of 45 (40–50) days. The distance from the distal flange of the stent to the anal verge ranged from 15 to 20 cm.

Clinical and technical success was initially achieved in all 8 cases (100%). However, two patients had external stent migration, one on postoperative day 3 and the other on day 14 after initial stent placement. Both of these patients had placement of a larger stent (23 mm stent diameter) and on follow-up complete resolution of the stricture was noted. Complete resolution of the anastomotic stricture or leak was achieved in all 8 cases (100%). Recurrence of the stricture after stent removal was not noted in any of these five patients. However, all 5 patients had a follow-up flexible sigmoidoscopy 3 months after stent removal. Three of the 5 patients had a recurrence of the anastomotic stricture that required placement of a CSEMS. Unfortunately, the anastomotic stricture was so severe in 2 of these patients in

Table 1: Patient demographics, anastomotic/stent characteristics, adverse events, and clinical outcomes.

Patient	Age/sex	Primary disease process	End to end anastomosis location	Anastomotic stricture or leak	Stent type*	Stent size#	Days stent left in place	Procedure or postoperative adverse events	Technical success	Clinical success	Follow-up flexible sigmoidoscopy
1	62/M	Sigmoid/rectal CA	Colorectal	Leak	FC WallFlex	23 mm × 10.5 cm	50	No	Yes	Yes	4 months
2	63/F	Sigmoid CA	Colorectal	Leak	FC WallFlex	23 mm × 10.5 cm	50	No	Yes	Yes	4 months
3	64/F	Diverticulosis in sigmoid colon	Colorectal	Leak	FC WallFlex	23 mm × 10.5 cm	45	No	Yes	Yes	4 months
4	33/M	Sigmoid CA	Colorectal	Stricture	FC WallFlex	18 mm × 15.3 cm	40	Stent migrated externally (3 d); 23 mm × 12.5 cm placed	Yes	Yes	3 months
5	57/M	Rectal CA	Colorectal + fistula	Stricture	FC WallFlex	18 mm × 15.3 cm	40	No	Yes	Yes; but later required anastomotic revision	3 months; recurrence of stricture; unable to place another stent
6	58/F	Rectal CA	Colorectal	Stricture	FC WallFlex	18 mm × 15.5 cm	40	No	Yes	Yes	3 months; recurrence of stricture; 23 mm × 15.5 cm stent placed and stricture resolved
7	47/M	Diverticulitis in sigmoid colon	Colorectal	Stricture	FC WallFlex	18 mm × 15.3 cm	50	Stent migrated externally (14 d); 23 mm × 15.5 cm placed	Yes	Yes; but later required anastomotic revision	3 months; recurrence of stricture; unable to place another stent
8	63/M	Diverticulitis in sigmoid colon	Colorectal	Stricture	FC WallFlex	18 mm × 15.5 cm	50	No	Yes	Yes	3 months

*Esophageal stent (FC: fully covered).
#Shaft diameter (mm) × length (cm).

whom stent placement was not technically feasible. In the long term, 2 of the 5 (40%) patients with recurrence of the anastomotic stricture eventually failed endoscopic placement of another stent. These two patients eventually required an exploratory laparotomy with colorectal anastomosis revision approximately 6 months later. Therefore, in the anastomotic stricture subgroup, 60% of patients had resolution of the stricture. The other patient with recurrence of the stricture had a 23 mm × 15.5 cm stent placed with resolution of the stricture noted upon removal of the stent and also on follow-up flexible sigmoidoscopy 3 months afterwards. Anastomotic leak completely resolved in the three patients in our series. Two patients had mild rectal pain after the initial stent placement which was treated with oral analgesic. Endoscopic stent removal was successful in all cases.

6. Discussion

Covered self-expanding esophageal metal stents (CSEMS) are commonly used and proven successful for the temporary decompression of a malignant obstruction or as palliative therapy when surgery is not warranted [10–12]. CSEMS are flexible stents that allow some bowel wall movement that helps the stent conform to the bends in the bowel. Stent placement can allow for luminal contents to be diverted from the defect site and facilitate natural closure and resolution of the defect, thus preventing extraluminal fluid collection and infection. The use of SEMS may be associated with a longer lasting dilatation and a lower rate of recurrence in cases of anastomotic stricture or leak [13]. Furthermore, this minimally invasive technique can prevent the need for invasive procedures. There has been limited experience reported in the current literature regarding the use of this technique for colorectal anastomotic strictures, leaks, or fistulas. The reported adverse events of stent insertion include mucosal overgrowth, stent migration, and obstruction.

Currie et al. performed a systematic review on 122 patients that had a self-expandable stent in the management of benign colorectal obstruction [14]. The predominant etiology was diverticulitis (54%) followed by anastomotic stricture (33%). Technical success was achieved in 94% and clinical success in 87% of patients. Overall, the perforation rate was 12% and the reobstruction rate was 14%. Migration of the stent occurred in 20% of cases. The most common reasons for clinical failure were perforation in 10 patients, persisting obstruction in the presence of a technically successful stent in 8 patients, and excessive anal pain after insertion of the stent in 3 patients [14]. Their analysis revealed that diverticulitis had a greater risk of developing complications during stenting, possibly due to the underlying inflammation and scarring [14]. It has been suggested that there is an increased risk of migration with self-expandable metal stents due to the use of covered and uncovered metal prostheses, which lack the required flexibility, in fibrotic and noncompliant benign strictures [14].

Vanbiervliet et al. reported on 43 patients that had fully covered self-expanding metal stents for benign colonic strictures [15]. The most common etiology was anastomotic strictures in 40 (93%) patients. The stents were placed and removed approximately 4–6 weeks later. Clinical success was achieved in 35 (81%) patients. Migration of the stent was observed in 27 (63%) patients. The median duration of stenting was 21 days. Their analysis showed that stents >20 mm in diameter migrated less often. Recurrence of stricture along with obstructive symptoms was observed in 23 (53%) patients. This study concluded that fully covered self-expandable metal stents for treatment of symptomatic benign colonic strictures are safe and effective, despite a high rate of spontaneous migration [15].

Abbas reported on 2 cases of an anastomotic stricture causing bowel obstruction in postoperative patients which were treated successfully with CSEMS placement [16]. Kim et al. reported a technical success of 100% and clinical success of 80% for the use of CSEMS for anastomotic leaks [6]. There was one of the five patients that had clinical failure but only had the stent placed for 20 days. This may not have been enough time to allow the anastomotic leak to completely heal. Sixty percent of their cases had postoperative adverse events of rectal pain and 40% had migration of the stent. Song et al. reported that rectal pain occurs in >60% of cases if the placement of the stent is within 5 cm of the anal verge [17].

The main limitation of this study is that it is a retrospective design with a small number of patients in this series. We therefore recommend further investigation of this minimally invasive technique in a large prospective controlled trial, given the potential benefits of this procedure. The recommended diameter for colonic stenting is 24 mm since it was determined as a cutoff regarding the migration risk. Nevertheless, our migration rate is lower than that observed in other studies; this could potentially be related to the severity of the stricture at the time of stent placement. Our study contributes to the available data on the use of esophageal CSEMS for management of postoperative colorectal leaks or strictures. Long term follow-up is required to evaluate the effectiveness and outcome of the procedure. We suggest a prospective comparative study (CSEMS versus dilation) to clearly establish the role of stenting in the treatment of the stricture. Furthermore, the use of CSEMS as a minimally invasive option and the avoidance of surgical intervention are very attractive in the treatment of anastomotic strictures or leaks. In conclusion, we recommend the use of CSEMS in the management of colorectal anastomotic leaks or strictures is feasible and is associated with high technical and clinical success.

Abbreviations

CSEMS: Covered self-expandable esophageal metal stents
MAC: Monitored anesthesia care
IRB: Institutional review board.

Disclosure

All participating authors in this study declare no financial, professional, or personal conflicts. No grant support was received for this case report. All authors were involved in paper preparation and literature review.

Authors' Contribution

Chad J. Cooper participated in study design/planning, data collection/analysis, paper preparation/editing, and medical literature search. Angel Morales and Mohamed O. Othman participated in study design/planning, surgical and endoscopic procedures, and paper preparation/editing.

References

[1] B. D. Shogan, E. M. Carlisle, J. C. Alverdy, and K. Umanskiy, "Do we really know why colorectal anastomoses leak?" *Journal of Gastrointestinal Surgery*, vol. 17, no. 9, pp. 1698–1707, 2013.

[2] N. A. Hirst, J. P. Tiernan, P. A. Millner, and D. G. Jayne, "Systematic review of methods to predict and detect anastomotic leakage in colorectal surgery," *Colorectal Disease*, vol. 16, no. 2, pp. 95–109, 2014.

[3] P. G. A. van Boeckel, K. S. Dua, B. L. A. M. Weusten et al., "Fully covered self-expandable metal stents (SEMS), partially covered SEMS and self-expandable plastic stents for the treatment of benign esophageal ruptures and anastomotic leaks," *BMC Gastroenterology*, vol. 12, article 19, 2012.

[4] C. J. DiMaio, M. P. Dorfman, G. J. Gardner et al., "Covered esophageal self-expandable metal stents in the nonoperative management of postoperative colorectal anastomotic leaks," *Gastrointestinal Endoscopy*, vol. 76, no. 2, pp. 431–435, 2012.

[5] D. Fraccalvieri, S. Biondo, J. Saez et al., "Management of colorectal anastomotic leakage: differences between salvage and anastomotic takedown," *The American Journal of Surgery*, vol. 204, no. 5, pp. 671–676, 2012.

[6] P. H. Kim, H.-Y. Song, J.-H. Park, J. H. Kim, H. K. Na, and Y. J. Lee, "Safe and effective treatment of colorectal anastomotic stricture using a well-defined balloon dilation protocol," *Journal of Vascular and Interventional Radiology*, vol. 23, no. 5, pp. 675–680, 2012.

[7] K. L. Suchan, A. Muldner, and B. C. Manegold, "Endoscopic treatment of postoperative colorectal anastomotic strictures," *Surgical Endoscopy and Other Interventional Techniques*, vol. 17, no. 7, pp. 1110–1113, 2003.

[8] L. Amrani, C. Ménard, S. Berdah et al., "From iatrogenic digestive perforation to complete anastomotic disunion: endoscopic stenting as a new concept of "stent-guided regeneration and re-epithelialization"," *Gastrointestinal Endoscopy*, vol. 69, no. 7, pp. 1282–1287, 2009.

[9] L. Feo and D. M. Schaffzin, "Colonic stents: the modern treatment of colonic obstruction," *Advances in Therapy*, vol. 28, no. 2, pp. 73–86, 2011.

[10] A. Lamazza, E. Fiori, A. V. Sterpetti, A. Schillaci, D. Scoglio, and E. Lezoche, "Self-expandable metal stents in the treatment of benign anastomotic stricture after rectal resection for cancer," *Colorectal Disease*, vol. 16, no. 4, pp. O150–O153, 2014.

[11] A. Repici, D. Reggio, C. De Angelis et al., "Covered metal stents for management of inoperable malignant colorectal strictures," *Gastrointestinal Endoscopy*, vol. 52, no. 6, pp. 735–740, 2000.

[12] K. Tominaga, M. Yoshida, I. Maetani, and Y. Sakai, "Expandable metal stent placement in the treatment of a malignant anastomotic stricture of the transverse colon," *Gastrointestinal Endoscopy*, vol. 53, no. 4, pp. 524–527, 2001.

[13] A. Mahajan, M. Rothermich, M. Gaidhane, and M. Kahaleh, "Esophageal self-expandable metal stent for an anastomotic colorectal stricture," *Endoscopy*, vol. 43, no. 2, pp. E415–E416, 2011.

[14] A. Currie, C. Christmas, H. Aldean, M. Mobasheri, and I. T. M. Bloom, "Systematic review of self-expanding stents in the management of benign colorectal obstruction," *Colorectal Disease*, vol. 16, no. 4, pp. 239–245, 2013.

[15] G. Vanbiervliet, P. Bichard, J.-F. Demarquay et al., "Fully covered self-expanding metal stents for benign colonic strictures," *Endoscopy*, vol. 45, no. 1, pp. 35–41, 2013.

[16] M. A. Abbas, "Endoscopic management of acute colorectal anastomotic complications with temporary stent," *Journal of the Society of Laparoendoscopic Surgeons*, vol. 13, no. 3, pp. 420–424, 2009.

[17] H.-Y. Song, J. H. Kim, K. R. Kim et al., "Malignant rectal obstruction within 5 cm of the anal verge: is there a role for expandable metallic stent placement?" *Gastrointestinal Endoscopy*, vol. 68, no. 4, pp. 713–720, 2008.

Permissions

All chapters in this book were first published in DTE, by Hindawi Publishing Corporation; hereby published with permission under the Creative Commons Attribution License or equivalent. Every chapter published in this book has been scrutinized by our experts. Their significance has been extensively debated. The topics covered herein carry significant findings which will fuel the growth of the discipline. They may even be implemented as practical applications or may be referred to as a beginning point for another development.

The contributors of this book come from diverse backgrounds, making this book a truly international effort. This book will bring forth new frontiers with its revolutionizing research information and detailed analysis of the nascent developments around the world.

We would like to thank all the contributing authors for lending their expertise to make the book truly unique. They have played a crucial role in the development of this book. Without their invaluable contributions this book wouldn't have been possible. They have made vital efforts to compile up to date information on the varied aspects of this subject to make this book a valuable addition to the collection of many professionals and students.

This book was conceptualized with the vision of imparting up-to-date information and advanced data in this field. To ensure the same, a matchless editorial board was set up. Every individual on the board went through rigorous rounds of assessment to prove their worth. After which they invested a large part of their time researching and compiling the most relevant data for our readers.

The editorial board has been involved in producing this book since its inception. They have spent rigorous hours researching and exploring the diverse topics which have resulted in the successful publishing of this book. They have passed on their knowledge of decades through this book. To expedite this challenging task, the publisher supported the team at every step. A small team of assistant editors was also appointed to further simplify the editing procedure and attain best results for the readers.

Apart from the editorial board, the designing team has also invested a significant amount of their time in understanding the subject and creating the most relevant covers. They scrutinized every image to scout for the most suitable representation of the subject and create an appropriate cover for the book.

The publishing team has been an ardent support to the editorial, designing and production team. Their endless efforts to recruit the best for this project, has resulted in the accomplishment of this book. They are a veteran in the field of academics and their pool of knowledge is as vast as their experience in printing. Their expertise and guidance has proved useful at every step. Their uncompromising quality standards have made this book an exceptional effort. Their encouragement from time to time has been an inspiration for everyone.

The publisher and the editorial board hope that this book will prove to be a valuable piece of knowledge for researchers, students, practitioners and scholars across the globe.

List of Contributors

Piyapan Prueksapanich, Pradermchai Kongkam and Rungsun Rerknimitr
Department of Medicine, Faculty of Medicine, King Chulalongkorn Memorial Hospital, Chulalongkorn University, Bangkok 10330, Thailand

Phonthep Angsuwatcharakon
Department of Medicine, Faculty of Medicine, King Chulalongkorn Memorial Hospital, Chulalongkorn University, Bangkok 10330, Thailand
Department of Anatomy, Faculty of Medicine, King Chulalongkorn Memorial Hospital, Chulalongkorn University, Bangkok 10330, Thailand

Thawee Rattanachu-ek
Center of Excellence, Laparoscopic Endoscopic Surgery, Department of Surgery, Rajavithi Hospital, Bangkok 10400, Thailand

Jaksin Sottisuporn
NKC Institute of Gastroenterology and Hepatology, Faculty of Medicine, Prince of Songkla University, Songkhla 90110, Thailand

Mihir S. Wagh, Disaya Chavalitdhamrong, Koorosh Moezardalan, Shailendra S. Chauhan, Anand R. Gupte, Michael J. Nosler, Chris E. Forsmark and Peter V. Draganov
Division of Gastroenterology, Hepatology and Nutrition, University of Florida, 1600 SWArcher Road, Room HD 602, Gainesville, FL 32610, USA

Daniel Boixeda-Miquel and Agustin Albillos
Gastroenterology Service, University Hospital Ramon y Cajal, 28801 Madrid, Spain

Enrique Vazquez-Sequeiros and Jose Ramon Foruny-Olcina
Gastroenterology Service, University Hospital Ramon y Cajal, 28801 Madrid, Spain
Gastroenterology Service, University Hospital Quiron, Madrid, Spain

Manuel Van Domselaar, Fernando González-Panizo and Diego Juzgado-Lucas
Gastroenterology Service, University Hospital Quiron, Madrid, Spain

Michael J. Levy
Developmental Endoscopy Unit, Gastroenterology Division, Mayo Clinic, Rochester, MN, USA

Tomoyuki Yada and Naomi Uemura
Department of Gastroenterology, Kohnodai Hospital, National Center for Global Health and Medicine, 1-7-1 Kohnodai, Ichikawa, Chiba 272-8516, Japan

Chizu Yokoi
Department of Gastroenterology, National Center for Global Health and Medicine, 1-21-1 Toyama, Shinjuku-ku, Tokyo 162-8655, Japan

Itsuko Asada-Hirayama, Shinya Kodashima, SatoshiMochizuki, Maki Konno-Shimizu, RieMikami-Matsuda, ChihiroMinatsuki, Chiemi Nakayama, Yu Takahashi, Nobutake Yamamichi and Kazuhiko Koike
Department of Gastroenterology, Graduate School of Medicine, The University of Tokyo, 7-3-1 Hongo, Bunkyo-ku, Tokyo 113-8655, Japan

Mitsuhiro Fujishiro and Keiko Niimi
Department of Endoscopy and Endoscopic Surgery, Graduate School of Medicine, The University of Tokyo, 7-3-1 Hongo, Bunkyo-ku, Tokyo 113-8655, Japan

Satoshi Ono
Center for Epidemiology and Preventive Medicine, The University of Tokyo, 7-3-1 Hongo, Bunkyo-ku, Tokyo 113-8655, Japan

Mohammad F. Madhoun, Sam Hong, William M. Tierney and John T. Maple
Division of Digestive Diseases and Nutrition, University of Oklahoma Health Sciences Center, 920 Stanton L. Young Boulevard, WP1345, Oklahoma City, OK 73104, USA

Sachin Wani
Division of Gastroenterology and Hepatology, University of Colorado, Anschutz Medical Campus, and Veterans Affairs Medical Center, Aurora, Denver, CO, USA

Shajan Peter, Ji Young Bang, Klaus Mönkemuller, Shyam Varardarajulu and C. Mel Wilcox
Division of Gastroenterology and Hepatology, University of Alabama at Birmingham, Birmingham, AL 35294-0012, USA

Julia K. LeBlanc, Michelle Juan, Lee McHenry, Stuart Sherman, Kathy McGreevy, Mohammad Al-Haddad and John DeWitt
Division of Gastroenterology and Hepatology, Indiana University Medical Center, 550 North University Boulevard, UH 4100, Indianapolis, IN 46202, USA

Index

A

Achalasia, 54-56, 59-61
Adrenal Gland, 14, 17
Angioectasias, 68-73

B

Biliary Cannulation, 2, 120, 125-126, 167, 171

C

Capsule Location Index, 107-111, 113
Celiac Disease, 88-89, 91-93, 208, 211
Celiac Plexus Neurolysis, 48-49, 51-53
Chemoradiotherapy, 28, 30, 33
Choledecholithiasis, 153
Colonoscope, 2, 75, 151
Colorectal Cancer, 101, 105-106, 114-116, 118-119, 146-147, 150-152
Computed Tomography-, 13
Confocal Laser Endomicroscopy, 42, 46-47
Cystogastrostomy, 181-185
Cytopathologic Diagnosis, 14

D

Diagnostic Yield, 13-17, 66, 68, 70-71, 81, 86, 92, 107, 110-113, 213
Duodenoscope, 2, 8, 154, 168, 174

E

Elastography, 203-207
Endobronchial Ultrasound, 14, 62-63, 65-67
Endomicroscopy, 42-43, 45-47, 91-92
Endoscopic Diagnosis, 23, 26, 33
Endoscopic Papillary, 34-35, 37, 39-41, 187, 194
Endoscopic Perforation, 2, 58
Endoscopic Sclerotherapy, 74-75, 77, 79
Endoscopic Submucosal Dissection, 19, 24-27, 160-161, 163-166
Endoscopic Therapy, 7, 19, 21-23, 25, 109, 111, 185, 192, 201
Endoscopic Treatment, 5, 7-11, 19, 26, 69, 80, 159, 181, 220
Endoscopic Ultrasound, 13, 15-18, 26, 42, 48-49, 51-53, 94, 99, 132, 167, 169, 171-173, 179-180, 182, 185, 193, 195-197, 199-200, 203, 205-207
Esophageal Mucosa, 29
Esophageal Squamous Cell Carcinoma, 28-29, 31, 33

G

Gastric Cancer, 19-27, 161, 165-166
Gastroesophageal Reflux, 54, 59
Gastrointestinal Content, 1, 5
Gastrointestinal Endoscopy, 1, 5-6, 12, 17, 25-27, 33, 40, 46-47, 52-53, 61, 71-72, 80, 86, 88, 92-93, 99, 103, 106, 112-113, 115, 118, 126, 131-132, 137-138, 152, 158-159, 165-166, 179, 185, 192, 206, 220

H

Hemorrhage, 17, 51, 58, 74-75, 77, 126-127, 139, 169, 193, 199-200
High Diagnostic, 107, 109, 111-113
Histoplasma Capsulatum, 62-63
Hydrogen Peroxide Irrigation, 181-185

I

Iatrogenic Perforation, 1-2, 5
Internal Hemorrhoid, 74-75
Intestinal Angioectasias, 68-69, 71, 73
Intramucosal Cancer, 23

L

Large Bile Duct Stone, 34
Lugol Chromoendoscopy, 28-33
Lung Metastasis, 13, 15

M

Magnification Endoscopy, 88-89, 91-93
Malignancy, 14-17, 33, 44-45, 63, 65-66, 94-95, 97-99, 101, 114, 161, 176, 179, 204, 211-212
Malignant Biliary Obstruction, 133, 135-138, 167, 171-175, 177-180, 192, 216
Mechanical Lithotripsy, 34-35, 37-41, 156
Mediastinal Lung Mass, 14
Mediastinoscopy, 13, 15-18, 65

N

Narrow Band Imaging, 20, 22, 25, 28-29, 31-33, 88-89, 91-93, 103
Nasobiliary Catheter, 154, 186-187, 189, 191-192
Neoplasia, 25-26, 28-29, 31-33, 46, 78, 92, 152, 160, 162, 165

O

Obscure Gastrointestinal Bleeding, 68, 71-73, 81-83, 85-87, 111-112
Ovesco Clip, 1-5

P

Pancreatic Cancer, 48-49, 51-53, 94-99, 135, 137-138, 190
Pancreatic Necrosectomy, 181-183, 185
Pancreatic Pathology, 94-95, 97, 99
Pancreatic Pseudocyst, 127-132, 181-182
Pancreaticobiliary System, 42-43, 45-47

Pancreaticoduodenectomy, 94-95, 97, 99
Peritoneal Space, 5
Peroral Endoscopic Myotomy, 54-56, 59, 61
Polyp Pathology, 100-103, 105
Postcolonoscopy, 100-101, 103, 105, 118
Postendoscopic Resection, 23

R
Radiation Proctopathy, 139, 141, 143, 145

S
Self-expandable Metal Stents, 7, 12, 215, 219-220
Small Cell Lung Cancer, 16-17
Spiral Enteroscopy, 107-113
Subacute Pulmonary Histoplasmosis, 62-63, 65, 67
Submucosal Dissection, 19, 24-27, 29, 55, 60, 160-161, 163-166

T
Tannic Acid, 74, 77, 79
Therapeutic Yield, 107-109, 111-113
Thoracoscopy, 13, 15
Transmural Drainage, 127, 129, 131, 169
Transpancreatic Precut Sphincterotomy, 120-126

U
Ultrasonography, 17, 19-20, 26, 99, 127, 141, 172-173, 179-180, 187, 190